Advancing Neuropsychology Through Population Health

Margaret Lanca · Robert Fallows
Editors

Advancing Neuropsychology Through Population Health

From Concept to Implementation

Springer

Editors
Margaret Lanca
Cambridge Health Alliance
Cambridge, MA, USA

Robert Fallows
Samaritan Medical Group
Albany, OR, USA

ISBN 978-3-032-22456-9 ISBN 978-3-032-22457-6 (eBook)
https://doi.org/10.1007/978-3-032-22457-6

This Springer imprint is published by the registered company Springer Nature Switzerland AG
The registered company address is: Gewerbestrasse 11, 6330 Cham, Switzerland

ML

To my loving husband Richard: Thank you for your constant support and enduring friendship. You keep me laughing every day.

To my children, Aidan and Brianna: You are the reason I want to make a small difference in the world and the highlight of my day.

And to my parents, Manuel and Fernanda. Thank you for having the courage to immigrate to a new land and seek a better life. You have shown me what is possible with hard work, tenacity, and dedication.

RF

To my wife and best friend, Tiffany: Being in a football family, I can definitely say that life is a full contact sport – and that there is absolutely no one I would rather have on my team than you. Thank you for your continuous support and love.

To my children, RJ and Ethan: Your humor, love, and compassion toward others inspires me to be the best dad possible, and to do my best to make our communities and healthcare the best I can.

To my family: From my parents to grandparents, my siblings, and Godparents, the values and wisdom you have bestowed upon me are hopefully well represented in this book.

Foreword

A Paradigm Shift in Clinical Neuropsychology

Clinical neuropsychology's history has experienced unusually high levels of growth and impact over its first 75 years. With the development of its organizations, such as the International Neuropsychological Society, the National Academy of Neuropsychology, and the Society of Clinical Neuropsychology, and its numerous journals, such as Neuropsychology, Archives of Clinical Neuropsychology, and The Clinical Neuropsychologist, a strong science and profession emerged. The science was initially exclusively focused on determining whether symptomology's etiology was "organic or functional"; for example, was it dementia or depression. This bifurcated dichotomy was measured exclusively with tests (e.g., the Finger Tapping Test) borrowed from other specialties (e.g., vocational psychology) and used cutoff scores. If a score was above a predetermined cutoff, sometimes mediated by such variables as age and educational attainment, then the patient was diagnosed as having "brain damage."

The advent of more advanced neuroradiological techniques, such as CT Scans and MRIs, as well as the development of behavioral neurology, provided the impetus to develop more sensitive and specific interpretations of measured data. T scores and percentiles, among other statistical measures, slowly replaced the dichotomous bifurcation by providing more careful analyses of measured deficits. And, until recently, the focus was clearly on one tail of the performance curve, impairment. More recently, the concept of positive psychology provided the foundation for appreciating and measuring the other tail of the performance continuum, the wellness side. Nevertheless, the focus remained, for the first three quarters of a century, on a singular, individual perspective of brain functioning.

Curiously, some of the most potent and revered theoretical foundations of clinical neuropsychology offered a socio-historical-cultural perspective that situated an individual's brain functioning within a larger context. Alexander Luria, arguably the founder of clinical neuropsychology, was influenced by his mentor, Lev Vygotsky, who indicated that understanding an individual must occur inside a larger context.

Appreciating the individual as well as the larger context, from familial to community, to cultural, while integrating it within a longitudinal and historical context, was hypothesized as the only way to appreciate how these "deficits" could be interpreted comprehensively. Indeed, these "deficits" should be mitigated by appreciating their function within a context, which can sometimes shift the deficit into an adaptation. The measurement was viewed as nothing more than an error in understanding how the brain works, both within a person and in a larger context. Interestingly, without referencing Luria and Vygotsky, the American Psychological Association (APA) approved the revision of its Multicultural Guidelines in 2017. To be multiculturally sensitive, the association indicated that individuals should be understood within concentric circles that began with an individual's personal experience, evolved through the interpretation of larger contexts, and eventually were encircled by a global perspective on that interpretation or attribute, whether it was neuropsychological (executive functioning) or psychological-affective. Everything was socio-historical-cultural.

Clinical neuropsychology, despite its unprecedented growth and impact across health in general and psychology in particular, has not fundamentally evolved to embrace this broader perspective. Psychology's first specialty, despite its success, has not embraced a larger, more community-based paradigm. Clinical neuropsychology has remained a profession and a science of a brain within a person.

In doing so, we have evolved deeply, but inside a bubble that does not generalize to the world around us. Regardless of our intentions, clinical neuropsychology has progressed far, but in a manner that seeks to understand and serve the few, often the privileged—the most endowed individuals of the most endowed countries. There is no future to a science and a profession limited to the few. This challenge has been most recently played out in the difficulties of interpreting and implementing the newest guidelines for the education and training of clinical neuropsychologists. Despite the experience in Minneapolis in 2022, which wholeheartedly endorsed a diverse, inclusive, and equitable specialty, the interpretation of what occurred that one week in Minnesota has been mitigated by narrow interpretations of what clinical neuropsychology should be.

These interpretations look backward rather than forward. This perspective does not endorse a shift in national and international demographics, does not endorse the value of serving all, and does not endorse external validation. Our constructs should reflect the beauty and power that a global perspective of clinical neuropsychology would bring to our foundational perspective.

To achieve such a paradigm shift, clinical neuropsychology, in its 75th year, must accept and endorse that the future of the specialty can only be realized by replacing the understanding of one brain, one person, with knowledge of one brain and one person within a larger perspective. By doing so, the paradigm shift brings hope and expansion of clinical neuropsychology.

This significant volume presents the first scholarly effort to initiate that shift. The authors and ideas presented provide a template for the future of clinical neuropsychology. May this effort mark the beginning of a new era for a more powerful, robust, diverse, equitable, and inclusive specialty. In doing so, the ideas borne out from this effort will continue to keep clinical neuropsychology not only as a leader in health-care in psychology but as a beacon for the inclusion in all things neurocognitive as leading the charge for bringing psychology to address critical issues ranging from a social justice to helping integrate neuropsychology into the charge of infusing the ideas of our brain science and practice to understanding the greater challenges facing today's complex and turbulent world.

Antonio E. Puente, PhD
2017 President American Psychological Association
Wilmington, USA

Preface

Even prior to the COVID pandemic of 2020, many neuropsychologists in healthcare systems were faced with the question of how to meet the increasing need for services. Wait lists were growing not just in the adult space, but within pediatrics as well, as research was mounting showing how essential neuropsychological services are to patient care and outcomes. Alongside this shift in demand came a heightened awareness of disparities in healthcare and in neuropsychology, most acutely for the need to create more sophisticated data normative solutions to move beyond race-based norming. Further, research on health disparities created a call to action to understand these factors and how to address them. Built environment, adverse childhood events, and social determinants of health are but a few drivers that have clear impact on cognitive health, which has a complex and measurable interaction with quality of life, health literacy, and health outcomes over individual lifetimes.

This book tries to capture these challenges to help the reader better appreciate how population health represents a promising framework for shifting neuropsychological science and practice. In the first section of the book, the reader is provided with a general introduction on population health but also shares possible solutions for how it can be tailored to neuropsychology. A focus on upstream, preventative care is emphasized with special attention to health equity, as the current US healthcare delivery system is critiqued and new financing models for healthcare are reviewed. Section two focuses on the practice environment broadly. A model for care for adult and pediatric populations is elaborated; however, the importance of cognitive health is addressed without the neuropsychologist directly involved in the care delivery discussion of cognition as the 6th vital sign. Section three concludes this book with a focus on leading for population health-based change leveraging technology and implementation science, providing a strong glimpse into the future of digital tools, next generation neuropsychology training, and a call to action for research and upstream preventative work.

Neuropsychology undoubtedly finds itself at a crossroads, and we posit throughout this text that population health can be an answer to our evolution. Successfully adopted, the neuropsychologist's job will expand from sole consult and evaluation to program design and implementation for measuring broad populations' cognitive abilities and adapting care to meet the needs of diverse individuals.

Cambridge, USA Margaret Lanca
Albany, USA Robert Fallows

Acknowledgments

A common theme emerged in our early conversations about editing this book. Reaching out to some of our trusted colleagues in this space, we listened to their apprehension and even fear that the future viability of their practice could be viewed as "too brief." Many of the pioneers in neuropsychology population health have taken educated risks in their careers to address the inequities within our profession. Our gratitude goes out to them, and the impact of their work is immense. The contributing authors in this book all represent a bright light for our field in evolving neuropsychology practice and science, so that the benefits of attending to cognitive health can be realized by all. In addition to our authors, we would like to express our thanks to Springer, and to our editor Catherine Thom, for believing in this book, and our vision to connect with those beyond neuropsychology—population health leaders, other healthcare specialties, and policy makers.

Margaret Lanca
My heartfelt gratitude goes to my co-editor, Robert Fallows. Working colleagues with similar interests living on opposite sides of the country, we knew each other little when he approached me with this brainchild of co-editing a book. We launched into this project and never looked back. He has become a trusted and admired colleague and the best part of this project. I could not have asked for a better partner.

I am indebted to my former and current Chiefs of Psychiatry at Cambridge Health Alliance (CHA), Philip Wang and Carl Fulwiler who opened my eyes to population health and patiently mentored me as I immersed myself in learning. Their vision and commitment to ensuring that every single person not only has equal access to healthcare but to better care is unparalleled and has deeply impacted my own view and hope for better healthcare for all. To my CHA Population Behavioral Health Innovation team, Kate Zona, Ana Progovac, Norah Mulvaney-Day, Lisa Rosenfeld, and Rajen Aldis for their wisdom and dedication to implementation science; working on an inter-disciplinary team has been the most rewarding part of this work. I am especially thankful to my partner in crime in population health at CHA for the past six years, Kate Zona. We took a leap of faith when we embarked on this less traveled road, guided by our enduring belief that measurement-based care will enhance clinical practice. Her even keeled and steadfast approach has made this experience invaluable through challenging times as well as the small gains.

And finally, to my neuropsychology Forensic High Tea group turned swanky dinners gang of respected neuropsychology colleagues and even better friends: Karen Postal, Nancy Hebben, Cheryl Weinstein, and Betsy Leritz whose constant enthusiasm for neuropsychology always leave me invigorated; they have each become mentors to me. Karen was the first to encourage me to write a book on my work in primary care neuropsychology over 10 years ago. Little did she know it would evolve into a field of work. I think she would have been proud—and I also dedicate this book in loving memory of her.

Robert Fallows

I wish to extend gratitude to Maggie for her partnership over the past 7 years. Our independently published papers on primary care based neuropsychology came out within a year of each other. Shortly after that, email conversations about our work flourished into an amazing partnership in the space of population health. She has been a fantastic collaborator and her work in the field of neuropsychology and at Cambridge Health Alliance serves as a strong guidepost for me.

I also wish to extend my heartfelt thanks to Samaritan Health Services. They took a risk in 2012 by asking a newly graduating fellow to start a neuropsychology service for their semi-rural healthcare system. Along the way, they have shown patience and excitement for the changes to not just neuropsychology, but behavioral health practice, which I have endeavored to implement. Special acknowledgements go out to Dr. Bob Turngren, Dr. Brent Godek, and Julie Osgood who have served as leaders in this space, as well as personal mentors for me in this work.

Contents

Editors and contributors

About the Editors

Margaret Lanca, PhD is the Director of Neuropsychology and Cognitive Wellness and Director of Population Behavioral Health Innovation at Cambridge Health Alliance. She is also Assistant Professor of Psychology in Psychiatry at Harvard Medical School. In the Division of Population Behavioral Health, she oversees the implementation of measurement-based care in psychiatry and participates in new initiatives geared toward improvement of patient-centered care. In Neuropsychology, Maggie directs the neuropsychology service and oversees the neuropsychology post-doctoral fellow training program. Her clinical work is specialized in the provision of multicultural neuropsychological assessments and understanding the factors influencing the assessment of patients of diverse backgrounds, such as early literacy and working effectively with medical interpreters. Her research has focused on improving neuropsychology assessments through investigation of clinical outcomes. She innovated neuropsychological brief neuropsychological assessments in primary care, cognitive stabilization intervention during covid-19, and guidelines for the provision of teleneuropsychology during covid-19. She is Past President of the Society of Clinical Neuropsychology, Division 40 of the American Psychological Association, Massachusetts Psychological Association and Massachusetts Neuropsychological Society. She is also a Fellow of the American Psychological Association, Division 40 (Society of Clinical Neuropsychology).

Robert Fallows, PsyD, MSHA, ABPP is a board certified neuropsychologist and the senior medical director for behavioral health at Samaritan Medical Group within Samaritan Health Services in Oregon. In addition to adopting neuropsychology to a population health-based model in geriatrics and sports medicine, he has been focused on upstream suicide prevention efforts and de-siloing behavioral health services—making behavioral health improvement every healthcare leader's responsibility. He has adopted collective impact and implementation science to drive change within the broader healthcare community, serving as a co-founding member of the Regional

Behavioral Health Council and co-chairing the Coast to Cascades Community Wellness Network. He is a fellow of the National Academy of Neuropsychology and has held several leadership roles with that organization, including conference program chair in 2024 and DistanCE chair. He has been an advocate for training in helping to found the psychology training program at Samaritan as associate program director and also served on the American Psychological Association's Division 40 education advisory committee.

Contributors

Alexandra. L. Clark, Ph.D.
Department of Psychology, The University of Texas at Austin, TX, USA
alexandra.clark@austin.utexas.edu
Molly Colvin, PhD, ABPP-CN
Associate Professor of Psychology, Harvard Medical School
Mass General Brigham, Department of Psychiatry, Boston, USA
mcolvin@mgh.harvard.edu
Heather Cuevas, PhD, APRN, ACNS-BC, FAAN
School of Nursing, The University of Texas at Austin, TX, USA
hcuevas@mail.nur.utexas.edu
Robert Fallows, PsyD, MSHA, ABPP
Samaritan Medical Group, Corvallis, OR, USA
rfallows@samhealth.org
Sanne Franzen, PhD
Department of Neurology & Alzheimer Center
Erasmus MC University Medical Center, Rotterdam, The Netherlands
s.franzen@erasmusmc.nl
Trevor A. Hall, PsyD, ABPdN
Divisions of Pediatric Psychology & Pediatric Critical Care
Oregon Health & Science University
Doernbecher Children's Hospital
halltr@ohsu.edu
Abbey M. Hamlin, M.A.
Department of Psychology, The University of Texas at Austin, TX, USA
abbeyh@utexas.edu
Margaret Lanca, Ph.D.
Department of Psychiatry, Cambridge Health Alliance, Cambridge, MA, USA
Department of Psychiatry, Harvard Medical School, Boston, MA, USA
mlanca@challiance.org
margaret_lanca@hms.harvard.edu
Victoria Leyva M.A.
Department of Psychology, The University of Texas at Austin, TX, USA
victoria.leyva@austin.utexas.edu

Caleb Pearson, PsyD, ABPP
Departments of Neurology, Neurosurgery, and Psychiatry
University of Kansas Medical Center, Kansas City, KS, USA
cpearson2@kumc.edu
Neil H. Pliskin, Ph.D., ABPP
Departments of Psychiatry and Neurology
University of Illinois College of Medicine, Chicago, IL, USA
npliskin@uic.edu
Antonio Puente, PhD.
Department of Psychology, University of North Carolina Wilmington
Shifali Singh, Ph.D.
Department of Neuropsychology, McLean Hospital, Belmont, MA, USA
Institute for Technology in Psychiatry, McLean Hospital, Belmont, MA, USA
Digital Neuropsychology and Brain Health Laboratory, Belmont, MA, USA
Department of Psychiatry, Harvard Medical School, Boston, MA, USA
ssingh@mclean.harvard.edu
Scott A. Sperling, Psy.D., ABPP
Center for Neurological Restoration, Neurological Institute
Section of Neuropsychology, Department of Neurology, Cleveland Clinic Lerner College of Medicine of Case Western Reserve University
sperlis@ccf.org
Elena Tsoy, PhD
Department of Neurology, University of California San Francisco, San Francisco, California, USA
Global Brain Health Institute, University of California San Francisco, San Francisco, California, USA
elena.tsoy@ucsf.edu
Sara Weisenbach, Ph.D., ABPP
Department of Neuropsychology, McLean Hospital, Belmont, MA, USA
Mood and Cognition in Aging Laboratory, Belmont, MA, USA
Department of Psychiatry, Harvard Medical School, Boston, MA, USA
sweisenbach@mclean.harvard.edu
Caroline Vaile Wright PhD
Senior Director of Health Care Innovation,
American Psychological Association, Washington, DC, USA
cwright@apa.org

Part I
Neuropsychology in the Era of Population Health: Frameworks, Value, and Equity

Chapter 1
Reframing Neuropsychology Through the Lens of Population Health: A Conceptual Overview

Margaret Lanca and Robert Fallows

Executive Summary

This chapter situates neuropsychology within the broader transformation of US healthcare toward population health management. Population health emphasizes equitable improvement of health outcomes across defined groups by addressing social, behavioral, and environmental determinants that account for most modifiable contributors to health. The chapter reviews the evolution of this framework highlighting how aligning health policy, financing, and healthcare delivery can improve prevention and chronic-disease management. Four foundational pillars—care management, quality and safety, public health, and health policy—are presented as interlocking systems for achieving sustainable health equity. Within this landscape, neuropsychology is reframed within population health management through its innovations and greater emphasis to detect, prevent, and manage cognitive decline. The chapter calls for expanding neuropsychological services into primary care and community settings, integrating social determinants data, and leveraging digital technologies for scalable, equity-oriented assessment. By adopting a population-health lens, neuropsychology can advance brain-health promotion, improve early detection, and demonstrate measurable value within value-based healthcare systems.

M. Lanca (✉)
Department of Psychiatry, Cambridge Health Alliance, Cambridge, MA, USA
e-mail: margaret_lanca@hms.harvard.edu

Department of Psychiatry, Harvard Medical School, Boston, MA, USA

R. Fallows
Samaritan Medical Group, Corvallis, OR, USA
e-mail: rfallows@samhealth.org

M. Lanca and R. Fallows (eds.), *Advancing Neuropsychology Through Population Health*, https://doi.org/10.1007/978-3-032-22457-6_1

What Is Population Health?

The healthcare industry is increasingly adopting a population health management (PHM) model to drive healthcare and address critical gaps in care delivery. This movement has been supported by various healthcare stakeholders including the American Medical Association's (AMA) formal endorsement of public health as part of medical responsibility, its integration to medical training, and academic medical centers' increased institutionalization of population health in medical research and health services research (Basu et al, 2019; Wise, 2000). The American Psychological Association (APA) also affirmed psychology's commitment to advancing population health, with a multi-tiered approach to enhance health equity, well-being, safety, and resilience across entire communities and societal groups (APA, 2022), and has joined with other organizations to drive change (CEO Alliance for Mental Health, 2024).

There are numerous definitions of population health, but common among them is a focus on equitable improvement of health outcomes by analyzing and managing key drivers of health across groups, aiming to enhance quality of life and patient experiences all the while reducing per capita costs. While medical care is essential, it accounts for only about 10% to 20% of modifiable contributors to health outcomes (see Fig. 1.1). The remaining factors are predominantly social determinants of health (SDOH), which include economic stability, education, social and community context, healthcare access and quality, and the neighborhood and built environment. Collectively, these SDOH can influence up to 30–55% of health outcomes (World Health Organization, 2023). Behavioral factors, such as tobacco use, alcohol consumption, diet, and physical activity, also play a significant role, potentially accounting for approximately 34% of health outcomes. Environmental conditions, including access to clean air and safe housing, further impact health, though their exact contribution varies. For instance, the physical environment alone may account for about 3% of health outcomes (Office of the Assistant Secretary for Planning & Evaluation, 2022). These insights underscore the necessity of a multifaceted approach to healthcare that extends beyond clinical services. Healthcare policy and healthcare delivery have been historically siloed entities, but there is greater appreciation that there needs to be increased collaboration to improve the overall health of a population. By addressing social, behavioral, and environmental determinants, healthcare systems can more effectively improve overall population health and reduce disparities.

Factors that Promote Health of a Population

Healthcare spending and reimbursement structures. The US healthcare system is complex and faces numerous challenges. Despite excelling in certain medical advancements, the system often falls short in delivering consistent, high-quality care and is burdened by exceptionally high costs. In 2023, national health expenditures (NHE) reached $4.9 trillion, accounting for 17.6% of the Gross Domestic Product

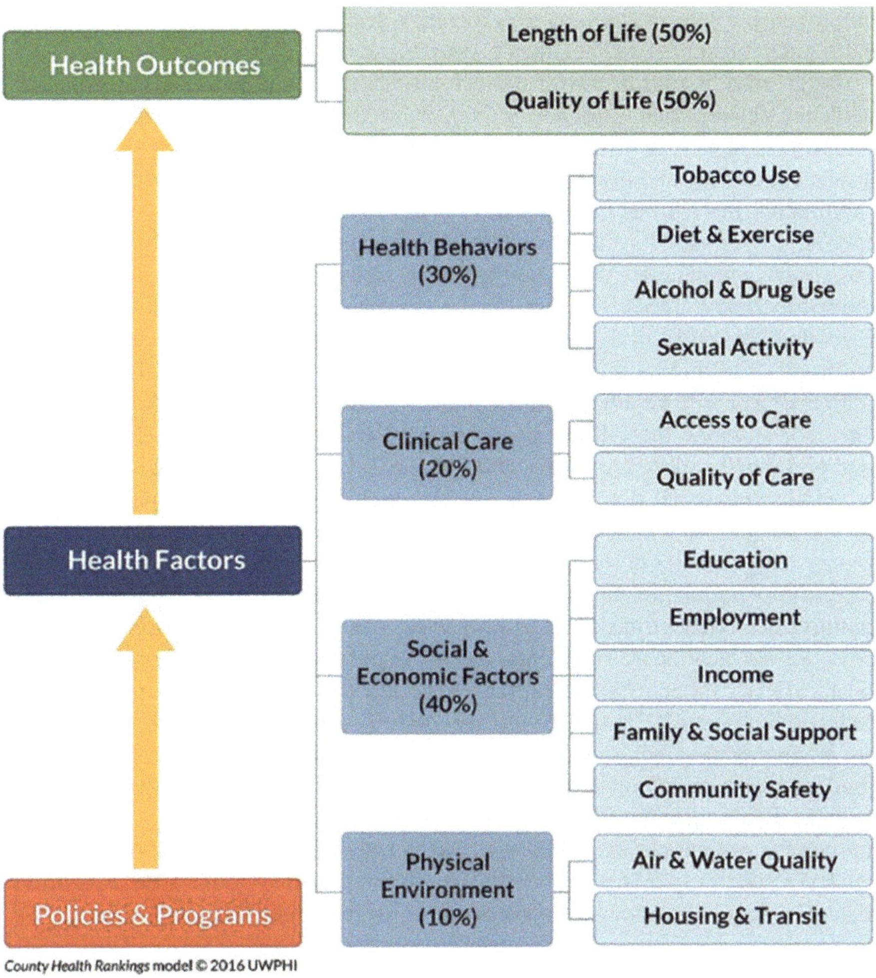

Fig. 1.1 County Health Rankings & Roadmaps Model of Health demonstrating the differential contribution of policies and health factors on health outcomes

(GDP). Projections indicate that by 2032, this figure could approach 20% of GDP. The complexity of the US healthcare system contributes to these challenges. Issues such as lack of insurance coverage, high costs of services, and suboptimal outcomes are well-documented. Policies have been implemented to address these issues, yet significant challenges persist (Levitt & Altmann, 2023). Despite higher healthcare spending, US health outcomes are not necessarily better than those in other high resourced countries. The US performs worse in some common health metrics like life expectancy and infant mortality and safety during childbirth (Peter G. Peterson Foundation, 2023). These factors emphasize that total investment in healthcare is not necessarily the principal driver for health outcomes and underscores the need for comprehensive reforms to enhance efficiency, reduce costs, and improve equitable health outcomes in the US healthcare system.

The primary way to improve the overall health of a population is to finance a healthcare delivery that is not solely focusing on treating illness but rather funding a system that addresses the needs of healthy and ill individuals, encompassing acute and chronic conditions, and involving both clinical services and public health initiatives. Traditionally the US has funded a fee-for-service (FFS) model that predominantly supports a "sick care" system, incentivizing healthcare that is sought during acute illnesses or emergencies. While caring for the sick remains essential, achieving true community health necessitates an equal emphasis on health promotion and disease prevention. This shift in delivery will require a transition in the financing of healthcare from a FFS model to a value-based care (VBC) model, which aligns provider reimbursement with health outcomes, preventive care, and care coordination (Gondi et al., 2022) which the US has begun to do. VBC emphasizes proactive management of defined patient groups by stratifying risk, targeting chronic disease control, and addressing social determinants, all of which begins at the primary care level and extends into specialty care. There is growing evidence showing that enhancing primary care capacity correlates with lower mortality, underscoring primary care's centrality to population health improvement (Basu et al., 2019). Industry survey findings have reflected this shift toward VBC. For example, it has been shown that across all US healthcare payments, approximately 60% of spending in 2023 was tied to a VBC model. Outland (2022) reported that the Centers for Medicare & Medicaid Services (2023) (CMS) has successfully tied approximately 90% of Medicare payments to value, with approximately 40% structured under advanced value-based programs including downside risk arrangements. Leao and colleagues (2023) reviewed the performance of VBC models within networks of care and demonstrated improved coordination and outcomes, particularly in two-sided risk arrangements, which are becoming increasingly prevalent in integrated systems. VBC is still in its infancy in the US but showing some promise for improving healthcare.

Social determinants of health. Expanding the focus of provision of healthcare to early intervention and disease prevention requires a fuller understanding of public health policies. Historically distinct from healthcare delivery, these policies are designed to improve community health and fundamentally serve as preventive healthcare. Coordinating health policy and healthcare delivery is important, because it can improve proactive care through prevention, early identification of disease, chronic disease management, and addressing social health inequities. With respect to the latter, the US Department of Health and Human Services (HHS) published, *Healthy People 2030*, a comprehensive framework for improving the nation's health over a 10-year period (2020–2030). It reinforces the importance of eliminating health disparities and achieving health equity (Healthy People Planning, 2019) to ensure that all Americans have equal opportunity to be healthy through equal access to healthcare education, childcare, transportation, housing, etc. Other comprehensive frameworks tying together health outcomes with social drivers have emerged such as *Vital Conditions* (Rippel Foundation, 2025), which outlines seven interdependent domains necessary for population level thriving. In addition to housing, lifelong learning, basic requirements for health and safety, and reliable transportation, this framework emphasizes the influence of the ecosystem, engagement with nature, meaningful and healthy work, and a sense of belonging, including civic engagement. Unlike other social determinants models, the Vital Conditions Framework offers a concise, actionable, and consensus-based structure for systems change. It emphasizes upstream investments in these domains that move beyond urgent services to foster long-term equity and well-being. Community health centers and multisector coalitions apply the model to align planning, resource allocation, and evaluation across sectors to advance population health.

Regardless of the SDOH framework, coordination of health policy and healthcare that addresses SDOH can result in better health outcomes. Gundersen and Ziliak (2015), for example, found that food-insecure seniors experience limitations in activities of daily living compared to food-secure seniors who are fourteen years older, indicating accelerated physical decline. This type of disconnected public health policy and health delivery system not only results in lower health outcomes but also greater costs through increased patient utilization in a solely FFS environment. However, when health policy and healthcare delivery share SDOH priorities within an advanced payment model (i.e., using VBC models) improvement is possible. Specifically, an accountable care organization appreciates that medical care achieved in a clinical setting can be lost when a patient returns home to sub-standard living conditions and other SDOH stressors that result in decompensation of health and costly readmission rates.

Integrating SDOH factors into care delivery enhances patient engagement and improves health outcomes. Patients facing greater psychosocial stressors may be less likely to participate in care management programs or follow complex medication treatment regimes. To address these disparities, healthcare systems increasingly embed SDOH data into electronic health records (EHRs), enabling clinicians to identify and respond to patients' social needs. Capturing information on housing stability, food insecurity, and transportation barriers allows for the development of personalized treatment plans and discharge instructions that consider both medical and social factors. The American Academy of Family Physicians (2022) advocates for the use of ICD-10 "Z" codes to standardize SDOH documentation, while Cantor and Thorpe (2018) emphasize that such integration supports targeted interventions to mitigate health disparities and provide holistic, patient-centered care.

There are numerous ways a hospital system can assess patient SDOH, though largely through self-report surveys. However, other community programs, such as outreach teams dispatched to conduct home visits for at-risk patients are also used. These teams assist with connecting patients to essential non-clinical resources by assessing their individual needs, providing health education, and linking patients to critical social services (e.g., utility assistance, transportation, lead abatement programs, and nutritional support initiatives like Meals on Wheels or the Women, Infants, and Children (WIC) program). By embracing these strategies, healthcare systems can move toward a more equitable and effective model of care that acknowledges and addresses the complex interplay of social factors influencing health.

Pillars of Population Health

Population health is based on four pillars that are foundational for improving the overall health of a community that, when combined with the above healthcare delivery factors, allow more people an equitable opportunity to sustain health. These are: (1) care management, (2) quality and safety, (3) public health, and (4) health policy (Fabius et al., 2021). Adequately addressing these pillars is especially important since only 55% of US adults receive the recommended preventative and acute care, and care for chronic conditions (McGlynn et al., 2003).

Care management. Care management involves collective efforts by patients, providers, public health, employers, insurers, and policymakers to work together to improve health and wellness. Coordinated care is especially important given the increase in chronic health conditions. Since advancements in healthcare have led to increased life expectancy, longer lifespans have also resulted in a higher prevalence of chronic diseases. Chronic diseases, defined as conditions lasting a year or more and requiring ongoing medical attention or limiting daily activities, are now the leading causes of death and disability worldwide (World Health Organization, 2020). According to the Centers for Disease Control and Prevention (CDC), in 2018, approximately 51.8% of adults had at least one chronic condition, and 27.2% had multiple chronic conditions (Watson et al., 2022). The most common chronic diseases include heart disease, cancer, chronic lung disease, stroke, Alzheimer's disease, diabetes, and chronic kidney disease. Therefore, knowing how to prevent health decline through promotion of healthy aging strategies, and learning how to manage one's chronic conditions can extend lifespans and good quality of life.

Coordinated care programs focus on prevention, early detection, and effective management of chronic conditions. Key components of successful care management programs include patient education, regular monitoring of patient conditions, personalized care plans through assignment of each patient to a care coordinator, and multidisciplinary care teams being responsible for the care of a patient. Coordinated care begins with regular screening of health conditions and once identified, health literacy enhancement/motivational interviewing/behavioral interventions for specific conditions at the outset of treatment. Interventions for health literacy are particularly important component in chronic care management because treatment decisions made collaboratively by patients and their providers, a process known as shared medical decision making, may play a significant role in outcomes (Hughes et al., 2018) (see Chapter 2 on how this can be applied to neuropsychology).

These chronic conditions not only diminish quality of life but also contribute significantly to healthcare costs. The cost of chronic disease to the American medical system accounts for more than $1 trillion every year (Waters & Graf, 2018). To address the burden of chronic diseases, care management programs have been developed, particularly in primary care and in integrated care delivery systems deploying population health service organizations. By emphasizing self-management and proactive care, care management programs have reduced hospitalizations, improved quality of life, and decreased healthcare costs. A review by Koikai and Khan (2023) found that self-management strategies for heart failure patients led to reduced mortality and hospitalizations, and were cost-effective, particularly when innovative approaches like smartphone applications were employed to improve therapy adherence. Similarly, a study by Jovicic et al. (2006) concluded that improved self-management in heart failure patients increased compliance, promoted quality of life, advanced clinical outcomes, reduced hospital readmissions, and decreased hospitalization costs. In a meta-analysis by Checa et al. (2022), nurse-led case management reduced all-cause hospital admissions and heart failure hospitalizations, improved quality of life at medium-term follow-up, and could be cost-effective in high-income countries. Collectively, these studies underscore the efficacy of self-management and care management programs in enhancing patient outcomes and reducing healthcare expenditures.

Quality and Safety. Quality and safety improvement programs are essential components of population health management, aiming to enhance healthcare delivery by minimizing errors and optimizing patient outcomes within healthcare organizations. These programs necessitate active collaboration among healthcare providers, patients, and quality improvement to continuously examine and refine healthcare structures, processes, and workflows and to identify and mitigate potential sources of errors. Effective coordination among these stakeholders is pivotal in achieving quality and safety in healthcare. Moreover, substantial efforts by local, state, and national public health organizations have been directed toward supporting and advancing quality improvement initiatives within local healthcare entities.

Implementing structured methodologies is fundamental to the success of quality improvement initiatives. Techniques such as Failure Modes and Effects Analysis (FMEA), Plan-Do-Study-Act (PDSA) cycles, Lean Six Sigma methodologies, and Root Cause Analysis (RCA) have been effectively employed to enhance healthcare quality and safety and these techniques can be used by neuropsychologists as well to improve systems in their clinic, department, etc. (see Chapter 9) on how this can be applied to neuropsychology). These strategies help to identify and resolve system inefficiencies and errors within healthcare processes, thereby improving patient outcomes. For instance, PDSA cycles enable iterative testing of changes to determine their impact on quality improvement. Lean Six Sigma methodologies focus on reducing process variation and eliminating waste, respectively, leading to more efficient and reliable healthcare delivery. RCA is employed retrospectively to analyze adverse events and identify underlying causes to prevent recurrence. Chassin and Loeb (2013) highlighted the importance of adopting these structured approaches to achieve substantial improvements in patient safety and healthcare quality. Their research emphasizes that healthcare organizations implementing these methodologies have observed significant reductions in medical errors and enhanced overall patient care.

Engaging patients and their families in their healthcare is also a critical aspect of quality improvement. The Agency for Healthcare Research and Quality (AHRQ) developed a guide to promote engagement, emphasizing that active participation of patients and families can lead to measurable improvements in safety and quality. This approach fosters a collaborative environment where patients feel empowered to contribute to their care decisions, enhancing the overall effectiveness of healthcare delivery.

Collaborative efforts among healthcare stakeholders are crucial for the success of quality improvement programs. The Partnership for Patients (PfP) initiative, for example, exemplifies this type of collaboration, bringing together physicians, nurses, hospitals, employers, patients, and advocates to improve the quality, safety, and affordability of healthcare for all Americans. This initiative, launched by the U.S. Department of HHS in 2011, is a national quality improvement program aimed at enhancing patient safety and reducing healthcare costs. The impact of the PfP has been significant. According to reports, from 2010 to 2014, there were approximately 2.1 million fewer patients harmed, resulting in an estimated 87,000 lives saved and nearly $20 billion in cost savings. These outcomes highlight the effectiveness of collaborative efforts in achieving substantial improvements in patient safety and healthcare quality (Agency for Healthcare Research & Quality, 2015).

In summary, quality and safety improvement programs are integral to enhancing population health through improved health delivery models and resulting in cost savings. The active involvement of healthcare providers, patients, and quality improvement teams, supported by structured methodologies and collaborative efforts, is essential for the continuous improvement of healthcare delivery systems. Support from public health organizations further bolsters these initiatives, ensuring that local healthcare entities have the necessary resources and guidance to implement effective quality improvement strategies.

Public health and public policy. Since 80–90% of the health of a population derives from outside the four walls of a healthcare facility, government-led programs at the local, state or federal levels are essential to bettering the health of a population and addressing health disparities. One of the government's roles is to establish comprehensive public health policies and then facilitate the implementation of programs aimed at mitigating community-wide health problems. Different countries carry this out in different ways though, with many European countries adopting the philosophy of the Beveridge Report, listing healthcare and other social services as a constitutional right. Although not the same in the US, social service programs such as nutritional assistance programs like the Supplemental Nutrition Assistance Program (SNAP) aim to alleviate food insecurity, a significant SDOH, thereby addressing disparities related to nutrition and chronic diseases. These public health policies and programs are not only directed at improving education and health behaviors but are also targeted at improving societal infrastructures are also determine population health. Community-based initiatives such as culturally tailored interventions, community health worker programs, and policies targeting social determinants such as housing and education have been instrumental in advancing health equity (Jack, 2021).

More robust policy measures are needed to improve health equity. Programs like the integration of Health in All Policies (HiAP) and Health Impact Assessments (HIAs), which address social determinants and reduce health disparities have not always led to significant changes in social determinants or reductions in health disparities.

In conclusion public health and public health policy are integral to identifying and addressing the complex interplay of factors that contribute to health disparities and disease burdens. Through targeted policy efforts and community-based strategies, it is possible to implement effective interventions that promote health equity and improve population health outcomes.

Healthcare Delivery Imperatives

To enhance population management, healthcare delivery models must prioritize the following: (1) a focus on the promotion of health and wellness of a defined population within a specific geographic area (not just treatment of illness); (2) the adoption of reimbursement structures that incentivize long-term health maximization at minimal cost; and (3) the development of data infrastructures that support care delivery and reimbursement by identifying and monitoring targeted populations, managing care processes, and evaluating quality and utilization metrics (Scherpbier et al., 2021). The integration of SDOH data into EHRs, for example, has proven effective in identifying care gaps among vulnerable populations. By leveraging comprehensive data, healthcare systems can proactively address the multifaceted needs of their communities. Technological advancements are also instrumental in expanding access to care and facilitating early disease detection, particularly through community outreach and primary care centers.

Although beyond the scope of this chapter to examine the details of each of these priorities, the American Hospital Association's Foster G. McGaw Award recent award winner provides a translational example exemplifying each of these main factors. In 2024, the Boston Medical Center (BMC) (2024) was awarded prestigious national honor, which recognizes hospitals that excel in community health improvement and equity. In 2021, BMC launched its Health Equity Accelerator (HEA), a system-wide initiative combining actionable research, integrated clinical care, and community engagement across five domains with high racial health disparities: (1) maternal and child health, (2) infectious disease, (3) behavioral health, (4) chronic conditions (e.g., diabetes), and (5) oncology/end-stage renal disease. Multidisciplinary teams co-designed interventions with community partners and research collaborators, targeting inequities such as preeclampsia among Black mothers. Interventions included expanding a doula program, producing patient education materials, and deploying remote hypertension monitoring, resulting in reduced maternal readmission rates. As part of community-embedded and data-driven initiatives, BMC hosted 47 multi-lingual pop-up vaccination events during the pandemic, bolstered by school, church, and YMCA partnerships. As a result, vaccination rates among primary care patients rose to approximately 82% for first dose and 75% fully vaccinated within one year. These measurable improvements were the result of trusted community relationships and aligned outreach strategies.

In summary, these strategies underscore the importance of creating a comprehensive healthcare delivery system that integrates SDOH, leverages technology, and fosters trusted community relationships. In doing so healthcare systems are better equipped to achieve sustainable improvements in equity, access, and long-term outcomes. The example of BMC illustrates how aligning data-driven interventions with culturally responsive community engagement can produce measurable reductions in health disparities. More broadly, such models demonstrate that investment in prevention and equity-oriented care delivery that not only strengthens community trust but also lays the groundwork for more resilient, cost-effective health systems.

Neuropsychology and Population Health

The discipline of neuropsychology stands at an exciting pivotal juncture, propelled by the growing acknowledgment of cognitive health as a cornerstone for quality of life and sustained autonomy throughout the human lifespan (Randolph, 2018) and the growth of population health management that can extend neuropsychology's reach. Cognitive well-being is increasingly recognized not only for its intrinsic value but also for its role in mitigating socioeconomic burdens, thereby becoming a priority in public health agendas (de Havenon et al., 2024; Medalia & Ehrlich, 2017). The CDC inaugurated the *Healthy Brain Initiative* (HBI) in 2005 in a concerted effort to embed cognitive health within public health frameworks. This early initiative endeavored to promote brain health, confront cognitive impairments, and support caregivers through collaborations. Its prominence is related to the later release of Healthy People 2030 by the CDC. The latest iteration of the HBI Road Map for 2023–2027 further accentuates health equity and the cultivation of partnerships to enhance cognitive health outcomes (Alzheimer's Association & CDC, 2023; National Association of Chronic Disease Directors, 2023).

The urgency of these public health endeavors is underscored by projections indicating a significant escalation in cognitive disorders among the elderly. Recent studies forecast that the annual incidence of dementia in US adults will surge from approximately 514,000 cases in 2020 to nearly 1 million by 2060 (Fang et al., 2025). Moreover, the lifetime risk of developing dementia post-55 years of age is estimated at 42%, with a pronounced prevalence among Black adults, highlighting imperative health equity considerations. This burgeoning prevalence not only intensifies the demand for adept cognitive management within healthcare systems but also amplifies the necessity for coordinated health strategies. The economic ramifications are equally profound. As of 2015, the annual per capita cost for Alzheimer's patients was estimated at $19,144.36, culminating in a national expenditure of approximately $167.74 billion. Projections for 2050 suggest these costs could escalate to an estimated $1.89 trillion, reflecting the intensifying economic strain of cognitive impairments on societal resources (Nandi et al., 2024). Importantly, the financial burden of Alzheimer's disease represents only a fraction of the overall economic impact of dementia, as other major neurocognitive disorders (e.g., vascular dementia, Lewy body dementia), along with central nervous system conditions (e.g., traumatic brain injury) and systemic medical illnesses that disrupt cognitive functioning, contribute significantly to escalating healthcare costs.

Neuropsychology delivery imperatives. This amplified cognitive focus underscores the imperative for holistic public health strategies and healthcare initiatives that address the socioeconomic determinants of cognitive decline to curtail both its prevalence and associated economic impacts. For neuropsychologists, this translates into an increased demand for cognitive assessments both upstream in primary care and community settings, as well as downstream in medical specialties. Neuropsychologists are already integrated across healthcare environments, including inpatient and outpatient hospital specialties (e.g., neurology, psychiatry, surgery, rehabilitation), primary care, and community-based private practices. This widespread presence facilitates the delivery of neuropsychological services across healthcare settings. Yet the field will need to evolve further by adopting greater proactive, preventative roles within interdisciplinary teams, leveraging its unique expertise to support assessment of early detection, risk reduction, and cognitive health promotion at the population level. To do this, neuropsychological services will need to expand more vigorously upstream (see Chapters 5 and 6 on how this can be applied to both adult and pediatric practices).

Early detection of diseases, such as mild cognitive impairment, can significantly improve outcomes by reducing adverse outcomes such as loss of autonomy and mitigate high healthcare costs associated with late-stage interventions (Whelan et al., 2022). Neuropsychological assessments play a crucial role in the early identification of cognitive decline, facilitating appropriate management strategies. Bondi et al. (2014), for example, demonstrated that MCI participants diagnosed using neuropsychological criteria had greater diagnostic precision and a higher progression rate to dementia compared to conventional diagnostic methods, underscoring the effectiveness of neuropsychological assessments in early detection.

By intervening at the earliest stages of cognitive decline, healthcare providers can prevent the progression to more severe conditions, thereby enhancing patients' quality of life. As such, neuropsychological assessments in primary care, particularly brief neuropsychological assessments (BNA) and repeatable cognitive screens can improve the early identification of cognitive issues, allowing for timely and targeted interventions. Cognitive assessments are vital not only for identification of cognitive disease such as dementia, but cognitive health is susceptible to impairment adversely affected by both central nervous system disorders as well as systemic medical conditions of the most common chronic diseases (e.g., heart disease, cancer, chronic lung disease, stroke, epilepsy and chronic kidney disease) throughout the lifespan. Cognitive dysfunction from these chronic illnesses can be profound and disrupt daily activities, occupational performance, caregiving responsibilities, and academic achievement. Cognitive deficits can also lead to substantial financial and psychological burdens on patients and healthcare systems (see Chapter 8).

Greater cognitive screening and BNAs in primary care can also have secondary benefits downstream. With the greater focus on cognitive health, and the aging American population, there has been a surge in the demand of neuropsychological referrals, which has led to extended wait times for neuropsychological evaluations. Expansion of cognitive assessments in primary care to identify cognitive disorders can reduce unnecessary referrals to the medical specialties while supporting the goal of population health by making neuropsychological services more accessible to a broader population.

Cognitive health promotion. In tandem with increased assessments in primary care, neuropsychology delivery models must continue to expand and drive cognitive health and wellness promotion. Neuropsychologists possess specialized expertise that can be used to educate individuals about cognitive health, as well as assess the benefits and risks associated with cognitive functions across various medical conditions. Dotson (2022), for example, offered a comprehensive guide to promoting cognitive health across the lifespan, particularly in older adults with education on the biological and lifestyle factors that can influence brain aging, including physical activity, mental stimulation, social engagement, sleep, and emotional health and emphasis on proactive strategies for maintaining brain function and preventing cognitive decline, while also addressing health disparities and accessibility challenges. Similarly, Braun (2021) delineated a practical, evidence-based approach to improving cognitive functioning and overall brain health with a seven-day plan that integrates primary lifestyle strategies (i.e., nutrition, physical activity, mental stimulation, stress management, sleep, and social connection). These types of cognitive wellness programs can be expanded to scale by partnering with care management programs to include patient education of cognitive health, regular monitoring of patient cognition, and personalized care plans that consider how to manage cognitive dysfunction.

Advances of technology in neuropsychology. As mentioned, one of tenets healthcare delivery in population health is to improve technology and data structures. Technological innovations can be leveraged by neuropsychology for its own advances. The implementation of digital cognitive tools for effective screening, such as phone apps and tablet-based assessments, for example, can help to increase screening efficiency by allowing for frequent, low-burden data collection. This increases ecological validity and provides clinicians with a continuous stream of cognitive performance data, rather than a single clinic-based snapshot. Digital tools can also expand access to underserved populations, improving the potential for cognitive data collection at a large scale and across diverse demographics, which feeds back into more representative datasets.

More broadly, the effective use of technology has the potential to improve patient outcomes. Integrating cognitive assessment findings directly into electronic medical record (EMR) can allow clinicians to monitor cognitive status alongside medical, behavioral, and SDOH data. By linking cognitive data with SDOH, neuropsychology can develop context-sensitive norms that account for environmental and systemic influences on cognition, reducing bias and improving interpretive accuracy. Traditional neuropsychological norms are often based on small, non-representative samples. Digital platforms can collect large, demographically diverse datasets, improving the representativeness of normative data across age, race/ethnicity, language, education, and socioeconomic status. With cloud-based systems, normative data can be updated in near real time as new populations are tested, enabling living norms rather than static reference tables that may become outdated.

A longitudinal record of brain health can also facilitate earlier detection of cognitive decline through big data and AI analytics. For example, aggregating cognitive performance data across large populations enables predictive modeling, helping to identify individuals at higher risk for conditions such as dementia, traumatic brain injury sequelae, or cognitive complications from chronic illness. AI can also improve triage models by flagging concerning patterns in real time. Instead of comparing an individual to a broad group norm, machine learning approaches can generate individualized expected performance profiles, improving diagnostic sensitivity for subtle cognitive changes over time and creating individual patient benchmarks, the cornerstone of personalized medicine.

Technological advances can also improve health equity by making cognitive assessments more accessible to diverse populations and increasing access to care, particularly through telehealth and rural outreach initiatives. COVID-19 not only accentuated the importance of cognitive health, but it also catalyzed a paradigm shift toward digital neuropsychology and tele-neuropsychology (Bilder et al., 2020; Postal et al., 2020; Singh & Germine, 2021). Overall, leveraging technology in a healthcare system can help identify care needs, track the healthcare delivery, and determine best practices. Data management systems, as well population health initiatives from data aggregation, can manage analytics programs with cognitive data to drive better outcomes.

Conclusions

With healthcare costs in the US continuing to increase and health outcomes being among the worst of resourced countries, the imperative for adopting a population health framework is apparent. Incorporating neuropsychological expertise into population health strategies is essential for addressing the complex interplay between cognitive health and overall well-being. By doing so, healthcare systems can better identify at-risk populations for cognitive decline and cognitive disorders, implement targeted interventions, and ultimately reduce health disparities related to cognitive impairments. This integrative approach aligns with the broader goals of public health to enhance quality of life and promote equitable healthcare outcomes for all individuals.

Neuropsychology is uniquely positioned to benefit from and contribute to the broader population health movement. For neuropsychology, this means extending its reach beyond traditional comprehensive neuropsychological evaluations in specialty care into upstream settings such as primary care, community health centers, and getting involved in public health preventive care initiatives. By integrating briefer neuropsychological assessments into routine healthcare encounters and collaborating with healthcare and community stakeholders for cognitive screening, neuropsychologists can facilitate earlier detection of cognitive decline, reduce unnecessary specialty referrals, and enhance access to underserved populations. Embedding SDOH data into neuropsychological practice will allow for greater holistic treatment for both cognitive functioning and the environmental and social factors influencing health. Moreover, as healthcare financing shifts toward VBC, neuropsychology can demonstrate value by aligning its services with goals of reducing hospitalizations, improving quality of life, and lowering costs. Technological innovations, including digital assessment tools, will be invaluable drivers of reaching these goals. Finally, by adopting a population health lens, neuropsychology can not only address the growing burden of dementia and other cognitive disorders but also promote brain health across the lifespan, providing much-needed education to traditionally hard-to-reach populations, which can ultimately reduce disparities and reinforce cognitive well-being as a cornerstone of public health.

References

Agency for Healthcare Research and Quality. (2015). *Saving lives and saving money: Hospital-acquired conditions update: Interim data 2014* (AHRQ Publication No. 15–0020). U.S. Department of Health & Human Services. https://www.ahrq.gov/hai/pfp/interimhacrate2014.html

Alzheimer's Association & Centers for Disease Control and Prevention. (2023). *Healthy brain initiative: State and local road map for public health*, 2023–2027. https://www.alz.org/getmedia/94815e3a-0764-4b73-a0fb-cce66afd5730/healthy_brain_initiative_road_map_2023_2027.pdf

American Academy of Family Physicians. (2022). *Social determinants of health (SDOH) and ICD-10 codes.* https://www.aafp.org/family-physician/patient-care/social-determinants-of-health/sdoh-icd-10-codes.html

American Hospital Association. (2024, July 18). *Boston Medical Center awarded the 2024 AHA Foster G. McGaw Prize.* https://www.aha.org/press-releases/2024-07-18-boston-medical-center-awarded-2024-aha-foster-g-mcgaw-prize

American Psychological Association. (2022). *Psychology's role in advancing population health.* https://www.apa.org/about/policy/population-health-statement.pdf

Basu, S., Berkowitz, S. A., Phillips, R. L., Bitton, A., Landon, B. E., & Phillips, R. S. (2019). Association of primary care physician supply with population mortality in the United States, 2005–2015. *JAMA Internal Medicine, 179*(4), 506–514. https://doi.org/10.1001/jamainternmed.2018.7624

Bilder, R. M., Postal, K. S., Barisa, M., Aase, D. M., Cullum, C. M., Gillaspy, S. R., Harder, L., Kanter, G., Lanca, M., Lechuga, D. M., Morgan, J. M., Most, R., Puente, A. E., Salinas, C. M., & Woodhouse, J. (2020). Interorganizational practice committee recommendations/guidance for teleneuropsychology (TeleNP) in response to the COVID-19 pandemic. *The Clinical Neuropsychologist, 34*(7–8), 1314–1334. https://doi.org/10.1080/13854046.2020.1767214

Bondi, M. W., Edmonds, E. C., Jak, A. J., Clark, L. R., Delano-Wood, L., McDonald, C. R., Nation, D. A., Libon, D. J., Au, R., Galasko, D. R., & Salmon, D. P. (2014). Neuropsychological criteria for mild cognitive impairment improves diagnostic precision, biomarker associations, and progression rates. *Journal of Alzheimer's Disease, 42*(1), 275–289. https://doi.org/10.3233/JAD-140276

Braun, M. (2021). *Boost your brain: A 7-day plan to enhance memory, focus, and well-being.* William Morrow.

Cantor, M. N., & Thorpe, L. (2018). Integrating data on social determinants of health into electronic health records. *Health Affairs, 37*(4), 585–590. https://doi.org/10.1377/hlthaff.2017.1252

CEO Alliance for Mental Health. (2024). *A unified vision for transforming mental health and substance use care.* https://ceoallianceformentalhealth.org/wp-content/uploads/2024/06/CEO-Alliance_Unified-Vision-3.1-Pathways-6.14.24.pdf

Centers for Medicare & Medicaid Services. (2023). *National health expenditure data.* https://www.cms.gov/Research-Statistics-Data-and-Systems/Statistics-Trends-and-Reports/NationalHealthExpendData

Chassin, M. R., & Loeb, J. M. (2013). High-reliability health care: Getting there from here. *The Milbank Quarterly, 91*(3), 459–490. https://doi.org/10.1111/1468-0009.12023

Checa, C., Canelo-Aybar, C., Suclupe, S., Ginesta-López, D., Berenguera, A., Castells, X., Brotons, C., & Posso, M. (2022). Effectiveness and cost-effectiveness of case management in advanced heart failure patients attended in primary care: A systematic review and meta-analysis. *International Journal of Environmental Research and Public Health, 19*(21), 13823. https://doi.org/10.3390/ijerph192113823

de Havenon, A., Stulberg, E. L., Littig, L., Wong, K.-H., Sarpong, D., Li, V., Sharma, R., Falcone, G. J., Williamson, J. D., Pajewski, N. M., Gottesman, R. F., Brickman, A. M., & Sheth, K. N. (2024). Socioeconomic and medical determinants of state-level subjective cognitive decline in the United States. *Alzheimer's & Dementia, 20*(11), 7567–7579. https://doi.org/10.1002/alz.14220

Dotson, V. M. (2022). *Keep your wits about you: The science of brain maintenance as you age.* American Psychological Association.

Fabius, R. J., Lawrence, C., Isaac, F., & Rachlin, R. (2021). *Population health: Creating a culture of wellness* (3rd ed.). Jones & Bartlett Learning.

Fang, E. F., et al. (2025). Dementia incidence trend analysis in the United States. *Journal of the American Geriatrics Society, 73*(1), 45–54. https://doi.org/10.1111/jgs.17345

Gondi, S., et al. (2022). Analysis of value-based payment and acute care use in a national population of Medicare Advantage beneficiaries. *JAMA Network Open, 5*(9), Article e2232180. https://doi.org/10.1001/jamanetworkopen.2022.32180

Gundersen, C., & Ziliak, J. P. (2015). Food insecurity and health outcomes. *Health Affairs, 34*(11), 1830–1839. https://doi.org/10.1377/hlthaff.2015.0645

Healthy People Planning. (2019). *Healthy people 2030 framework. U.S. Department of Health and Human Services.* https://health.gov/healthypeople/objectives-and-data/browse-objectives

Hughes, T. M., Merath, K., Chen, Q., Sun, S., Palmer, E., Idrees, J. J., Okunrintemi, V., Squires, M., Beal, E. W., & Pawlik, T. M. (2018). Association of shared decision-making on patient-reported health outcomes and healthcare utilization. *American Journal of Surgery, 216*(1), 7–12. https://doi.org/10.1016/j.amjsurg.2018.01.011

Jack, L., Jr. (2021). Advancing health equity, eliminating health disparities, and improving population health. *Preventing Chronic Disease, 18*, E79. https://doi.org/10.5888/pcd18.210286

Jovicic, A., Holroyd-Leduc, J. M., & Straus, S. E. (2006). Effects of self-management intervention on health outcomes of patients with heart failure: A systematic review of randomized controlled trials. *BMC Cardiovascular Disorders, 6*, 43. https://doi.org/10.1186/1471-2261-6-43

Koikai, J., & Khan, Z. (2023). The effectiveness of self-management strategies in patients with heart failure: A narrative review. *Cureus, 15*(7), Article e41863. https://doi.org/10.7759/cureus.41863

Leao, D. L. L., Pereira, A. M. A., Almeida, C. C., & Oliveira, M. D. (2023). The impact of value-based payment models for networks of care: A systematic review. *Population Health Management, 26*(3), 223–234. https://doi.org/10.1089/pop.2022.0141

Levitt, L., & Altmann, D. (2023). Persistent challenges in U.S. healthcare policy. *Health Policy Journal, 12*(3), 45–58. https://doi.org/10.1016/j.hpjo.2023.03.00

Magnan, S. (2017). Social determinants of health 101 for health care: Five plus five. *NAM Perspectives, 7*(10), 1–17. https://doi.org/10.31478/201710c

McGlynn, E. A., Asch, S. M., Adams, J., Keesey, J., Hicks, J., DeCristofaro, A., & Kerr, E. A. (2003). The quality of health care delivered to adults in the United States. *The New England Journal of Medicine, 348*(26), 2635–2645. https://doi.org/10.1056/NEJMsa022615

Medalia, A., & Ehrlich, M. F. (2017). Cognitive remediation in schizophrenia. *Oxford University Press*. https://doi.org/10.1093/med:psych/9780199395224.001.0001

Nandi, A., et al. (2024). Economic burden of Alzheimer's disease in the United States. *Alzheimer's & Dementia, 20*(1), 123–132. https://doi.org/10.1002/alz.13001

National Association of Chronic Disease Directors. (2023). *Healthy Brain Initiative*. https://chronicdisease.org/healthy-aging/resources-for-action/healthy-braininitiative/

Office of the Assistant Secretary for Planning and Evaluation. (2022). *Social determinants of health*. U.S. Department of Health and Human Services. https://aspe.hhs.gov/topics/health-health-care/social-determinants-health

Outland, B. E. (2022). Reforming physician payments to achieve greater equity and value. *Annals of Internal Medicine, 175*(3), 418–419. https://doi.org/10.7326/M21-4484

Peter G. Peterson Foundation. (2023). *U.S. healthcare spending and outcomes*. https://www.pgpf.org/blog/2023/03/how-does-the-us-healthcare-system-compare-to-other-countries

Postal, K. S., Bilder, R. M., Barisa, M., Aase, D. M., Cullum, C. M., Gillaspy, S. R., Harder, L., Kanter, G., Lanca, M., Lechuga, D. M., Morgan, J. M., Most, R., Puente, A. E., Salinas, C. M., & Woodhouse, J. (2020). Interorganizational practice committee recommendations/guidance for teleneuropsychology (TeleNP) in response to the COVID-19 pandemic. *Archives of Clinical Neuropsychology, 35*(7–8), 1314–1334. https://doi.org/10.1080/13854046.2020.1767214

Randolph, C. (2022). The future of neuropsychology: Emphasizing cognitive health. *Neuropsychology Review, 32*(4), 567–580. https://doi.org/10.1007/s11065-022-09512-3

Randolph, J. J. (Ed.). (2018). *Positive neuropsychology: Evidence-based perspectives on promoting cognitive health*. Springer.

Rippel Foundation. (2025). *Vital conditions for health and well-being*. https://rippel.org/vital-conditions/

Scherpbier, A., Walsh, K., & Skoufalos, A. (2021). Healthcare delivery models for population health management. *Population Health Management, 24*(5), 563–570. https://doi.org/10.1089/pop.2020.0238

Singh, S., & Germine, L. (2021). Technology meets tradition: A hybrid model for implementing digital tools in neuropsychology. *International Review of Psychiatry, 33*(4), 382–393. https://doi.org/10.1080/09540261.2020.1835839

Waters, H., & Graf, M. (2018). *The costs of chronic disease in the U.S.* (1st ed.). Milken Institute. https://milkeninstitute.org/sites/default/files/reports-pdf/ChronicDiseases-HighRes-FINAL_2.pdf

Watson, K. B., Carlson, S. A., Loustalot, F., Town, M., Eke, P. I., Thomas, C. W., & Greenlund, K. J. (2022). Chronic conditions among adults aged 18–34 years—United States, 2019. *Morbidity and Mortality Weekly Report, 71*(30), 964–970. https://doi.org/10.15585/mmwr.mm7130a3

Whelan, R., Barbey, F. M., Cominetti, M. R., Yassa, M. A., Ziegler, G., Zanto, T. P., Fjell, A. M., et al. (2022). Developments in scalable strategies for detecting early markers of cognitive decline. *Translational Psychiatry, 12*, 473. https://doi.org/10.1038/s41398-022-02237-w

Wise, B. (2000). New AMA policies on public health. *JAMA, 283*(9), 1216. https://doi.org/10.1001/jama.283.9.1216

World Health Organization. (2020). *Noncommunicable diseases: Key facts* [Fact sheet]. https://www.who.int/news-room/fact-sheets/detail/noncommunicable-disease

World Health Organization. (2023). *Social determinants of health*. https://www.who.int/health-topics/social-determinants-of-health

Chapter 2
Applying a Population Health Framework to Neuropsychological Practice

Margaret Lanca and Robert Fallows

Executive Summary
This chapter outlines a neuropsychological population health framework that integrates neuropsychology at all levels of healthcare, from the community to the health system. It emphasizes the need for a population-focused approach to neuropsychology, discussing pathways to achieve greater access to cognitive assessments and greater integration of cognitive health at all levels of healthcare. The chapter highlights the expanding role of neuropsychologists, particularly in identifying at-risk populations within otherwise healthy communities, underscoring the importance of early detection and intervention. The chapter then transitions to the applications of neuropsychological practices within population health. It examines current practices in neuropsychology, pointing out how they diverge from traditional population health methods. A significant focus is placed on the evolving needs of diverse and changing demographics. Additionally, the chapter envisions a neuropsychology-focused population health framework, outlining its own pillars and guiding principles that will be explored further throughout the book. This vision aims to integrate neuropsychology more deeply into population health management, ensuring that cognitive health is prioritized alongside physical and mental health in community and healthcare settings.

M. Lanca (✉)
Department of Psychiatry, Cambridge Health Alliance, Cambridge, MA, USA
e-mail: margaret_lanca@hms.harvard.edu

Department of Psychiatry, Harvard Medical School, Boston, MA, USA

R. Fallows
Samaritan Medical Group, Corvallis, OR, USA
e-mail: rfallows@samhealth.org

M. Lanca and R. Fallows (eds.), *Advancing Neuropsychology Through Population Health*, https://doi.org/10.1007/978-3-032-22457-6_2

Why Population Health and Why Does Neuropsychology Need to Get Involved?

Introduction

Population health is viewed as a promising solution for closing key gaps in healthcare delivery systems both abroad, but specifically within the United States (US). It addresses the healthy and the unhealthy, the acutely ill and the chronically ill, and the clinical delivery system in the public sector and private sector. Population health is, at its core, an organizing framework for achieving health equity—that is, ensuring that every person has a fair and just opportunity to attain their highest level of health. While traditional healthcare models focus on treating illness after it occurs, population health seeks to address the root causes of why some groups experience poorer health outcomes, shorter lifespans, and greater disease burden than others. The goal is to improve the health of all individuals to create thriving communities and a productive workforce. It does so by expanding the scope of care beyond the clinic walls to consider the social, environmental, and economic determinants that shape health long before an individual seeks medical attention (Braveman et al., 2022).

One factor that is particularly critical to healthcare providers and clinical neuropsychologists alike is the cost of chronic disease to the US medical system, with more than $1 trillion spent every year for chronic health conditions alone as estimated in 2016 (Waters & Graf, 2018). With the advancements in healthcare, life expectancy has increased, and with longer lifespans there is also a higher prevalence of chronic disease. According to the Centers for Disease Control (CDC) in 2018, approximately 51.8% of adults had at least one chronic condition and 27.2% had multiple chronic conditions (Boersma et al, 2020). The most common chronic diseases include heart disease, cancer, chronic lung disease, stroke, Alzheimer's disease, diabetes, and chronic kidney disease. Adults with multiple morbidity accounted for 93% of Medicare spending and two-thirds of overall healthcare costs. Chronic diseases increasingly drain resource utilization and place fiscal pressure on aging populations. Therefore, better management of chronic conditions can extend lifespans and good quality life. However, this focus must run in tandem with better health prevention programs and early identification of illness before it becomes severe or chronic. Overall, the current healthcare system struggles to address the health problems at the tip of the healthcare iceberg. Health conditions are highly prevalent, and massive health disparities exist. Healthcare is fragmented, few people receive minimally acceptable care, and there is a high burden of disability of health disorders. We are slow to detect and late to intervene across all populations of people, but especially in those historically minoritized by the healthcare system. Consequently, all of these lead factors to poor health outcomes and high rate of mortality, for which some pay a higher cost than others.

To address these poor health outcomes, population health factors such as predefined healthcare priorities (e.g., prevention work, expanded Information Technology (IT) infrastructure), social determinants, and healthcare spending establish the foundation (and guide the likelihood of success) of the healthcare delivery system, upon which the pillars of population health management are built upon (see Fig. 2.1). Healthcare spending and reimbursement structures need to be carefully crafted to finance a delivery system that addresses the needs of both healthy and sick individuals. However, traditional fee for service models in the US have predominantly supported a "sick system" incentivizing healthcare that is primarily sought during when people are acutely sick. However, achieving true community health necessitates an equal emphasis on health promotion, disease prevention and care continuity, rather than episodic treatment. By aligning financial incentives around these outcome metrics rather than volume (i.e., number of patient visits) alone, a more equity-focused population model is engrained. Such a system may also hold appeal to both insurance companies and the individuals they insure. Specifically, addressing "adverse selection" has undoubtedly been a challenge within the Affordable Care Act. That is, health insurance companies need healthy individuals in their risk pool to create balance; however, many healthy individuals have balked at the idea of being required to maintain health insurance when they are not "sick." By not focusing on volumes of sick individuals alone but also addressing outcome metrics with a focus on keeping people healthy, individuals may see more benefit in maintaining some base of health insurance.

Addressing social determinants of health (SDOH) is also foundational to shape population health, and constant attention is required to improve assessment of SDOH across communities and target programs to address them. Notably, these programs must be rooted in the communities they serve and delivered from a trauma-informed, bottom-up approach. If not attended to or poorly implemented, the ground gained in clinical settings can be lost when a patient returns home, leading to costly, stressful, and avoidable treatments and re-admission rates. In essence, population health recognizes that inequities in healthcare access, quality, and outcomes are not inevitable—they are design problems within systems. Therefore, achieving health equity is not a side effect of population health; it is the central mission.

The primary pillars of population health are then built upon this foundation, and include clinical care management, quality and safety, and public health and policy (public health and policy collapsed into one here for design purposes given similar governmental origin) (Fig. 2.1) (Fabius, 2021). The impetus for care management is based on the critical need to improve upon care coordination, and that clinical management and effective self-management must be actively promoted. As will discussed across other chapters, achieving high levels of self-management is a significant challenge given both the growing gap between the average patient's health literacy and advances in medical science, as well as the cognitive challenges that many chronic health conditions introduce. Quality and safety improvement rely on both providers and patients together examining the structure and organization of healthcare delivery and improving processes that can lead to error. Supportive local state and national public health efforts must complement the quality and safety work being done at local healthcare institutions and coordination is necessary. Safety does

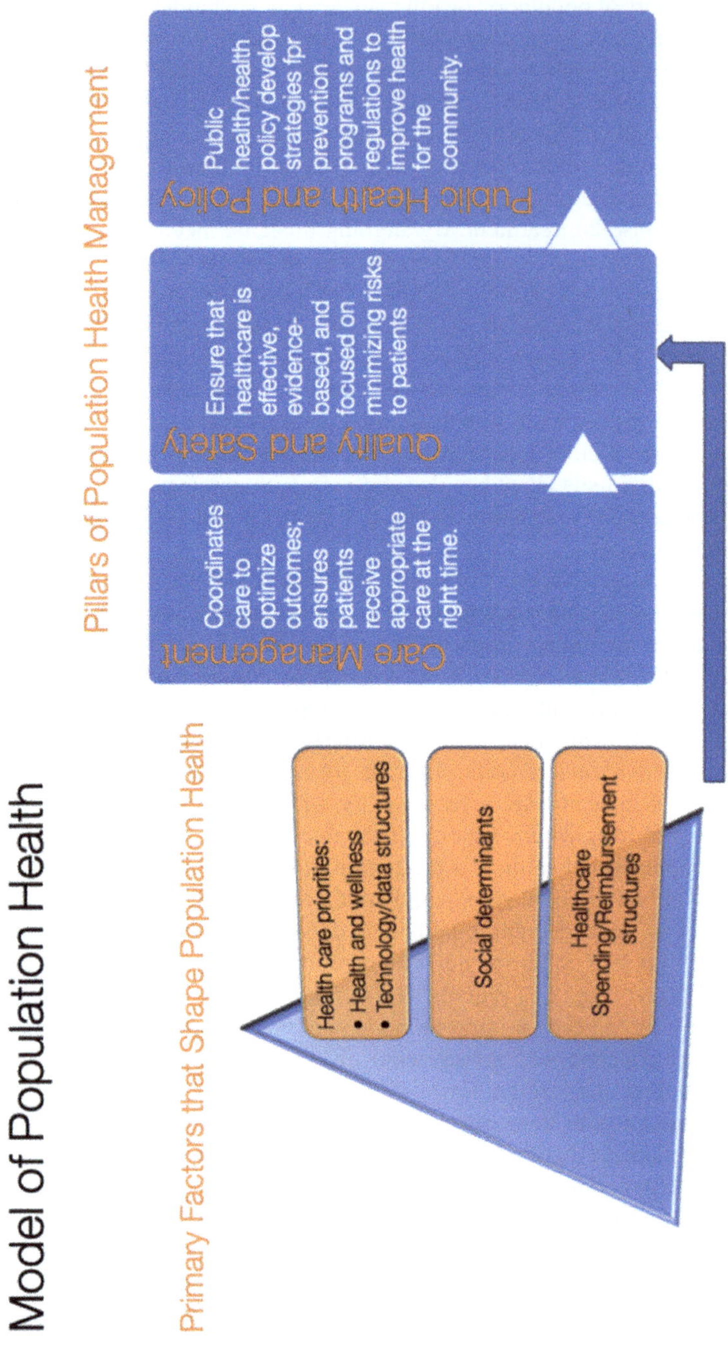

Fig. 2.1 Model framework that illustrates the primary factors that shape population health driving the primary pillars of population health management

not happen by accident, but through a near obsession with failure and use of implementation science (IS) techniques to identify and close gaps. Policies and interventions are designed not just to improve average health outcomes, but to narrow the gaps between those who are most and least advantaged. For instance, initiatives that create safe walking environments, expand early childhood programs (including a focus on reducing risk of adverse childhood experiences (ACEs)), or provide equitable access to preventive screenings directly advance population health goals by leveling opportunities for wellness. Successful execution of these three pillars will allow many more people to receive evidence-based care and health-related services.

Connecting Public Health and Clinical Care

In population health management, there is an expansion of healthcare from the sole focus being on the individual patient to understanding the needs and caring for the population. The push in healthcare reform and movement toward population health is to look beyond the local healthcare clinic or hospital to consider the targeted population and consider three main goals: (1) prevention; (2) early detection; and (3) intervention. This requires collaboration with public health through implementation of targeted public policies with community stakeholders to drive health initiatives. Prevention to a large degree happens outside of traditional healthcare service delivery. Within healthcare delivery, it may look like a vaccine within a primary care clinic, breast cancer screening, or free condoms at the front desk; however, in the community, prevention may look like a collaboration between a public health department and a minority congregation at a church to improve engagement in preventative screening (e.g., who isn't going to the health clinic and how can we encourage them?) or a campaign to repair and improve homes or sidewalks in a low income housing area (e.g., whose environment predisposes them to more risk?).

To achieve this goal of greater prevention and early detection, there needs to be greater collaboration between community and public health with traditional clinical care. Population health lies at the intersection of both the work of community and public health with healthcare provision. As shown in Fig. 2.2, this intersection is representative of the collaboration between these entities that traditionally have been siloed. At the community level, there has been increased efforts for large healthcare organizations to develop relationships with interest holders in the community and also to embed primary care clinics in community settings (e.g., School Based Health Centers [U.S. Department of Education, 2025]) to improve access to healthcare and greater collaboration with community interest holders. With evolving population health, the intersection of these two entities needs to expand. These partnerships improve communication to healthcare organizations and increase awareness about the needs of communities. Many healthcare organizations now have Chief Community Officers and/or Population Health Service Organizations to oversee, manage, and develop system-wide community health strategies. It results in extending healthcare upstream with a greater emphasis on primary care being at the center of a patient's

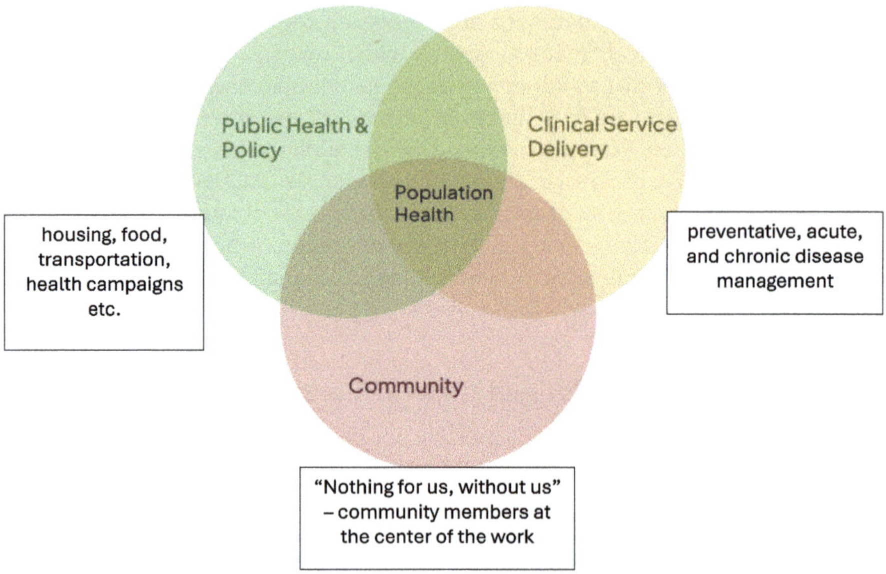

Fig. 2.2 Representation of the relationship between public policy and public health and clinical services in a population health model

overall coordination of care, as well as greater coordination with community stakeholders, instead of patients seeking and driving their own healthcare needs, especially through specialty care without coordination at the primary care level.

Neuropsychology Population Health

Neuropsychology can be well positioned to provide care both upstream in the community and primary care as well as downstream in specialty care, already being well represented at all facets and levels of healthcare. As can be seen in Fig. 2.3, neuropsychologists have traditionally worked in private clinics embedded in communities (e.g., concussion clinics, behavioral health clinics, neurology clinics, and forensic/court settings) as well as multiple levels of health systems. More recently, there has been an influx of neuropsychologists working in primary care and of course, most traditionally, neuropsychologists are well represented in specialty care like psychiatry, neurology, rehabilitation, as well as inpatient surgical care. There has been growing efforts to have clinicians represented in community settings such as schools (e.g., teen health centers), and this is an area where neuropsychologists may already present. What is lacking are existing systems that improve bidirectional collaboration between healthcare systems, and smaller community-level health provision (e.g., private clinics) with community entities that can facilitate access to care, and health education programs. Second, the coordination of care across the different levels and systems could also be improved in ways that could benefit neuropsychology practice (e.g., sharing of prior neuropsychological reports and medical records). This is one area where healthcare needs to improve in general, so that patients can cross healthcare systems and levels and choose to share their electronic medical record (EMR) more easily (e.g., without the burden of physically obtaining medical records and transporting them across systems). As an example, several states have a secure statewide network that facilitates the transmission of healthcare data and health information among providers, hospitals, and other healthcare entities as allowed by applicable state and federal laws. States are continuing to promote HIEs (Health Information Exchanges) with state-level policy, funding or governance support. This is particularly important with the increased numbers of patients with multiple medical conditions who seek various medical specialists, and especially for those who are unable to coordinate and advocate for care on their own (including many patients with cognitive impairment).

Population-focused neuropsychology can improve health outcomes by increasing prevention efforts, increasing access to neuropsychology and expanding early cognitive intervention among other initiatives. Direct examples of care include developing prevention programs at the community level such as designing and implementing a cognitive wellness program which taps into neuropsychology expertise of cognitive health. Another example of direct care could include participating in the development and implementation of cognitive screening programs at the clinic level or in the community by leveraging technology advances (e.g., tablet-based cognitive screenings). Other examples might be more indirect though, including working with

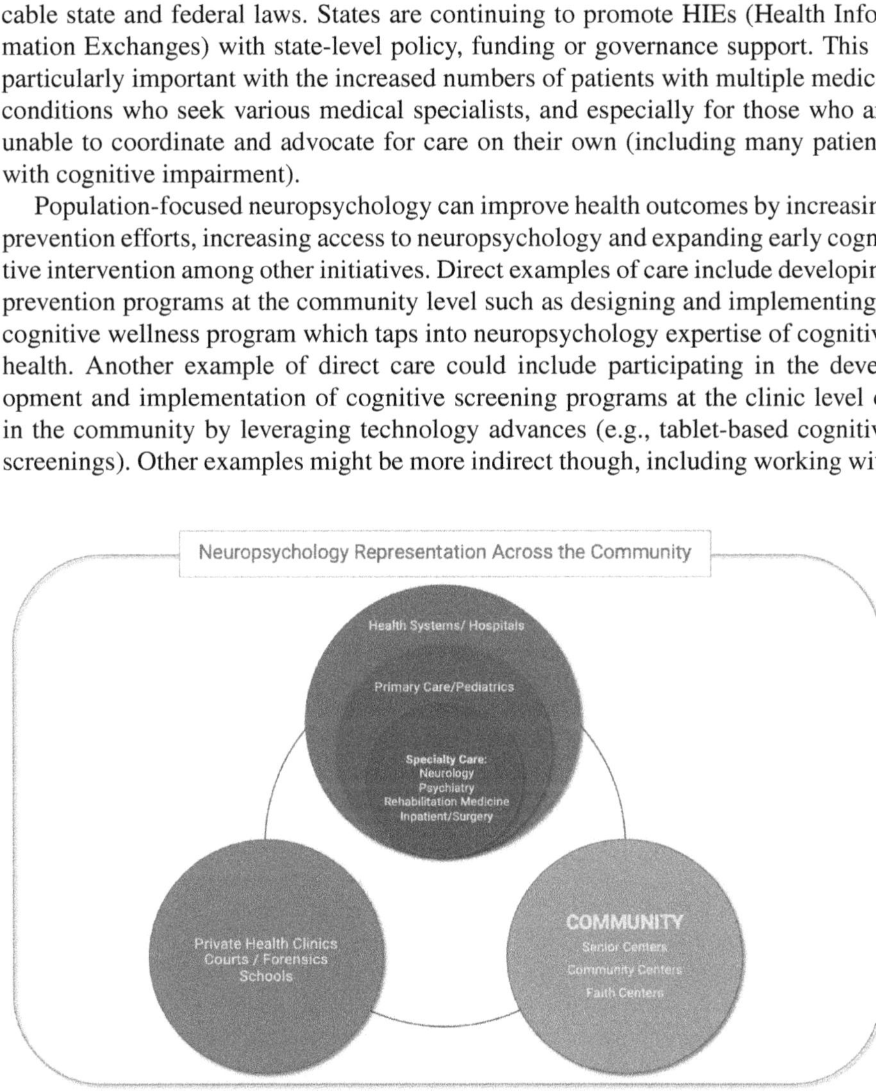

Fig. 2.3 Neuropsychology representation at various levels of healthcare and in the community

EMR specialists to integrate cognitive test results and health literacy scores such that each patient has a health information communication strategy specific to them. An example of how this may play out could include an endocrinologist seeing a patient with diabetes who has an A1c of 13.3%, but the EMR reflects low health literacy and executive dysfunction (from cognitive screening). The plan could then be co-developed with the patient and tailored with the assistance of artificial intelligence to include a greater breakdown of treatment steps (e.g., instead of "use glucometer daily, log results, and adjust insulin bolus," it could state "set a reminder on phone for just before breakfast to check blood sugar, write the number in the log, and then use the table to see how much insulin you need—call our diabetes nurse with any questions").

Increased efforts toward cognitive health education and neuropsychology at the community level can also help communities to understand when and how neuropsychology can be helpful to them. At the clinic level, there is a need to improve neuropsychology triage models so that critical ill patients could be seen more swiftly, and all patients can access neuropsychology assessments for their designated level of care (e.g., cognitive screening, brief neuropsychological assessments or more comprehensive assessments). This type of prevention work can also be facilitated by improved reimbursement models that incentivizes prevention care as many types of prevention work are not currently reimbursable for psychologists.

Thinking Upstream in Population-Focused Neuropsychology

Health prevention forms the scaffolding of population health strategy, from shaping environments before disease ever emerges (primordial) to managing chronic illness and its ripple effects (tertiary) (AbdulRaheem, 2023; Kisling, & Das, 2022). Primordial prevention addresses the underlying social, economic, and environmental conditions that determine population health before specific risk factors even develop. It's about altering the context that breeds risk—such as policy, equity, and environment rather than individual behavior. Examples of primordial strategies include designing walkable communities to reduce sedentary lifestyles, regulating air quality to prevent cardiovascular and neurodevelopmental disorders, and addressing SDOH (e.g., education, housing, income inequality) with programs and subsidies. Primordial interventions have resulted in innovations such as the development of affordable, culturally appropriate grocery stores with healthy foods in urban food deserts. In a neuropsychology context, primordial strategies can focus on reducing early-life adversity, toxic stress, and poverty exposure all of which elevate lifetime risk for cognitive decline and mental health disorders. Highlighting the need for these interventions, a large population health driven study recently demonstrated that childhood maltreatment results in significant cognitive changes which are sustained into late midlife across multiple domains (Maxfield et al., 2025). Primordial strategies are typically the focus of public health. However, a case can certainly be made to increase healthcare, and neuropsychology's engagement in large-scale primordial interventions.

Primary, secondary, and tertiary strategies in turn, are the clear focus for healthcare providers in collaboration with public health. Table 2.1 compares prevention strategies for medicine and neuropsychology. Primary prevention aims to prevent the onset of disease or injury by reducing exposure to risk factors or increasing resilience before disease occurs. Population health primary endeavors include immunization programs, obesity reduction programs, smoking cessation programs, and nutrition campaigns. In a neuropsychology context, this can include cognitive health education for middle-aged adults to prevent dementia, public education on brain health, stress management, sports concussion prevention, and sleep hygiene before cognitive decline begins. Secondary prevention focuses on early detection and timely intervention to halt or slow disease progression in its initial stages. This is where screening and measurement-based care (MBC) are critical. There are already multiple nationwide programs for blood pressure screening for hypertension, depression, and suicide-risk screening in primary care, and cognitive impairment screening in aging populations. Expanding on these programs for cognitive health can include screening for mild cognitive impairment or traumatic brain injury risk factors to intervene before functional decline. Finally, tertiary prevention manages established disease to prevent complications, reduce disability, and improve quality of life. The focus shifts from prevention to rehabilitation and optimization. Critical tertiary strategies in medicine include cardiac rehabilitation for post-myocardial infarction, chronic disease management programs for diabetes, integrated behavioral health for stroke survivors. In a neuropsychology context, this can be seen in cognitive rehabilitation for stroke, traumatic brain injury, or progressive dementia to maintain function and reduce caregiver burden.

As an example of how population health management can be put into practice to assist neuropsychologists, let us consider the work being done at a local community healthcare organization in Cambridge MA, namely Cambridge Health Alliance (CHA). At this institution achieving community well-being through population health is a focus, and there is a Community Health department whose work is geared to understanding the communities it serves, reducing health inequities and barriers to care, and providing greater connections to these communities. Periodically the department conducts Community Health Assessments, which serve to support a Community Health Improvement Plan (i.e., CHIP). These assessments entail gathering state-level statistics and combining them with focus groups conducted with local community residents, and one-to-one interviews with community leaders. These community members are not all patients to the healthcare system but residents of surrounding communities in its catchment area. Meeting with community stakeholders and residents is important to getting a better understanding of the community health challenges and barriers to healthcare. The goal of these assessments is to understand the community better, foster community relationships by bridging the divide between healthcare and communities, and to initiate programs based on community-identified health needs and priorities (CHIP) (Cambridge Health Alliance, 2025). As shown in Fig. 2.4, statistics are gathered on the demographics of the servicing towns

Table 2.1 Comparison of levels of prevention for physical and cognitive health

Levels of prevention strategies in population health			
Level of strategy	Primary strategies	Secondary strategies	Tertiary strategies
Physical health	Improve overall health of individuals by promoting healthy environments & cultures	Early detection of disease; reduce barriers to early treatment; improving outcome and reducing disease chronicity	Minimize disease complications and comorbidities through EBT and coordination of continuity of care; progress monitoring
	E.g., tobacco reduction, nutrition, exercise	E.g., detecting early-stage breast cancer	E.g., chronic care monitoring for disease specific indicators
Cognitive health	Improve overall cognitive health of individuals	Early detection of cognitive disorders; reduce barriers to early treatment; improving outcomes and reducing disease chronicity	Minimize complications of cognitive disorders
	E.g., cognitive determinants of health, and cognitive wellness education	E.g., Early cognitive screening/brief neuropsyc assessments/repeated assessments	Increased regular screening/ assessments to update treatment recommendations

including racial, ethnic, and linguistic diversity, all of which are known indicators of health outcomes, as well as other SDOH indicators such as food and housing insecurity. These statistics help to clarify which towns have higher rates of food insecurity and housing insecurity, for example, lower rates of healthcare, as well as residents who speak languages other than English in their home. Statistics are also gathered (as shown in Fig. 2.4) on major health outcomes for key illnesses/ disorders such as cancer, chronic disease, mental health, and substance use disorders. As this figure shows there are significant disparities across towns compared to the Massachusetts average across various health outcomes. These statistics are then combined with information from focus groups and individual interviews to better understand the barriers to care for local residents. The information is then used to develop and improve existing programs that connect patients to much-needed services (CHIP). The Health Improvement Team, for example, works with healthcare providers, residents, community-based organizations and city leaders to assess health status, determine priorities, build action plans, and provide leadership around health issues that impact the community. Examples of programs developed by this department in concert with local community officials include HIV prevention services, sexual and reproductive health services, trauma and community violence services, and youth initiatives.

At the provider healthcare level, CHA also conducts a biannual SDOH screening for every patient. Figure 2.5 demonstrates a streamlined example of an SDOH measure conducted at this facility, though many published screens exist including

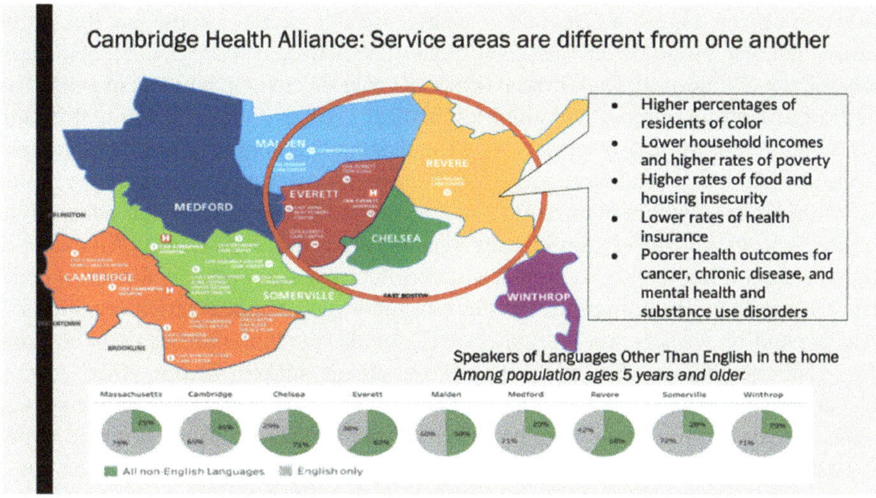

The burden of chronic disease, poor mental health, substance use, and sexual and reproductive health concerns is not distributed equally across our communities.

Health Indicator	MA	Cambridge	Chelsea	Everett	Malden	Medford	Revere	Somerville	Winthrop
Cancer deaths	136.2	109.6	141.7	129.7	145.8	127.1	125.6	133.0	136.1
Heart disease deaths	127.8	102.2	140.6	123.7	126.7	113.6	112.2	133.5	117.4
Diabetes deaths	16.3	15.5	18.4	21.2	19.3	17.0	17.5	19.2	14.2
Asthma ED visits	355.3	220.6	479.7	518.2	358.7	253.2	317.0	321.9	199.3
COPD hospitalizations	168.3	107.5	273.8	242.7	176.1	142.7	196.9	154.8	125.8
Mental health-related ED visits	2,039.7	2,780.9	3,444.0	2,435.2	2,913.4	1,611.4	1,864.6	2,030.3	1,485.3
Substance use-related ED visits	1,140.8	2,049.1	2,455.8	1,613.8	2,077.6	950.2	1,270.9	1,295.3	932.3
Preterm births	9.0%	7.3%	9.6%	9.8%	8.2%	8.0%	8.7%	8.0%	7.0%
Gonorrhea incidence	122.0	131.7	249.2	181.3	176.3	128.5	179.2	151.2	153.8
Syphilis incidence	20.1	24.7	53.6	46.7	38.1	24.2	38.9	32.5	24.2
HIV incidence	6.9	4.6	13.3	13.7	12.8	5.9	11.1	4.2	–
All-cause mortality	692.8	542.0	832.5	670.3	688.1	610.0	607.3	639.4	668.5

Among these 12 selected health indicators, rates tend to be higher (worse) in Chelsea, Everett, Malden, and Revere, compared to state averages.

Lower (better) than MA average
Similar to MA average
Higher (worse) than MA average

Indicators are expressed as age-adjusted rates per 100,000, except for preterm births, which is expressed as percentage of live births.
Color coding is based on percentage difference from the state average, calculated as above, below, or within 5%. Color coding does not imply statistical significance.
Data Sources: Massachusetts Registry of Vital Records and Statistics, 2019-2023 5-Year Aggregates; Massachusetts Department of Public Health (DPH), Bureau of Infectious Disease and Laboratory Sciences, 2019-2023 5-Year Aggregates; Center for Health Information and Analysis, Massachusetts Acute Hospital Case Mix Database, 2017-2021 5-Year Annual Averages.

Fig. 2.4 Population level statistics for sample healthcare organization

the PREPARE ® Screening Tool, which was developed to standardize assessment of social determinants of health across clinical settings (National Association of Community Health Centers, 2024) and has been published in multiple languages. If a patient triggers a positive SDOH screen, they are immediately offered to speak with a health specialist to connect them with local social services. This SDOH information is then included in the EMR so that providers can review the screening results at medical visits. Neuropsychologists at this institution review SDOH findings for patients prior to a clinical encounter to better understand the psychosocial stressors impacting the patient. This kind of information helps the neuropsychologist to appreciate the patient psychosocial stressors better to inform evaluations, which is well known to impact cognition. Beyond normative data though, we know that this information can also guide better treatment plans. The neuropsychologist can also capitalize on the Community Department initiated programs to help patients in need. The scope of utilization of these community statistics is still evolving. Certainly this kind of data can be enormously useful for better understanding cognitive health outcomes . At the clinical level, catchment area statistics are also useful for the neuropsychologist to understand which communities have greater disease burden and what might be other community-level stressors for a patient from that community. An example could be examining rates of dementia across different towns or the incidence of pediatric concussions. By doing this, the neuropsychologist can help target community-level prevention work focused on intervening on drivers that increase dementia risk (e.g., sedentary factors driven by built environment, lack of healthy food access, etc.) or helping to drive population interventions (e.g., free bike helmets for kids or coach education on safer tackling practices in youth football). Another useful population tool for the clinic neuropsychology director is to assess whether the neuropsychology clinic patient demographics are representative of the overall hospital level demographics and or servicing area demographics. Health inequities are pervasive throughout healthcare and a savvy neuropsychology director cannot solely be focused on filling providers' schedule by just relying on who shows up but needs to intentionally address barriers that results in inequitable access across those communities they serve.

Upstream Access, Downstream Impact: Strengthening Cognitive Health Through Equitable Neuropsychological Pathways

While there is growing recognition of array of diseases that impact cognitive functioning (Schretlen et al., 2025) and a greater need for cognitive evaluations, timely access to neuropsychological services remains problematic with wait lists of 10–12 months not being uncommon (Cass et al., 2020; Han et al., 2014). Delays in neuropsychological assessment can inevitably lead to worse patient and family/caregiver outcomes in neurodegenerative and acquired conditions. Considering that central nervous system disorders are the leading cause of global disease burden (GBD 2021 Nervous System Disorders Collaborators, 2024), some degree of wait-lists is to be expected. However, the role of siloed neuropsychology practices and comprehensive neuropsychological batteries (> six hours) has come under question as neuropsychologists face the need to adapt to a growing demand.

Neuropsychological assessment and practice models have been proposed to help expedite neuropsychological access, such as the development of shorter neuropsychological batteries in multiple sclerosis (BICAMS; Benedict et al., 2012), report

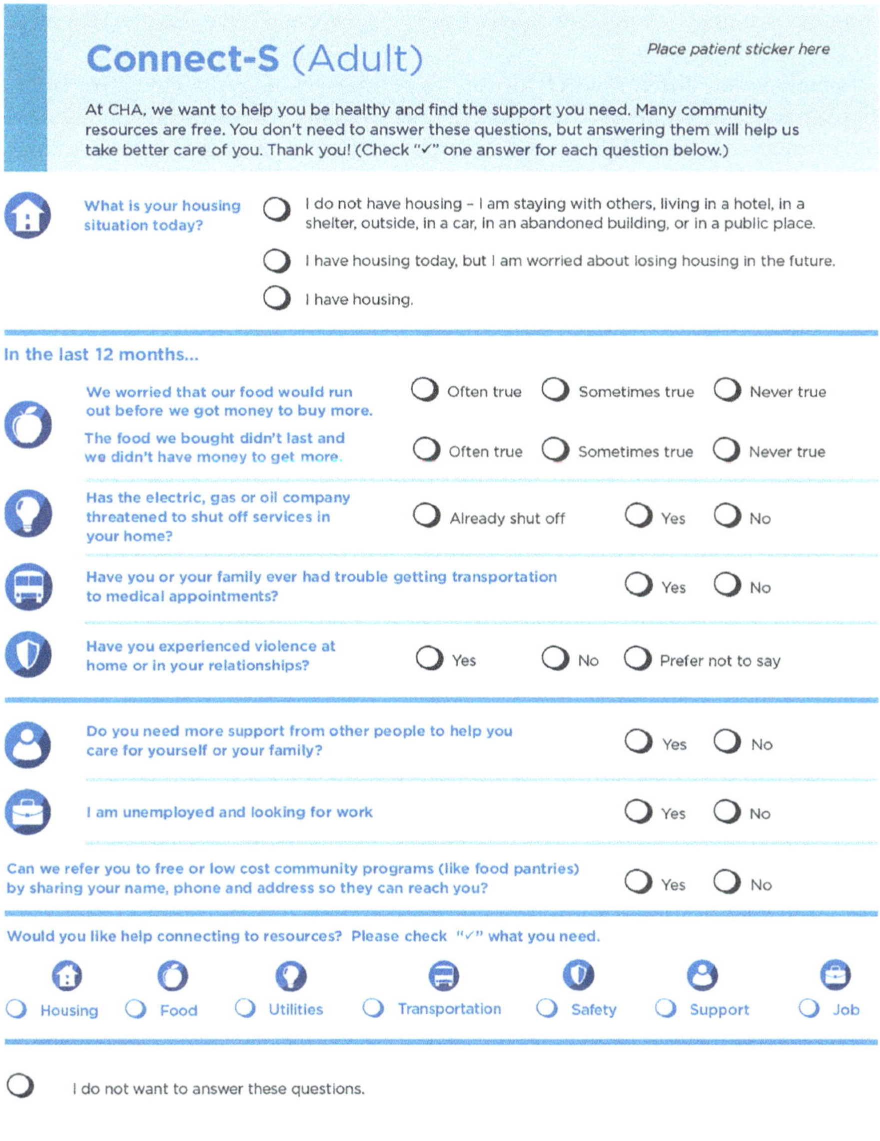

Connect-S (Adult)

Place patient sticker here

At CHA, we want to help you be healthy and find the support you need. Many community resources are free. You don't need to answer these questions, but answering them will help us take better care of you. Thank you! (Check "✓" one answer for each question below.)

What is your housing situation today?
- I do not have housing – I am staying with others, living in a hotel, in a shelter, outside, in a car, in an abandoned building, or in a public place.
- I have housing today, but I am worried about losing housing in the future.
- I have housing.

In the last 12 months...

We worried that our food would run out before we got money to buy more.	Often true	Sometimes true	Never true
The food we bought didn't last and we didn't have money to get more.	Often true	Sometimes true	Never true
Has the electric, gas or oil company threatened to shut off services in your home?	Already shut off	Yes	No
Have you or your family ever had trouble getting transportation to medical appointments?		Yes	No
Have you experienced violence at home or in your relationships?	Yes	No	Prefer not to say
Do you need more support from other people to help you care for yourself or your family?		Yes	No
I am unemployed and looking for work		Yes	No
Can we refer you to free or low cost community programs (like food pantries) by sharing your name, phone and address so they can reach you?		Yes	No

Would you like help connecting to resources? Please check "✓" what you need.

Housing Food Utilities Transportation Safety Support Job

I do not want to answer these questions.

GR20_200

Fig. 2.5 Example of SDOH screen at Cambridge Health Alliance (CHA)

templates for shorter write-ups (Interorganizational Practice Committee, n.d.), re-allocation of office staff for target screening and triage (Cass et al., 2020), computerized screening approaches (Rao, 2018), and integration of neuropsychology into care teams (Glen et al., 2019). With respect to integration, one such model of care within a stroke program demonstrated the ability to decrease average wait times over 78%

while maintaining high patient satisfaction ratings through integration (Han et al., 2014).

Implementing different levels of care in neuropsychology is imperative from a population health perspective because it aligns specialty services with patient accessibility, efficiency, and clinical need. Neuropsychology can no longer remain solely in tertiary referral settings; rather, a stepped model ensures that screening, brief assessments, and full evaluations are deployed in a cost- and needs-appropriate fashion. Integrating screening and stepped care can reduce delays, lower "lost to follow up" rates, and expand capacity (e.g., the Inter-Organizational Practice Committee guidelines on neuropsychology service levels). The imperative rests on three pillars: equity (ensuring underserved populations gain access), efficiency (matching intensity of service to risk), and outcome-oriented care (earlier identification of cognitive issues yields better functional outcomes).

Lanca (2018) described the neuropsychology clinical care level as a tier model in which patients received a brief neuropsychological assessment (BNA) embedded in primary care settings. The BNA allowed for shorter focused cognitive testing and a standard neuropsychological clinical interview by a neuropsychologist or neuropsychology resident, and actionable recommendations to the patient and to the referring provider on the same day of service—all delivered without the full battery length and referral delay typical of specialty clinics. The rationale is that many patients present with subtle cognitive concerns in primary care, and a full evaluation may not initially be required; instead, brief evaluation supports triage: either returning to primary care with monitoring, initiating interventions, or escalating to a full neuropsychological assessment as needed. Lanca framed this clinical care tier as mid-intensity and high value: it bridged the gap between simple cognitive screening and comprehensive neuropsychological testing, enhancing access while maintaining specialist oversight. Similar to a primary care model of making medical treatment decisions based on a "stepped care" approach (Sobell & Sobell, 1999), neuropsychological assessments were also conformed to this path. In a medical model of stepped care, the selection of treatment is directed such that medical treatment proceeds in a stepwise fashion from least intensive to most intensive. If the patient responds to the least invasive treatment, then treatment is maintained for as long as necessary, but if the patient's status remains the same or declines, then a more intensive level of treatment is implemented. The result is that more intensive treatments are reserved for more extreme problems (Sobell & Sobell, 2000). Many medical conditions (e.g., hypertension, diabetes) are treated in primary care using this approach, with the addition of specialist consultation at the higher steps of care as needed. As shown in Fig. 2.6, this "clinical care level" neuropsychology model situated neuropsychology within primary care, allowing rapid cognitive screening, targeted BNAs, and data-driven triage to full neuropsychological evaluations when indicated.

Recent evidence underscores that enhanced neuropsychological presence in primary care can improve access, efficiency, and outcomes. Fowler et al. (2015) investigated whether neuropsychological testing in primary care impacted physician-initiated interventions related to cognitive impairment or slowed the rate of cognitive impairment progression. Providing cognitive findings to primary care physicians

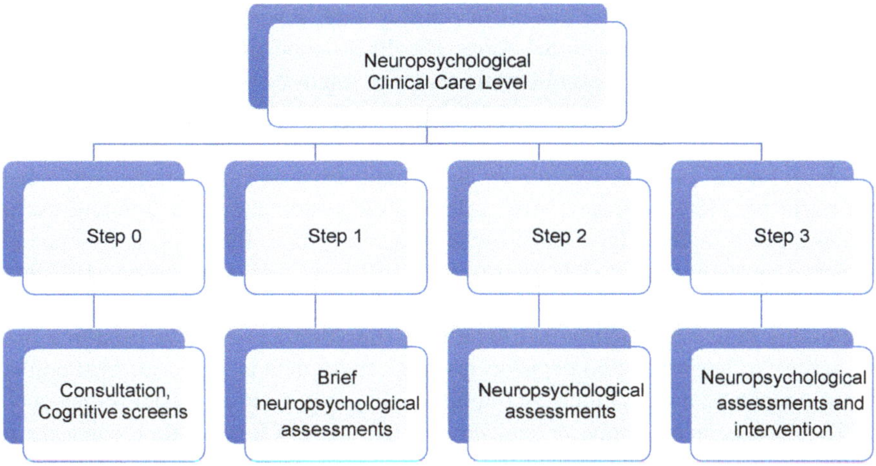

Fig. 2.6 Description of neuropsychological care at each stepped level. *Note* This figure was created by the author

resulted in more cognitive-related interventions, more documented discussions about cognition, more ordering of blood tests to rule out reversible causes and significantly more patients had a medication for cognition listed in their chart. In a follow-up paper Fowler et al (2025) underscored the importance of early detection practices for cognitive decline in primary care to improve outcomes for patients and caregivers. Verghese et al. (2024) showed that embedding brief cognitive assessments in primary care significantly increased downstream "care actions" (e.g., diagnosis, management, or referral). The Inter-Organizational Practice Committee's 2020–2021 guidelines further recommend tiered and hybrid delivery models—including teleneuropsychology—to preserve access and equity across risk levels. Collectively, these findings show that more frequent cognitive testing, even without full neuropsychological evaluations, can have tremendous clinical value for clinical care, and at the same time may reduce wait times for more comprehensive evaluations (by reducing the number of referrals with patients triaged to screening instead), and optimize resource allocation.

Measurement-Based Care (MBC) as a Population Health Tool in Neuropsychology

Full expansion of a stepped model of cognitive care entails that providers systematically conduct cognitive screening for patients (Level 0). In practice, at a primary care or specialty clinic, this would mean systematic periodic administrations of a screen that would be used to make clinical decisions about next level of care. The optimal cadence of administration is dictated by the clinical need. For example, for the average not-at-risk elder patient in primary care, a yearly cognitive screening, perhaps done in cadence with the Annual Wellness checkup might be most appropriate. In a Multiple Sclerosis clinic, the cadence might be more frequent for at-risk patients (being careful to define 'at risk' as including several different traditional neurological indicators, but also considering SDOH, psychological functioning, and non-neurological factors). Essentially, systematic cognitive screening is equivalent to a cognitive MBC program. MBC refers to the systematic collection and use of patient-reported and clinician-rated outcome data to guide clinical decision-making. In contrast to traditional models that rely primarily on clinician judgment, MBC integrates standardized, repeated outcome measures—such as symptom severity scales, functioning indices, or quality-of-life ratings—into routine care to be used in a clinical setting to inform shared decision-making. These data inform treatment adjustments in real time and facilitate continuous quality improvement (QI) (Fortney et al., 2017). MBC is increasingly recognized as a hallmark of high-quality, value-based healthcare (Lewis et al., 2019).

In general medicine, MBC aligns closely with population health frameworks. Systematic measurement of clinical indicators (e.g., HbA1c for diabetes, PHQ-9 for depression) has been shown to improve treatment adherence, clinical outcomes, and cost efficiency. For example, Greenhalgh et al. (2018) demonstrated that outcome monitoring systems promote communication, transparency, and patient engagement across healthcare settings. Additionally, MBC supports health systems' transition toward learning health systems, wherein aggregated outcome data identify trends and inform system-level improvements (IOM, 2015; Lewis et al., 2019). The challenge facing health systems using multiple MBC tools is finding meaningful integration of the data such that a provider's panel of patients can be appropriately triaged to receive the correct attention and care at the right time. This is ultimately one of the potential future benefits of artificial intelligence.

In behavioral health, MBC has growing empirical support. Fortney et al. (2017) found that MBC doubled the likelihood of clinical response and remission in depression compared to treatment-as-usual. Lambert et al. (2018) reported that providing clinicians with regular feedback on client progress reduced treatment dropout and improved psychotherapy outcomes. In large-scale studies of veterans and community mental health systems, MBC improved treatment fidelity and patient satisfaction (Scott & Lewis, 2015). Routine outcome monitoring is now endorsed by major organizations including the American Psychological Association (APA, 2021), the Joint Commission, and the Substance Abuse and Mental Health Services Administration (SAMHSA) as a core element of evidence-based care. Although the impact of cognitive MBC program is not yet understood, similar outcomes may be possible with increased patient engagement in their cognitive health.

Recent reviews highlight that MBC for behavioral health enhances efficiency and equity by identifying non-responders early, tailoring interventions to individual trajectories, and providing objective data for payers and policymakers (de Jong, 2021; Lewis et al., 2019). Implementation of MBC programs is complex and requiring attention at all organizational levels. Multiple implementation science (IS) studies have documented the facilitators and barriers of MBC in outpatient and inpatient settings (Lanca et al., 2025; Rosenfeld et al, 2024). Facilitators have been identified at all levels (i.e., program, clinician, and patient levels). Studies have shown that patients reported having greater insight into their symptoms, increased adherence to behavioral health treatment, and greater treatment satisfaction with systematic symptom reporting. Clinicians also reported increased understanding of the patient, increased therapeutical alliance, and enhanced clinical skills with the incorporation of MBC into treatment (Jensen-Doss et al., 2020). At the programmatic level, MBC has substantiated program efficacy and effectiveness; as such, it can be used to improve treatment fidelities and program flexibility with increased personalized care (Kilbourne et al., 2018). Multiple barriers have also been reported across patient, clinician, and organizational levels. Time restrictions is one of the greatest barriers to successful MBC implementations and increased innovations to reduce time burden is needed, such as rapid digital support tools and automated (not dependent on the provider ordering the tool) integration to EMR as opposed to paper-and-pencil version. This can be especially problematic for a cognitive MBC that may also include clinician administration, increasing the priority for tablet or app self-administration innovations. Organizational resources are also critical to support ongoing staff and clinician training and large-scale continuous monitoring of program fidelity. Organizational resources are also essential for ongoing implementation and QI work. At the patient level, reported barriers included time burden, a greater need and commitment to equity and technology accessibility, as well as greater understanding of individual patient challenges for those who may not tolerate MBC programs (e.g., the patient with chronic suicidality who is frustrated by use of tools such as the Columbia Suicide Severity Rating Scale at every visit).

Collectively, these findings indicate that MBC not only improves individual outcomes but also strengthens health system performance—bridging clinical practice, QI, and population health, but the implementation of MBC programs requires resources, especially IT resources, and IS expertise for greater success. To succeed at scale, cognitive MBC cannot simply be dropped into practice and assumed to function. It needs systematic embedding into workflows, continual clinician behavior feedback, data systems integration, and organizational/leadership buy-in. IS and QI provide the frameworks, methods, and metrics to translate evidence into routine, sustainable practice. Without them, MBC initiatives often remain pilot projects, with limited uptake, poor fidelity, and weak sustainability (Lewis et al., 2018). By applying IS/QI, organizations can map barriers, tailor strategies, monitor process metrics, and adapt interventions—thereby closing the research-to-practice gap (Davis & D'Lima, 2020). IS emphasizes that interventions succeed not merely because they are effective, but because they fit their context—including organizational readiness, leadership, and resources. Key IS principles include assessing determinants (barriers and facilitators), deploying targeted strategies (e.g., training, audit and feedback, clinical champions), and tracking implementation outcomes such as adoption, fidelity, and sustainability. These steps are reinforced through QI methods like Plan-Do-Study-Act (PDSA) cycles that allow rapid testing and refinement (Zamboni et al., 2020).

Applied to neuropsychology, these frameworks offer a blueprint for implementing cognitive screening/BNAs within an MBC model. An effective process begins with assessing the current state of cognitive screening/BNA workflows and clinician readiness, followed by identifying barriers (e.g., time constraints, IT limitations) and facilitators (e.g., leadership support). Next, implementation strategies—such as embedding brief cognitive measures into the EMR, training teams, and assigning champions—help integrate MBC into daily practice. Pilot programs should measure both implementation outcomes (screening rates, acceptability, referral efficiency) and clinical outcomes (earlier detection, improved care actions). Finally, iterative PDSA cycles refine procedures for broader scale-up and sustainability. In doing so, MBC evolves from a measurement activity into a learning health system process—one that continuously improves access, equity, and outcomes in cognitive and neuropsychological care (Davis & D'Lima, 2020; Lewis et al., 2018). Figure 2.7 provides an example of such an implementation, while Chapter 9 provides an illustrative example of change management and quality improvement techniques in action.

MBC for cognitive assessments holds potential for transforming clinical neuropsychology, bridging traditional assessment with modern population health and QI paradigms. Neuropsychology has long been strong in measurement, yet those measurements often remain episodic, collected during a single evaluation and rarely used to guide ongoing care. Cognitive MBC reimagines this process by embedding continuous, systematic feedback loops into neuropsychological practice. Through repeated and standardized outcome tracking—such as cognitive screens administered by health professionals (not necessarily a neuropsychologist), cognitive symptom inventories, functional ability scales, or cognitive performance indices through phone apps or tablet-based screening administration—MBC can enable neuropsychologists to monitor patient progress over time, evaluate intervention effectiveness, and adjust recommendations dynamically. In such a model, multidisciplinary teamwork is critical, including, QI and IS colleagues for implementation. At the functioning stage, the innovator neuropsychologist would direct the cognitive screening program and collaborate with and work with other disciplines, such as medical assistants who conduct the cognitive screening, master's level clinicians, and/or community health workers to help with the implementation of health improvement strategies. This approach moves the field of neuropsychology beyond static assessment toward a model of adaptive, data-informed clinical decision-making. At a systems level, a cognitive MBC programs enables learning health systems to identify disparities in access or recovery, and refine triage pathways (Institute of Medicine, 2015). Ultimately, MBC can transform neuropsychology from a consultative specialty to a continuous outcome science, aligning clinical insight with measurable progress and sustainable population health outcomes.

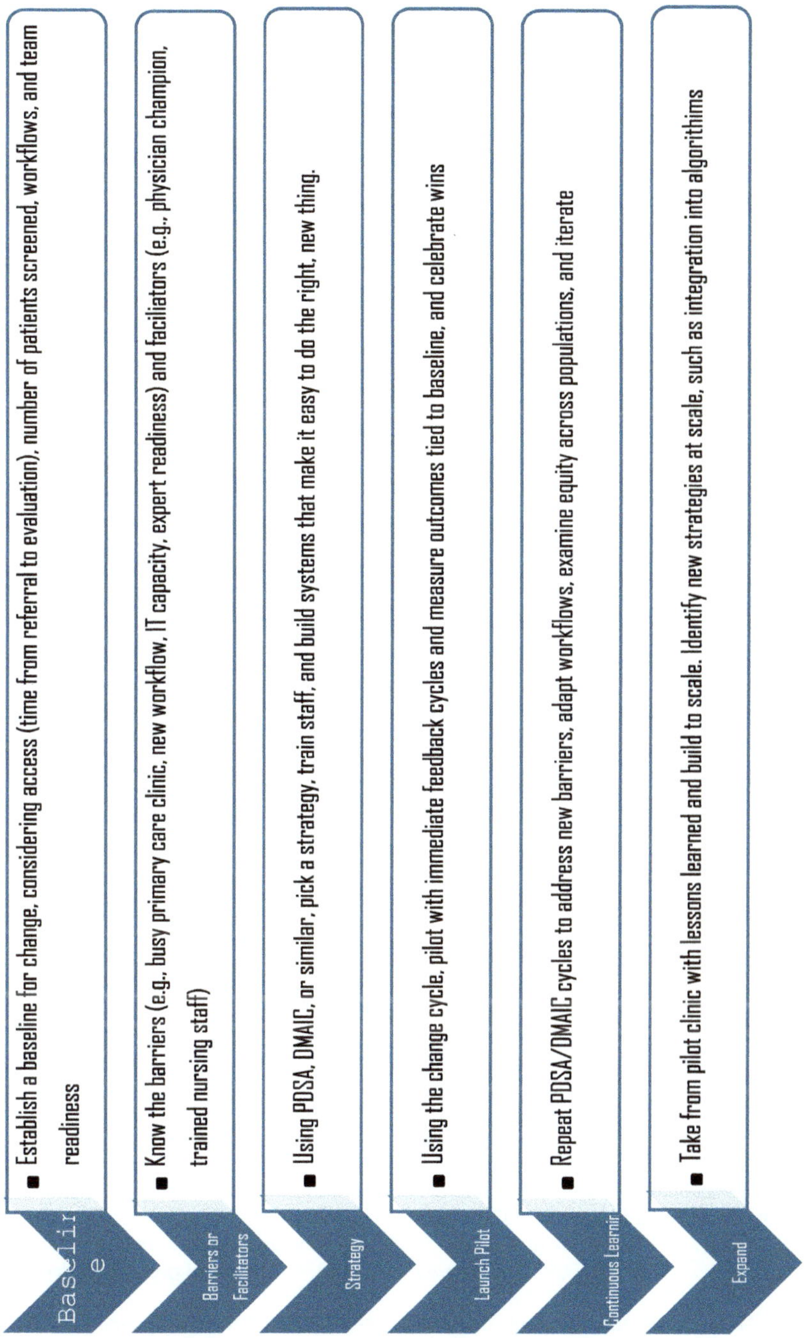

Fig. 2.7 Example applying implementation of cognitive screening MBC in neuropsychology

Summary

Population health offers a comprehensive framework for improving healthcare outcomes by emphasizing prevention, early detection, and coordinated intervention across community and clinical settings. The model seeks to bridge the divide between public health and healthcare delivery, targeting both the healthy and the chronically ill to achieve health equity and sustainability amid escalating healthcare costs. Neuropsychology's engagement in population health is essential because cognitive health intersects with nearly all chronic diseases that drive healthcare utilization and disability. Despite neuropsychology's presence across community, primary, and specialty care, fragmented systems and long wait times limit access, continuity, and early intervention. Adopting a population health approach allows neuropsychologists to expand their work "upstream," by expanding cognitive screening, innovating wellness programs, and cognitive education, while also optimizing "downstream" interventions and impacts in rehabilitation and tertiary care.

Implementing tiered levels of care—ranging from brief cognitive screenings to comprehensive neuropsychological evaluations—aligns specialty services with population health principles of equity, efficiency, and measurable outcomes. Embedding brief assessments within primary care enhances early detection and facilitates triage for complex cases, reducing delays and expanding reach. MBC further strengthens this model by integrating systematic outcome tracking into neuropsychological workflows, turning episodic evaluations into ongoing, data-informed care. However, scaling MBC requires deliberate application of IS and QI methods to ensure sustainability and fidelity (Lewis et al., 2018). These frameworks guide adaptation to clinical contexts, train teams, and use iterative feedback cycles—which can help transform neuropsychology into a learning health system. Ultimately, neuropsychology's integration into population health models positions the field to contribute directly to preventive cognitive health, early intervention, and system-level innovation in value-based care.

References

AbdulRaheem, Y. (2023). Unveiling the significance and challenges of integrating prevention levels in healthcare practice. *Journal of Preventive Medicine & Public Health, 13*(4), 850–859.

American Psychological Association. (2021). *Clinical practice guideline for the treatment of depression across three age cohorts.* APA.

Benedict, R. H., Amato, M. P., Boringa, J., Brochet, B., Foley, F., Fredrikson, S., Hamalainen, P., Hartung, H., Krupp, L., Penner, I., Reder, A. T., & Langdon, D. (2012). Brief international cognitive assessment for MS (BICAMS): International standards for validation. *BMC Neurology, 12*, 55. https://doi.org/10.1186/1471-2377-12-55

Boersma, P., Black, L. I., & Ward, B. W. (2020). Prevalence of multiple chronic conditions among U.S. adults, 2018. *Preventing Chronic Disease, 17*, 200130. https://doi.org/10.5888/pcd17.200130

Braveman, P., Arkin, E., Proctor, D., Kauh, T., & Holm, N. (2022). *What is health equity?* Robert Wood Johnson Foundation.

Cass, J., Fristad, M., Valleru, J., Gallup, J., & Butter, E. (2020). Improving wait times for pediatric neuropsychology services. *Evidence-Based Practice in Child and Adolescent Mental Health, 5*(2), 128–138.

Cambridge Health Alliance. (2025). *Regional wellbeing report 2025: A community health needs assessment*. Cambridge Health Alliance.

Davis, R. E., & D'Lima, D. (2020). Building capacity in dissemination and implementation science: A systematic review of the academic literature on teaching and training initiatives. *Implementation Science, 15*(1), Article 97. https://doi.org/10.1186/s13012-020-01051-6

de Jong, K. (2021). A decade of progress in routine outcome monitoring and feedback: Systematic review. *Psychotherapy Research, 31*(3), 281–292. https://doi.org/10.1080/10503307.2020.1760629

Fabius, R. (2021). Preventative strategies and pillars of population health. In *Population health: Creating cultures of wellness* (3rd ed., pp. 3–22). Jones & Bartlett Learning.

Fortney, J. C., Unützer, J., Wrenn, G., Pyne, J. M., Smith, G. R., Schoenbaum, M., & Harbin, H. T. (2017). A tipping point for measurement-based care. *Psychiatric Services, 68*(2), 179–188. https://doi.org/10.1176/appi.ps.201500439

Fowler, N. R., Partrick, K. A., Taylor, J., Hornbecker, M., Kelleher, K., Boustani, M., Cummings, J. L., MacLeod, T., Mielke, M. M., Brosch, J. R., Lee, J., Shobin, E., Galvin, J. E., Fillit, H., Udeh-Momoh, C., & Willis, D. R. (2025). Implementing early detection of cognitive impairment in primary care to improve care for older adults. *Journal of Internal Medicine, 298*(1), 31–45. https://doi.org/10.1111/joim.20098

Fowler, N. R., et al. (2015). Primary care cognitive testing improves dementia care actions. *Journal of the American Geriatrics Society, 63*(9), 1881–1887.

GBD 2021 Nervous System Disorders Collaborators. (2024). Global, regional, and national burden of disorders affecting the nervous system, 1990–2021: A systematic analysis for the Global Burden of Disease Study 2021. *The Lancet Neurology, 23*(4), 344–381. https://doi.org/10.1016/S1474-4422(24)00038-3

Glen, E. T., Hostetter, G., Ruff, R. M., Roebuck-Spencer, T. M., Denney, R. L., Perry, W., Fazio, R. L., Garmoe, W. S., Bianchini, K. J., & Scott, J. G. (2019). Integrative care models in neuropsychology: A national academy of neuropsychology education paper. *Archives of Clinical Neuropsychology : THe Official Journal of the National Academy of Neuropsychologists, 34*(2), 141–151. https://doi.org/10.1093/arclin/acy092

Greenhalgh, J., Gooding, K., Gibbons, E., Dalkin, S., Wright, J., Valderas, J., & Black, N. (2018). How do patient-reported outcome measures (PROMs) support clinician-patient communication and shared decision-making? *Patient Education and Counseling, 101*(4), 575–584. https://doi.org/10.1016/j.pec.2017.08.003

Han, D. Y., Anderson, A. J., Jones, J. E., Hermann, B. P., & Sattin, J. A. (2014). Neuropsychology in multidisciplinary stroke care: Clinical feasibility of the NINDS-CSN vascular cognitive impairment harmonization standards. *International Scholarly Research Notices*, 216024. https://doi.org/10.1155/2014/216024

Interorganizational Practice Committee. (n.d.). *Neuropsychology toolkit*. https://iopc.online/report-writing

Institute of Medicine. (2015). *Vital signs: Core metrics for health and health care progress*. National Academies Press.

Inter-Organizational Practice Committee (IOPC). (2021). Guidelines for tele- and hybrid neuropsychological care delivery. *Clinical Neuropsychologist, 35*(5), 1023–1038.

Jensen-Doss, A., Douglas, S., Phillips, D. A., Gencdur, Ö., Zalman, A., & Gomez, N. E. (2020). Measurement-based care as a practice improvement tool: Clinical and organizational applications in youth mental health. *Evidence-Based Practice in Child & Adolescent Mental Health, 5*(3), 233–250. https://doi.org/10.1080/23794925.2020.1784062

Kilbourne, A. M., Beck, K., Spaeth-Rublee, B., Ramanuj, P., O'Brien, R. W., Tomoyasu, N., & Pincus, H. A. (2018). Measuring and improving the quality of mental health care: A global perspective. World *Psychiatry, 17*(1), 30–38. https://doi.org/10.1002/wps.20482

Kisling, J., & Das, J. K. (2022). Optimizing population health nursing: Levels of prevention and beyond. In *Population health for nurses* (pp. 45–59). OpenStax.

Lambert, M. J., Whipple, J. L., & Kleinstäuber, M. (2018). Collecting and delivering progress feedback: A meta-analysis of routine outcome monitoring. *Psychotherapy, 55*(4), 520–537. https://doi.org/10.1037/pst0000176

Lanca, M. (2018). Clinical neuropsychology and population health: Expanding access through levels of care. *Archives of Clinical Neuropsychology, 33*(3), 269–278.

Lanca, M., Zona, K., Aldis, R., Carson, N., Fulwiler, C., Wang, P. S., Engineer, N., Mulvaney-Day, N., & Progovac, A. M. (2025). *Clinician perspectives on measurement-based care to inform pre-implementation training and workflow design on an adolescent psychiatric inpatient unit. Evidence-Based Practice in Child and Adolescent Mental Health.* Advance online publication. https://doi.org/10.1080/23794925.2025.2491064

Lewis, C. C., Boyd, M. R., Puspitasari, A. J., Navarro, E., Howard, J., Simon, G., & Kroenke, K. (2019). Implementing measurement-based care in behavioral health: A review. *JAMA Psychiatry, 76*(3), 324–335. https://doi.org/10.1001/jamapsychiatry.2018.3326

Lewis, C. C., et al. (2018). Implementing measurement-based care in behavioral health: A review. *JAMA Psychiatry, 76*(3), 324–335.

Maxfield, M., Courtney, K., Assuras, S., Manly, J. J., & Widom, C. S. (2025). Childhood maltreatment and cognitive functioning from young adulthood to late midlife: A prospective study. *Neuropsychology, 40*(2), 178–190. https://doi.org/10.1037/neu0001042

National Association of Community Health Centers. (2024). *PRAPARE® Screening Tool*. https://prapare.org/the-prapare-screening-tool/

Rao, S. M. (2018). Role of computerized screening in healthcare teams: Why computerized testing is not the death of neuropsychology. *Archives of Clinical Neuropsychology, 33*(3), 375–378. https://doi.org/10.1093/arclin/acx137

Rosenfeld, L., Progovac, A. M., Leff, S., Zhang, A., Tian, L., Huttlin, E., Wang, D., Fulwiler, C., Aldis, R., Wang, P., Stahr, J., Mulvaney-Day, N., Lanca, M., & Tepper, M. (2024). Remote measurement-based care to improve equity in psychiatry: Contrasting pre-implementation patient, provider, and administrative leader attitudes. *Learning Health Systems. Learning Health Systems, 8*(1), Article e10472. https://doi.org/10.1002/lrh2.10472

Schretlen, D. J., Finley, J. C. A., Del Bene, V. A., & Varvaris, M. (2025). The ubiquity of cognitive impairment in human illness: A systematic review of meta-analyses. *Archives of Clinical Neuropsychology, 40*(4), 863–877. https://doi.org/10.1093/arclin/acae113

Scott, K., & Lewis, C. C. (2015). Using measurement-based care to enhance any treatment. *Cognitive and Behavioral Practice, 22*(1), 49–59. https://doi.org/10.1016/j.cbpra.2014.01.010

Sobell, M. B., & Sobell, L. C. (1999). Stepped care for alcohol problems: An efficient method for planning and delivering clinical services. *Addiction, 94*(6), 767–775.

Sobell, M. B., & Sobell, L. C. (2000). Stepped care as a heuristic approach to the treatment of alcohol problems. *Journal of Consulting and Clinical Psychology, 68*(4), 573–579.

U.S. Department of Education. (2025, October). *School-based mental health services grant program*. https://www.ed.gov/grants-and-programs/grants-birth-grade-12/safe-and-supportive-schools/school-based-mental-health-services-grant-program#:~:text=Program%20Description,in%20LEAs%20with%20demonstrated%20need.

Verghese, J., Holtzer, R., Ayers, E., Sanders, A. E., Bower, L. M., Bennett, D. A., & for the 5-Cog Study Group. (2024). Effect of a brief cognitive assessment on dementia care in primary care: The 5-Cog randomized trial. *JAMA Network Open, 7*(3), e241234. https://doi.org/10.1001/jamanetworkopen.2024.1234

Waters, H., & Graf, M. (2018). *The costs of chronic disease in the U.S.* (1st ed.). Milken Institute. https://milkeninstitute.org/sites/default/files/reports-pdf/ChronicDiseases-HighRes-FINAL_2.pdf

Zamboni, K., et al. (2020). How and under what circumstances do quality improvement collaboratives lead to better outcomes? *Implementation Science, 15*, Article 27.

Chapter 3
Reimagining Neuropsychology in a Value-Based Healthcare System

Caroline Vaile Wright, Neil H. Pliskin, and Scott A. Sperling

Executive Summary
This chapter explores the transition of US healthcare toward value-based care (VBC) and its implications for neuropsychology. It traces the evolution from fee-for-service (FFS) and managed care models to VBC frameworks that reward quality, outcomes, and patient experience over service volume. The authors examine how neuropsychological services, historically constrained by limited reimbursement and administrative barriers, can adapt to evolving reimbursement systems such as CMS's Quality Payment Program. Emphasizing the need for cost-effectiveness data, technology integration, and quality measurement, the chapter outlines strategies for aligning neuropsychological practice with population health goals. Through innovative partnerships including integrated care, outcome-based research, and digital tools, neuropsychologists can play a pivotal role in improving access, efficiency, and outcomes across not only behavioral, but physical healthcare.

C. V. Wright (✉)
American Psychological Association, Washington, DC, USA
e-mail: cwright@apa.org

N. H. Pliskin
Departments of Psychiatry and Neurology, University of Illinois College of Medicine, Chicago, IL, USA
e-mail: npliskin@uic.edu

S. A. Sperling
Center for Neurological Restoration, Neurological Institute Section of Neuropsychology, Department of Neurology, Cleveland Clinic Lerner College of Medicine, Case Western Reserve University, Cleveland, OH, USA
e-mail: sperlis@ccf.org

M. Lanca and R. Fallows (eds.), *Advancing Neuropsychology Through Population Health*, https://doi.org/10.1007/978-3-032-22457-6_3

Introduction

The healthcare system in the United States (US) is in the midst of a major transformation that has affected all healthcare specialties, including clinical psychology/neuropsychology. Driving this transformation is the fact that healthcare spending in the US has steadily grown to represent a disproportionately large share of the nation's gross domestic product (GDP), raising concerns about sustainability and economic impact. As noted in Chapter 1, the rising healthcare expenditure is inconsistent with other high-income countries and does not lead to better outcomes. Rather, much of this growth reflects the rising costs of medical services, pharmaceuticals, and administrative overhead, as well as the aging population and increased prevalence of chronic diseases (Dieleman et al., 2020). Addressing the imbalance between healthcare consumption and overall economic productivity has therefore become a critical national policy priority.

A Shift in Payment Models Is Needed that Recognizes Cost Outcome Data

The shift from traditional fee-for-service (FFS) to alternative payment models (APMs)—including value-based payment (VBP), accountable care organizations (ACOs), and Medicaid managed-care/value-based arrangements—has pushed behavioral health toward greater integration with medical care, earlier intervention, and outcome-focused services, but with problematic results for access, quality, and specialty behavioral health services like neuropsychology. For neuropsychology specifically, the limits imposed by third-party payers for the number of hours considered acceptable for an evaluation conflict with traditional practice patterns that have emphasized long testing sessions, scoring, and interpretive reports. Indeed, the most readily available professional practice data suggest that many neuropsychologists are delivering services over multiple days or averaging over 10 h per evaluation (Sweet, Klipfel, et al., 2021). This traditional mode of time- and resource-intensive clinical assessment practice has come into increasing conflict with the current healthcare market calling for APMs, measurable cost reductions and population metrics that emphasize briefer and more sensitive diagnostic workups.

Recognizing the need for cost outcome data, several studies supported by the American Academy of Clinical Neuropsychology Foundation have demonstrated cost-effectiveness and clinical utility of cognitive assessment using briefer assessments models (VanKirk et al., 2013). Likewise, there are efforts underway to modernize and improve neuropsychological assessment, and to position the field to provide population metrics for conditions where earlier detection of conditions, such as Mild Cognitive Impairment (MCI), can be achieved through combined population data (National Neuropsychology Network; NNN; Loring et al., 2022). The goals of the NNN align with the move toward population health, including "transition to contemporary psychometric methods, large-scale item-level data collection, data sharing and harmonization through the NIH/NIMH Data Archive." By combining clinical assessments with information in the electronic health records as well as patient reported social determinants of health, innovative methods such as artificial intelligence algorithms can support clinicians in developing more robust prevention strategies and personalized treatment. This not only enhances clinical decision-making for individuals but also informs system-level changes that improve access, efficiency, and outcomes in mental and behavioral healthcare.

Background: Current Problematic Payment Model for Neuropsychology

Neuropsychological testing and evaluation services are essential to developing accurate diagnoses and treatment plans for individuals across the lifespan, including those with Alzheimer's disease and related dementias, stroke, epilepsy, traumatic brain injury, and neurodevelopmental disorders. Despite the medical necessity of neuropsychological services and the clear benefits of such services on a multitude of health outcomes (Begali, 2020; Bowie et al., 2008; Keefe et al., 2006; Pritchard et al., 2020; Spitz et al., 2012; Sieg et al., 2019; Vankirk et al., 2013), access to these services in the US is constrained by the structure of the US healthcare system. Access to care is strongly influenced by payers, be it in the public or private sector, and systemic inequities in access and coverage contribute to disparities in healthcare outcomes and higher overall state and federal costs.

Public and Private Healthcare Payer Systems

The US healthcare system is comprised of a diverse system of public and private providers and payers. Access to healthcare services in the US therefore varies depending on an individual's coverage, which itself is highly variable and dependent upon a multitude of factors, such as one's age, medical history, residence, and employment status. Public healthcare programs provide coverage for specific populations, such as the elderly, children, and those with low incomes. These programs are funded and operated by federal and state governments, and include Medicare, Medicaid, and the Children's Health Insurance Program.

Medicare is the federal health insurance program primarily serving adults ages 65 and older, who as a population are most likely to require neuropsychological testing and evaluation services given their higher risk of developing neurological disorders and cognitive decline. Medicare itself is consists of several components: (1) Part A provides coverage for inpatient hospital care, skilled nursing facility care, hospice, and some home health services, (2) Part B provides coverage for outpatient services, including those for physical and mental and behavioral health services, (3) Part C (Medicare Advantage) is a private insurance plan that encompasses Part A and B benefits, and often additional services, and (4) Part D provides coverage for outpatient prescription drugs. Importantly, while Medicare provides millions of Americans with healthcare coverage, it does not cover all specialized services, and out-of-pocket costs are not uncommon. Moreover, individuals are often faced with limited access to specialty providers, including clinical neuropsychologists, or extensive waitlists to obtain specialty care, given their network, geographical location, and/or the limited number of specialty providers who participate in Medicare secondary to constraints on reimbursement.

The private sector consists of employer-sponsored insurance plans and individual insurance plans that can be purchased through marketplaces. Private insurance coverage is typically provided via one of three models: (1) Health Maintenance Organizations (HMO), which require individuals to obtain care within a network of providers and obtain referrals for specialists, (2) Preferred Provider Organizations (PPO), which tend to offer greater access to out-of-network providers, at higher out-of-pocket costs, and (3) Point-of-Service Plans, which combine features of HMOs and PPOs. Private insurance plans often cover specialized healthcare services, including neuropsychological testing and evaluation services, but the type of coverage, coverage requirements, and amount of coverage vary considerably across plans. Individuals with private insurance are typically responsible for paying a deductible or co-pay, and obtaining a prior authorization before receiving specialized care, which can cause critical delays in obtaining diagnoses and treatment. High deductibles and co-pays, preauthorization requirements, and the limited number of providers who accept private insurance serve as barriers to care, which in turn exacerbate inequities in healthcare outcomes, particularly for vulnerable rural, minoritized, and low-income communities.

Fee-for-Service Payment Systems and Population Health

The fragmented FFS US healthcare system has marked consequences on population health. Barriers to neuropsychological testing and evaluation services cause delays in the diagnosis of cognitive impairment and/or dementia and identification of the etiology of said impairments. Though cures for neurodegenerative diseases do not yet exist, there are medications that have been shown to stabilize or improve the cognitive (Dubois et al., 2012; Henderson et al., 2016; Seppi et al., 2011; Wang et al., 2015), and neurobehavioral symptoms associated with dementia (Cummings et al., 2014; Seppi et al., 2011). The early detection of cognitive impairment is also necessary for gaining access to novel anti-amyloid antibody intravenous infusion therapies and participating in clinical trials that may yield benefit. Moreover, the results of neuropsychological evaluations often lead to the provision of nonpharmacological therapies, patient and care partner resources, and short- and long-term care supports. In the absence of a neuropsychological evaluation, these critical therapies and resources often go unprovided. This in turn contributes to disparities in the health, daily functioning, well-being, and quality of life of patients and care partners, between those who have timely access to neuropsychological services and those who do not. The economic toll also rises, as those with less access to specialized care and greater morbidities are more likely to present to the emergency department, be hospitalized, and be admitted earlier to nursing care facilities (Mittelman et al., 1996; Sieg et al., 2019; Vankirk et al., 2013).

Although creating equity in access to neuropsychological services cannot be solved by a single course of action, changes to public and private healthcare policies can yield significant population health benefits. Such changes include expanding coverage for neuropsychological testing and evaluation services (including for routine cognitive screenings and assessments for at risk populations), eliminating burdensome preauthorization requirements, providing permanent coverage for all neuropsychological services when provided via telehealth—and reimbursing for these telehealth services at the same non-facility rate as in-person services, and increasing the reimbursement rates of neuropsychological testing and evaluation services to incentivize provider participation.

In addition to reforms to healthcare policy and payer systems, efforts need to be made to ensure that neuropsychologists can capitalize on recent technological innovations to streamline assessments, detect early cognitive impairment, and improve patient care outcomes. Digital and remote cognitive assessment platforms offer the neuropsychologists opportunities to assess and monitor individuals' cognition, mood, and behavior outside of clinic, in naturalistic environments (Schmitter-Edgecombe et al., 2024a). Digital biomarkers, including passive (e.g., tracking sleep, activity, and speech) (Hantke et al., 2023; Schmitter-Edgecombe et al., 2024b, 2025) and active (Singh et al., 2023; Sliwinski et al., 2018) monitoring systems, have also shown promise in detecting early cognitive impairment, fluctuations in cognitive functioning, and correlates of cognitive change. The data obtained from these technological innovations can be used by neuropsychologists to enhance their understanding of individuals' level of cognitive and functional impairment and subsequently develop patient-centered interventions.

When scaled and supported via healthcare policies and systems, technological innovations have the capacity to improve population health outcomes. For example, digital and remote cognitive assessment can be integrated into standard models of preventive care. Artificial Intelligence and machine learning tools can also be integrated into preventive care models, to aid in the early detection of cognitive impairment via the assessment of specific speech and language patterns predictive (Kaser et al., 2024; Lopes da Cunha et al., 2024), and the identification of individuals at-risk of cognitive impairment via the integration and analysis of large and complex sets of demographic, cognitive, neurobehavioral, and medical data. However, before these innovations can be implemented in clinical practice and their potential benefits realized, new Current Procedural Terminology (CPT) codes will need to be developed and approved. CMS will then need to adopt these codes and recommended reimbursement values, thereby allowing physicians and qualified healthcare providers alike to integrate these services in their clinical practice. Similarly, it will be important to ensure that private payers adopt equitable coverage policies for these same services.

Managed Care and Payment Models

Managed care in the US has evolved over more than a century in response to economic, public health, and policy shifts, culminating in its dominance during the 1990s when most private insurers and public programs like Medicare and Medicaid adopted its principles (DeLeon et al., 1994). Although managed care remains central to US healthcare, it has continually faced scrutiny over cost containment, access, and quality of care. Examples of cost containment strategies within behavioral healthcare have historically included reduced reimbursement rates, mandated utilization reviews and session limits, reduced inpatient stays, use of nondoctoral providers, and patient co-pays and deductibles (Wright et al., 2019).

The impact of managed care on assessment has also been profound. Neuropsychological testing and assessment have historically been constrained by managed care policies designed to reduce costs. Although these various cost containment policies were initially successful, costs eventually rose again, suggesting that any cost savings achieved through methods such as session limits or reduced assessments had plateaued (Gasquoine, 2010; Sanchez & Turner, 2003). In response to unsuccessful attempts at containing costs, over the last decade or so, the healthcare landscape has started to embrace new reimbursement mechanisms to replace FFS. The most common are value-based programs, which reward healthcare providers with incentive payments for the quality of care, as opposed to quantity of care, they provide (Nordal, 2012).

Value-Based Care and Neuropsychology

Value-based care (VBC) is poised to become a leading reimbursement model for healthcare services, replacing FFS models, which have historically been the dominant mode of payment (Daub et al., 2020; Rothrock et al., 2024). Federal programs have strongly embraced the shift, with the Centers for Medicare and Medicaid Services (CMS) declaring their intention for 100% of Medicare beneficiaries participating in a VBC arrangement by 2030 (Centers for Medicare & Medicaid Services, 2021). However, any attempts at cost containment via effective value-based arrangements must define value beyond cost alone, and prioritize delivering high-value healthcare that improves outcomes and the patient's experience of care without causing undue burden and dissatisfaction to providers (Bodenheimer & Sinsky, 2014; Daub et al., 2020).

Implementing VBC demands a highly complex and challenging strategy, which includes substantial cultural and infrastructure shifts needed to move away from reporting FFS productivity metrics (e.g., length of testing or number of visits) to reporting direct and/or indirect assessments of quality to determine reimbursement (Rothrock et al., 2024). To complicate matters further, there are a range of VBC reimbursement models, depending on the needs of the clinical setting and services offered, including pay for performance, per member per month risk sharing, bundled payments, sub-capitation, and full capitation. Most examples of successful implementation of VBC models have focused on healthcare outside of behavioral health and neuropsychology, in particular primary care. That is, in part, due to the numerous challenges to scaling VBC in behavioral health, including solo or small group practice size, lack of administrative support, and lack of consensus on what to measure to determine whether quality services were delivered (Rothrock et al., 2024).

One of the biggest challenges for successful participation by psychologists and neuropsychologists, however, involves the lack of health information technology (HIT) readiness, in particular the ability to capture value-based quality metrics through an electronic health record (EHR) or data registry (Daub et al., 2020). In many ways, this challenge is unique within behavioral health relative to other areas of medicine. To promote the integration of EHRs in healthcare, in 2009 Congress implemented the Health Information Technology for Economic and Clinical Health Act (HITECH Act) (Snipes, 2016). The legislation authorized incentive payments to clinicians and hospitals to invest in EHR systems; however, psychologists, neuropsychologists, and other behavioral health providers were left out of the HITECH Act, preventing them from receiving financial incentives to build out HIT infrastructure, thereby putting them at a disadvantage particularly as reimbursement models continue to evolve.

That said, neuropsychology may be uniquely positioned given its increasing recognition as a valuable contributor to integrated care models, especially in primary care and geriatric settings, which are foundational to VBC (Glen et al., 2019). Bringing neuropsychological services into clinics that patients already visit—where care teams collaborate and learning opportunities overlap—can improve access to personalized treatment and enhance the overall care experience. Specific improved quality outcomes can include high patient satisfaction, improved patient care, increased rate of completed referrals, improved communication among providers and coordination of services, as well as a reduction in healthcare costs (Stelmokas et al., 2022). Donders (2020) has also noted cost savings when integrating neuropsychological evaluations into healthcare, as evidenced by reduced unnecessary imaging, fewer specialist referrals, and better-targeted interventions across various conditions. For example, TBI and stroke assessments can help tailor rehabilitation, reducing long-term disability costs, while an early and accurate dementia diagnosis can delay institutionalization and reduce caregiver burden (Prigatano & Pliskin, 2003).

Despite these noted potential opportunities, neuropsychology and neuropsychologists face barriers in VBC environments. For example, billing and reimbursement practices often lag behind innovative care models, potentially disincentivizing clinics from investing in integrated care teams. Accessing quality data can also be a challenge as there is often limited outcome data specific to neuropsychological services, available outcome measures are typically unstandardized, and may not include both objective (e.g., reduced hospitalizations) and subjective (e.g., improved patient satisfaction) markers of value (Prigatano & Pliskin, 2003). To address these barriers, there is a growing call for neuropsychologists and other researchers to engage in "value research," including cost-effectiveness studies and longitudinal outcome tracking (Glen et al., 2020). For VBC models to reach their full potential, healthcare providers and clinics will need to develop new skills, capacities, infrastructure, and systems for managing clinical, financial, and operational functions (Daub et al., 2020). Moreover, federal initiatives led by CMS and others will be critical to building infrastructure to support VBC by offering financial incentives to those providers initially excluded from the HITECH Act and supporting interoperability of EHRs to enable coordinated care. These efforts would in turn align with the goals of VBC including better outcomes, lower costs, and improved patient experience.

The Role of Quality Measures in VBC for Neuropsychologists

Value-based care relies on quality measures to ensure patients receive effective treatment, often focusing on influencing healthcare utilization (such as high cost emergency visits or hospital readmissions), clinical indicators linked to improved health (such as blood pressure control in patients with hypertension), and/or provider practices that support better patient outcomes (such as screening for depression) (Rothrock et al., 2024). This increased focus on patient outcomes has led measure developers and payors, such as CMS, to expand the library of quality measures available within VBC models with the intention to better support "a holistic, patient-centered approach to quality measurement" (Core Quality Measures Collaborative, 2020, p. 4). In addition to supporting a patient-centered approach, patient-reported outcomes (PROs), which provide information on the patient, provided by the patient, without interpretation, have a great deal of appeal by gaining information regarding whether quality care is being delivered via multiple domains such as symptom reduction, increased functioning, and positive experience of care (Basch et al., 2015; IOM, 2015).

However, many have raised concerns regarding the use of PROs in holding providers financially accountable for providing quality care (Wright et al., 2019). These concerns include the resource-intensive nature of collecting, reporting, and analyzing PRO data, and skepticism about their ability to impact care quality (Hoenders et al., 2014; Liptzin, 2009). Additional concerns include the use of patient-reported data for benchmarking purposes and to draw comparisons among groups of providers and/or facilities, particularly in light of the fact that many measures lack sensitivity to change or can adequately address differences among providers' caseloads (e.g., providers with more complex patient populations compared to others) (Hoenders et al., 2014). To address these concerns, many VBC arrangements incorporate process variables (e.g., that a testing referral was responded to by a provider within a designated time frame) that may influence outcomes and are measured as potential targets for change in addition to the focus on outcomes (Rothrock et al., 2024).

As behavioral health settings prepare to transition away from FFS toward VBC arrangements, leadership, direct service, and administrative support staff need to be knowledgeable about and on board with participation (Daub et al., 2020). This includes training providers in the implementation of quality measurement, ensuring organizations have the structural and leadership capacity to support change management and implementation of new systems, and including quality measures that are meaningful to both patients and providers to increase "buy-in" (Daub et al., 2020). Core strategies involve including all clinic employees in decision-making processes, offering ongoing supervision and continuous learning opportunities, and implementing programs that support employee well-being (Daub et al, 2020). Of note quality reporting can include aspects of measurement-based care (MBC), an evidence-based practice of using systematic assessment to inform clinical decision-making by sharing and using that data with patients; however, VBC participation does not necessarily require adherence to MBC best practices given its primary intention is to allow providers to meet the requirements of payors and/or other stakeholders (Rothrock et al., 2024).

Transitioning to VBC contracts may be even more challenging for neuropsychologists, whether in small independent practices or embedded in integrated care settings, due to the nature of their work (van Heugten et al., 2020). Assessments of cognitive functioning are typically accomplished by neuropsychologists performing a consultative role or to assist with differential diagnosis or treatment planning in some manner, making identifying appropriate quality measures quite difficult. Patient-reported outcome measures are often not relevant as most neuropsychologists typically do not follow patients for treatment after the evaluation is completed with the value of such services often being realized outside of the epoch of care provided for a given patient; noted exceptions may include settings (such as long-term care) where repeated cognitive screenings and the use of functioning measures may significantly influence ongoing care. As a result, process-based quality measures are necessary for the practice pattern of neuropsychologists to be represented. Yet there is no agreed upon core set of process-based quality measures to assess the work of neuropsychologists in existing VBC models.

As one potential alternative, King and colleagues (2022) developed a self-assessment audit tool to evaluate neuropsychological assessment quality with the intention of addressing variability in clinical practice. Recognizing that neuropsychological assessment may drift from gold standard practices without routine monitoring and audit, King et al. identified 39 standards based on best practices and expert consensus. Standards were grouped into process standards, and report style and content standards, with tailored core and supplementary standards within each group for diverse service settings. The researchers placed significant emphasis on holistic assessment, contextual interpretation, and clear communication in reports, with the aim to standardize practice and promote reflective quality improvement (King et al., 2022).

An additional area of focus in the quality improvement literature for neuropsychological assessment is validation of psychometric evaluations and test development (Facchin et al., 2025; Sweet et al., 2021). Quality neuropsychological assessment is dependent on regular psychometric validation of existing and new tests, including test–retest reliability, construct validity, ecological validity, and ensuring cultural relevance and accuracy. The more recent introduction of digital tools and real-life tasks offers promise in addressing limitations of traditional paper-and-pencil tests. For example, Karjaki and colleagues (2023) used digital voice recordings to evaluate cognitive status and successfully differentiated patients with dementia from those who had normal cognition, suggesting digital technologies may offer affordable, accessible ways to evaluate behavior and function.

Finally, with the rise of telehealth because of the COVID-19 public health emergency, studies have begun evaluating the psychometric reliability of online neuropsychological assessments and remote testing. Preliminary research suggests that remote tests show variable reliability, with some tasks such as sustained attention and picture recognition, performing particularly well; however, reliability may be affected by certain factors like age, technical proficiency, and whether the testing occurred in an unsupervised setting. Although additional research is warranted, early findings suggest remote cognitive assessments may be a useful and cost-effective alternative to in-person clinic-based assessment, making it an attractive option for inclusion in VBC contracts (Peterson et al., 2025).

Implementation Takeaway #1

Neuropsychologists are encouraged to assess their readiness to transition from a traditional FFS reimbursement model to one that promotes value-based care by focusing on six core areas: leadership, care delivery, health information technology, partnership, financial culture, and organizational culture. As a starting point, we offer a *Framework for Preparing for Value-Based Care in Neuropsychology* (see Table 3.1).

A Value-Based Care Model: CMS's Quality Payment Program and the Impact on Neuropsychology

The US federal government, and in particular, CMS, plays a critical role in healthcare in this country. With a combined 139 million beneficiaries, Medicare is the largest payer of inpatient hospital services for older adults, and Medicaid is the largest payer of mental health and long-term care services (CMS, 2017). Given rising healthcare costs, it's no surprise that CMS is leading efforts to implement VBC models

Table 3.1 Tasks for Preparing for Value-Based Care in Neuropsychology

1. Define the Value Proposition & Assess your Readiness Clarify how neuropsychological assessment contributes to the VBC goals: • Improved outcomes: Accurate diagnosis, tailored treatment, better functional recovery • Cost reduction: Avoid unnecessary imaging, reduce specialist referrals, optimize resource use • Patient experience: Enhanced understanding, empowerment, and satisfaction
2. Identify Target Populations Focus on populations where neuropsychological input has high impact: • Dementia and mild cognitive impairment • Traumatic brain injury • Stroke and other neurological conditions • ADHD and learning disorders • Behavioral health integration (e.g., depression with cognitive complaints)
3. Establish Key Metrics Use a mix of clinical, economic, and experiential metrics: Clinical Outcomes • Diagnostic accuracy • Functional status (e.g., ADLs, IADLs, return to work) • Treatment adherence and engagement Economic Outcomes • Reduction in imaging or specialist referrals • Avoided hospitalizations or ER visits • Cost savings from targeted interventions Patient-Centered Outcomes • Patient satisfaction and understanding • Caregiver burden reduction • Goal attainment
4. Integrate into Care Pathways Map where neuropsychological services fit within VBC workflows: • Pre-surgical evaluations • Post-acute rehabilitation planning • Behavioral health screening and triage • Cognitive monitoring in chronic disease management
5. Use Validated Tools and Standards Ensure assessments align with: • Evidence-based guidelines (e.g., AACN, NAN) • Performance validity testing • Culturally appropriate norms • Audit tools for quality assurance
6. Build Data & HIT Infrastructure Support outcome tracking with: • EHR integration for longitudinal data • Standardized documentation templates • Dashboards for clinical and financial metrics

(continued)

Table 3.1 (continued)

7. Engage Stakeholders and build relationships to obtain buy-in Include: • Primary care and specialty providers • Payers and health system leadership • Patients and caregivers • Quality improvement teams
8. Pilot and Scale Implementation or other Quality Improvement Study Start with a pilot in a high-impact area, then: • Collect baseline and post-intervention data • Refine workflows and documentation • Scale to other service lines or populations

(Wright et al., 2019). To begin, legislation was passed by Congress in 2015, which repealed the sustainable growth rate (SGR), a mechanism that had been in place since 1997 to control Medicare expenses. The SGR was replaced with a new Medicare payment program called the Quality Payment Program (QPP), which includes two payment models: the Merit-Based Incentive Program (MIPS) and Advanced Alternative Payment Models (APMs). Advanced APMs include Medicare providers managing a patient population under a shared-savings or bundled payment arrangement, which requires meeting strict certified technology and financial risk criteria. MIPS, on the other hand, applies payment adjustments to claims submitted on individual Medicare patients, and as such is often more applicable to neuropsychologists based on their typical billing patterns. All Medicare billing psychologists were added as eligible clinicians to the QPP program in 2019 (CMS, 2018).

To elucidate further, MIPS combines three former legacy programs—the Physician Quality Reporting System, the Value-Based Modifier, and Meaningful Use—into one large composite program. Four components make up this composite score: quality, promoting interoperability, improvement activities, and cost. Within the quality component, Medicare providers are required to submit six measures for every patient they see over a 12-month period. At least one quality measure must be an outcome measure (e.g., a patient-reported outcome measure) or a measure deemed "high priority" by CMS. The provider's quality performance is then scored and combined with the other three performance categories—promoting interoperability, improvement activities, and cost.

Those who score at or above the CMS-determined threshold will receive a zero or positive payment adjustment respectively, and those who score below receive a negative adjustment. Medicare payment adjustments appear two years after the MIPS participation period, so for those providers reporting to MIPS in 2025, they will see a ±9% payment adjustment in 2027 based on whether they fall above or below the performance threshold, respectively. In the final analysis, this very complicated VBC program offers high risk but potentially high reward for participating neuropsychologists. Given its complexity, CMS created an exemption to ease burden on small practices called the low-volume threshold (LVT), meaning that psychologists and other providers who see few Medicare patients and/or generate little reimbursement from those services are not required to participate in MIPS reporting. Since the inception of the program, it has become clear that many clinical psychologists, particularly those in independent practice, who bill Medicare fall under the LVT and are exempt, because they treat and bill too few Medicare patients. However, depending on the clinical setting (e.g., memory clinics) and patient population served (i.e., more patients aged 65 or older), neuropsychologists appear less likely to fall under the LVT and as such, are often subject to mandatory MIPS reporting.

To assist neuropsychologists in successfully meeting MIPS reporting requirements, in 2018, the American Psychological Association (APA) received approval from CMS as a qualified clinical data registry (QCDR) named the Mental and Behavioral Health Registry (MBHR). Clinical data registries and performance dashboards provide data visualizations and advanced analytics enabling the provider to see their quality performance and make service delivery adjustments in real time (Daub et al., 2020). Being a QCDR also allows APA, assisted by an advisory committee of quality measurement experts, to develop and propose meaningful quality measures to CMS that are specialty specific. This is particularly beneficial to neuropsychologists given the reporting challenges noted earlier due to the lack of measures, particularly outcome measures, as a result of the consultative nature of the work.

To that end, beginning in 2019 APA partnered with the National Academy of Neuropsychology (NAN) to develop a suite of neuropsychology measures that would better align with the consultative nature of their service delivery. Moreover, the partnership played a critical role in supporting joint advocacy to work with CMS to approve and maintain the developed quality measures. APA staff and NAN Professional Affairs and information Committee (PAIC) committee members followed best practices in measure development, and after measure specifications were developed, they were sent out for peer review with experts identified in the field in the particular measurement area. Feedback was then incorporated prior to submission to CMS.

For the 2025 MIPS reporting period (CMS, 2025), the MBHR includes four neuropsychology-specific measures developed as a result of this partnership: (1) *Cognitive Assessment with Counseling on Safety and Potential Risk* (MBHR11), (2) *Consideration of Cultural-Linguistic and Demographic Factors in Cognitive Assessment* (MBHR15), (3) *Comprehensive Cognitive Assessment Assists with Differential Diagnosis* (MBHR16), and (4) *Provision of Feedback Following a Cognitive or Mental Status Assessment with Documentation of Understanding of Test Results and Subsequent Healthcare Plan with Timely Transmission of Results* (MBHR18).

The Future for the CMS Quality Payment Program

Since its inception a decade ago, CMS has enacted multiple changes to the QPP program, including greater emphasis on aligning cost with quality in terms of contribution to overall performance. But the most significant changes announced recently by CMS are the intention to sunset MIPS and replace with a new mandatory reporting option, the MIPS Value Pathways (MVPs) (CMS, n.d.). MVPs, which include a focused core set of quality measures, improvement activities, and cost measures tailored to a specialty (e.g., neurology) or condition (e.g., lower extremity joint repair), represent CMS's desire to address providers' concerns regarding quality payment reporting burden. Given that at some undetermined point in the future, MVPs will be the only reporting option for neuropsychologists, APA and NAN subsequently collaborated and proposed the *Promotion of Optimal Neuropsychology Consultation MVP* in 2023. Following several years of joint advocacy to influence CMS staff, the Neuropsychology MVP was eventually posted for the 2026 MVP Candidate Feedback Period and was subsequently moved forward to rulemaking in the 2026 Medicare Physician Fee Schedule proposed rule. In their public comment letter, APA strongly supported CMS finalizing the MVP. The intent of the MVP is to create a cohesive and specialty-specific set of measures that promote optimal neuropsychological care across a lifespan patient population and improve quality of care and value in neuropsychological evaluations. For example, providing clarification of differential diagnosis or etiological factors of cognitive impairment or complaints for individuals who undergo cognitive assessment, will improve the quality of care for patients. Consideration of appropriate and relevant cultural-linguistic and demographic factors with individuals, who undergo cognitive assessment, will improve the quality of care and quality of life for patients through the provision of appropriate assessment methods. Further, provision of timely assessment results to patients, who undergo cognitive or mental status assessment, will improve the quality of treatment and management of mental health, as well as the quality of life for patients.

In addition to the goal of ensuring high quality care, it's important to reiterate that for Medicare providers who are currently required to participate in MIPS, MVPs will be the only reporting option at some point in the near future. That means that providers without a relevant MVP for their specialty will need to report on a core set of quality measures that may at best not be meaningful and at worst, not be applicable. This has important financial implications as the same Medicare payment adjustments currently applicable to MIPS participation, will be applied to MVP participation (i.e., a $\pm 9\%$ payment adjustment two years after the participation period depending on whether the provider falls above or below the performance threshold, respectively). Therefore, having a relevant MVP will be critical, particularly for specialty providers.

APA's partnership with NAN has helped ensure that neuropsychological care is better represented in Medicare's quality reporting system. Together, the two associations developed and advocated for measures that reflect the unique nature of neuropsychological services, leading to the inclusion of four specialty-specific measures in the 2025 reporting program. Looking ahead, the proposed Neuropsychology MVP aims to make care more personalized, culturally responsive, and effective—ultimately improving the lives of patients by ensuring timely, accurate assessments and better communication of results.

Final Takeaway

This chapter focused on current shifts in the US healthcare reimbursement system away from FFS and toward VBC and used CMS's QPP as one of the leading examples of this shift given its role as one of the largest national payors of services for older adults, mental health and long-term care. Although this may not feel very relevant to providers who do not bill Medicare, reimbursement and coverage decisions made by CMS often have a trickle-down effect on commercial payers. Although the authors are not aware of any large-scale VBC model being applied to neuropsychologists currently, this shift will make its way to behavioral health providers across settings eventually and as such, preparing for these changes is critical to our profession. For example, the greater emphasis on reimbursement for preventative services in VBC models (e.g., early detection and intervention because of cognitive screenings in high-risk populations), creates opportunities for expanding neuropsychologists' role beyond diagnostic assessment into proactive health management. By participating in VBC models, neuropsychologists can demonstrate measurable contributions to population health and position themselves as essential partners in integrated care teams.

References

Basch, E., Spertus, J., Dudley, R. A., Wu, A., Chuahan, C., Cohen, P., Goertz, C., et al. (2015). Methods for developing patient-reported outcome-based performance measures (PRO-PMs). *Value in Health, 18*, 493–504. https://doi.org/10.1016/j.jval.2015.02.018

Begali, V. L. (2020). Neuropsychology and the dementia spectrum: Differential diagnosis, clinical management, and forensic utility. *NeuroRehabilitation, 46*(2), 181–194. https://doi.org/10.3233/NRE-192965

Bodenheimer, T., & Sinsky, C. (2014). From triple to quadruple aim: Care of the patient requires care of the provider. *Annals of Family Medicine, 12*, 573–576. https://doi.org/10.1370/afm.1713

Bowie, C. R., Leung, W. W., Reichenberg, A., McClure, M. M., Patterson, T. L., Heaton, R. K., & Harvey, P. D. (2008). Predicting schizophrenia patients' real-world behavior with specific neuropsychological and functional capacity measures. *Biological Psychiatry, 63*(5), 505–511. https://doi.org/10.1016/j.biopsych.2007.05.022

Centers for Medicare and Medicaid Services (CMS). (2017). *Medicare and Medicaid basics*. https://www.cms.gov/Outreachand-Education/Medicare-Learning-Network-MLN/MLNProducts/Downloads/ProgramBasicsText-Only.pdf

Centers for Medicare and Medicaid Services (CMS). (2018). *Quality Payment Program Year 3 proposed rule overview*. https://www.cms.gov/Medicare/Quality-Initiatives-Patient-Assessment-Instruments/Value-Based-Programs/MACRA-MIPS-and-APMs/Overview-of-Proposed-Rule-for-Year-3-2019-slides.pdf

Centers for Medicare and Medicaid Services. (2021). *Innovation center strategy refresh*. https://innovation.cms.gov/strategic-direction-whitepaper

Centers for Medicare and Medicaid Services. (2025). *2025 Qualified Clinical Data Registry (QCDR) Measure Specifications*. https://qpp.cms.gov/resources/document/a1a4daa8-bf34-43b8-a493-026f4199fa36

Centers for Medicare and Medicaid Services. (n.d.). MIPS Value Pathways (MVPs). https://qpp.cms.gov/mips/mips-value-pathways

Core Quality Measures Collaborative. (2020, November 25). *Analysis of measurement gap areas and measure alignment.* National Quality Forum.

Cummings, J., Isaacson, S., Mills, R., Williams, H., Chi-Burris, K., Corbett, A., Dhall, R., & Ballard, C. (2014). Pimavanserin for patients with Parkinson's disease psychosis: A randomised, placebo-controlled phase 3 trial. *Lancet, 383*(9916), 533–540. https://doi.org/10.1016/S0140-6736(13)62106-6

Daub, S., Rosenzweig, C., & Schilkie, M. C. (2020). Preparing for a value-driven future. *Families, Systems, & Health, 38*, 83–86. https://doi.org/10.1037/fsh0000476

DeLeon, P. H., VandenBos, G. R., & Bulatao, E. Q. (1994). Managed mental health care: A history of the federal policy initiative. In R. L. Lowman & R. J. Resnick (Eds.), *The mental health professional's guide to managed care* (pp. 19–40). (Reprinted from *Professional Psychology: Research and Practice,* 22, 1991, pp. 15–25). https://doi.org/10.1037/10148-002

Dieleman, J. L., Cao, J., Chapin, A., et al. (2020). US health care spending by payer and health condition, 1996–2016. *JAMA, 323*(9), 863–884. https://doi.org/10.1001/jama.2020.0734

Donders, J. (2020). The incremental value of neuropsychological assessment: A critical review. *The Clinical Neuropsychologist, 34*(1), 56–87. https://doi.org/10.1080/13854046.2019.1575471

Dubois, B., Tolosa, E., Katzenschlager, R., Emre, M., Lees, A. J., Schumann, G., Pourcher, E., Gray, J., Thomas, G., Swartz, J., Hsu, T., & Moline, M. L. (2012). Donepezil in Parkinson's disease dementia: A randomized, double-blind efficacy and safety study. *Movement Disorders, 27*(10), 1230–1238. https://doi.org/10.1002/mds.25098

Facchin, A., Cavicchiolo, E., & Chan, E. (2025). Editorial: Neuropsychological testing: From psychometrics to clinical neuropsychology. *Frontiers in Psychology, 16*, 1549236. https://doi.org/10.3389/fpsyg.2025.154923

Gasquoine, P. G. (2010). Comparison of public/private health care insurance parameters for independent psychological practice. *Professional Psychology: Research and Practice, 41*, 319–324. https://doi.org/10.1037/a0020268

Glen, E. T., Hostetter, G., Ruff, R. M., Roebuck-Spencer, T. M., Denney, R. L., Perry, W., Fazio, R. L., Garmoe, W. S., Bianchini, K. J., & Scott, J. G. (2019). Integrative care models in neuropsychology: A national academy of neuropsychology education paper. *Archives of Clinical Neuropsychology, 34*(2), 141–151. https://doi.org/10.1093/arclin/acy092

Glen, T., Hostetter, G., Roebuck-Spencer, T. M., Garmoe, W. S., Scott, J. S., Hilsabeck, R. C., Arnett, P., & Espe-Pfeifer, P. (2020). Return on investment and value research in neuropsychology: A call to arms. *Archives of Clinical Neuropsychology, 35*(5), 459–468. https://doi.org/10.1093/arclin/acaa010

Hantke, N. C., Kaye, J., Mattek, N., Wu, C. Y., Dodge, H. H., Beattie, Z., & Woltjer, R. (2023). Correlating continuously captured home-based digital biomarkers of daily function with post-mortem neurodegenerative neuropathology. *PLoS ONE, 18*(6), Article e0286812. https://doi.org/10.1371/journal.pone.0286812

Henderson, E. J., Lord, S. R., Brodie, M. A., Gaunt, D. M., Lawrence, A. D., Close, J. C. T., Whone, A. L., & Ben-Shlomo, Y. (2016). Rivastigmine for gait stability in patients with Parkinson's disease (ReSPonD): A randomised, double-blind, placebo-controlled, phase 2 trial. *The Lancet Neurology, 15*(3), 249–258. https://doi.org/10.1016/S1474-4422(15)00389-0

Hoenders, R. H. J., Bos, E. H., Bartels-Velthuis, A. A., Vollbehr, N. K., van der Ploeg, K., de Jonge, P., & de Jong, J. T. V. M. (2014). Pitfalls in the assessment, analysis, and interpretation of Routine Outcome Monitoring (ROM) data: Results from an outpatient clinic for integrative mental health. *Administration and Policy in Mental Health and Mental Health Services Research, 41*, 647–659. https://doi.org/10.1007/s10488-013-0511-7

Institute of Medicine (IOM). (2015). *Psychosocial interventions for mental and substance use disorders: A framework for establishing evidence-based standards.* National Academies Press.

Karjadi, C., Xue, C., Cordella, C., Kiran, S., Paschalidis, I. C., Au, R., & Kolachalama, V. B. (2023). Fusion of low-level descriptors of digital voice recordings for dementia assessment. *Journal of Alzheimer's Disease, 96*, 507–514.

Kaser, A. N., Lacritz, L. H., Winiarski, H. R., Gabirondo, P., Schaffert, J., Cullum, C. M., et al. (2024). A novel speech analysis algorithm to detect cognitive impairment in a Spanish population. *Frontiers in Neurology, 15*, 1342907.

Keefe, R. S. E., Poe, M., Walker, T. M., & Harvey, P. D. (2006). The relationship of the Brief Assessment of Cognition in Schizophrenia (BACS) to functional capacity and real-world functional outcome. *Journal of Clinical and Experimental Neuropsychology, 28*(2), 260–269. https://doi.org/10.1080/13803390500360539

King, L., Hirst, R. E., Methley, A., Javed, H. M., Bowman, A. R., & Stevens, L. H. (2022). Improving the quality of neuropsychological assessment practice: The development of a self-assessment audit tool. *Archives of Clinical Neuropsychology, 37*, 814–825.

Liptzin, B. (2009). Quality improvement, pay for performance, and "outcomes measurement": What makes sense? *Psychiatric Services, 60*, 108–111. https://doi.org/10.1176/ps.2009.60.1.108

Lopes da Cunha, P., Ruiz, F., Ferrante, F., Sterpin, L. F., Ibáñez, A., Slachevsky, A., Matallana, D., Martínez, Á., Hesse, E., & García, A. M. (2024). Automated free speech analysis reveals distinct markers of Alzheimer's and frontotemporal dementia. *PLoS ONE, 19*(6), Article e0304272. https://doi.org/10.1371/journal.pone.0304272

Loring, D. W., Bauer, R. M., Cavanagh, L., Drane, D. L., Enriquez, K. D., Reise, S. P., Shih, K., Umfleet, L. G., Wahlstrom, D., Whelan, F., Widaman, K. F., Bilder, R. M., & NNN Study Group. (2022). Rationale and design of the national neuropsychology network. *Journal of the International Neuropsychological Society: JINS, 28*(1), 1–11. https://doi.org/10.1017/S1355617721000199

Mittelman, M. S., Ferris, S. H., Shulman, E., Steinberg, G., & Levin, B. (1996). A family intervention to delay nursing home placement of patients with Alzheimer disease. *JAMA, 276*(21), 1725–1731.

Nordal, K. C. (2012). Healthcare reform: Implications for independent practice. *Professional Psychology: Research and Practice, 43*, 535–544. https://doi.org/10.1037/a0029603

Office of the Assistant Secretary for Planning and Evaluation (ASPE). (2021, July). *Supporting value-based care transformation through interoperability and care coordination.* https://aspe.hhs.gov/sites/default/files/2021-07/value-based-care.pdf

Peterson, K. A., Leddy, A., & Hornberger, M. (2025). Reliability of online, remote neuropsychological assessment in people with and without subjective cognitive decline. *PLOS Digital Health, 4*(4), Article e0000682. https://doi.org/10.1371/journal.pdig.0000682

Prigatano, G., & Pliskin, N. (2003). *Clinical neuropsychology and cost outcome research: A beginning.* https://doi.org/10.4324/9781315787039

Pritchard, A. E., Sweeney, K., Salorio, C. F., & Jacobson, L. A. (2020). Pediatric neuropsychological evaluation via telehealth: Novel models of care. *The Clinical Neuropsychologist, 34*(7–8), 1367–1379. https://doi.org/10.1080/13854046.2020.1806359

Rothrock, N. E., Bott, M., Douglas, A., McKune, E. W., Owings-Fonner, N., Ross, D., Wright, C. V., et al. (2024). Understanding and preparing for value-based care: A primer for behavioral health providers. *Professional Psychology: Research and Practice, 55*, 68–78. https://doi.org/10.1037/pro0000537

Sanchez, L. M., & Turner, S. M. (2003). Practicing psychology in the era of managed care: Implications for practice and training. *American Psychologist, 58*, 116–129. https://doi.org/10.1037/0003-066X.58.2.116

Schmitter-Edgecombe, M., Brown, K., Chilton, R. C., Whiteley, N., & Greeley, D. (2024a). Naturalistic assessment of everyday multitasking in Parkinson's disease with and without mild cognitive impairment. *The Clinical Neuropsychologist, 38*(8), 1910–1930. https://doi.org/10.1080/13854046.2024.2325681

Schmitter-Edgecombe, M., Luna, C., Dai, S., & Cook, D. J. (2024b). Predicting daily cognition and lifestyle behaviors for older adults using smart home data and ecological momentary assessment. *The Clinical Neuropsychologist*, 1–25. Advance online publication. https://doi.org/10.1080/13854046.2024.2330143

Schmitter-Edgecombe, M., Luna, C., Beech, B., Dai, S., & Cook, D. J. (2025). Capturing cognitive capacity in the everyday environment across a continuum of cognitive decline using a smartwatch n-back task and ecological momentary assessment. *Neuropsychology, 39*(1), 28–43. https://doi.org/10.1037/neu0000984

Seppi, K., Weintraub, D., Coelho, M., Perez-Lloret, S., Fox, S. H., Katzenschlager, R., Sampaio, C., et al. (2011). The movement disorder society evidence-based medicine review update: Treatments for the non-motor symptoms of Parkinson's disease. *Movement Disorders, 26*(Suppl 3), S42–S80. https://doi.org/10.1002/mds.23884

Sieg, E., Mai, Q., Mosti, C., & Brook, M. (2019). The utility of neuropsychological consultation in identifying medical inpatients with suspected cognitive impairment at risk for greater hospital utilization. *The Clinical Neuropsychologist, 33*(1), 75–89. https://doi.org/10.1080/13854046.2018.1465124

Singh, S., Strong, R., Xu, I., Fonseca, L. M., Hawks, Z., Grinspoon, E., Germine, L. T., et al. (2023). Ecological momentary assessment of cognition in clinical and community samples: Reliability and validity study. *Journal of Medical Internet Research, 25*, Article e45028. https://doi.org/10.2196/45028

Sliwinski, M. J., Mogle, J. A., Hyun, J., Munoz, E., Smyth, J. M., & Lipton, R. B. (2018). Reliability and validity of ambulatory cognitive assessments. *Assessment, 25*(1), 14–30. https://doi.org/10.1177/1073191116643164

Snipes, C. (2016). The use of electronic health record in behavioral health quality improvement initiatives. In W. O'Donohue & A. Maragakis (Eds.), *Quality improvement in behavioral health* (pp. 193–206).

Spitz, G., Ponsford, J. L., Rudzki, D., & Maller, J. J. (2012). Association between cognitive performance and functional outcome following traumatic brain injury: A longitudinal multilevel examination. *Neuropsychology, 26*(5), 604–612. https://doi.org/10.1037/a0029239

Stelmokas, J., Cigolle, C., Rochette, A., Tolle-Fu, K., Surber, C., Bloor, L., & Lee, P. (2022). Integration of neuropsychological assessment and intervention services into a specialty geriatric medicine clinic. *Professional Psychology: Research and Practice, 53*, 483–493. https://doi.org/10.1037/pro0000394

Sweet, J. J., Heilbronner, R. L., Morgan, J. E., Larrabee, G. J., Rohling, M. L., Boone, K. B., Participants, C., et al. (2021a). American Academy of Clinical Neuropsychology (AACN) 2021 consensus statement on validity assessment: Update of the 2009 AACN consensus conference statement on neuropsychological assessment of effort, response bias, and malingering. *The Clinical Neuropsychologist, 35*(6), 1053–1106. https://doi.org/10.1080/13854046.2021.1896036

Sweet, J. J., Klipfel, K. M., Nelson, N. W., & Moberg, P. J. (2021). Professional practices, beliefs, and incomes of U.S. neuropsychologists: The AACN, NAN, SCN 2020 practice and "salary survey". *The Clinical neuropsychologist, 35*(1), 7–80. https://doi.org/10.1080/13854046.2020.1849803

van Heugten, C., Caldenhove, S., Crutsen, J., & Winkens, I. (2020). An overview of outcome measures used in neuropsychological rehabilitation research on adults with acquired brain injury. *Neuropsychological Rehabilitation, 30*(8), 1598–1623. https://doi.org/10.1080/09602011.2019.1589533

Vankirk, K. K., Horner, M. D., Turner, T. H., Dismuke, C. E., & Muzzy, W. (2013). CE hospital service utilization is reduced following neuropsychological evaluation in a sample of U.S. veterans. *The Clinical Neuropsychologist, 27*(5), 750–761. https://doi.org/10.1080/13854046.2013.783122

Wang, H.-F., Yu, J.-T., Tang, S.-W., Jiang, T., Tan, C.-C., Meng, X.-F., Wang, C., Tan, M.-S., & Tan, L. (2015). Efficacy and safety of cholinesterase inhibitors and memantine in cognitive impairment in Parkinson's disease, Parkinson's disease dementia, and dementia with Lewy bodies: Systematic review with meta-analysis and trial sequential analysis. *Journal of Neurology, Neurosurgery, and Psychiatry, 86*(2), 135–143. https://doi.org/10.1136/jnnp-2014-307659

Wright, C. V., Goodheart, C., Bard, D., Bobbitt, B. L., Butt, Z., Lysell, K., McKay, D., & Stephens, K. (2019). Promoting measurement-based care and quality measure development: The APA mental and behavioral health registry initiative. *Psychological Services*. https://doi.org/10.1037/ser0000347

Chapter 4
Promoting Health Equity in Neuropsychology as a Cornerstone of Population Health

Elena Tsoy and Sanne Franzen

Executive Summary
This chapter emphasizes the critical role of health equity in population health by exploring how social determinants of health (SDOH) influence both healthcare access and cognitive health outcomes. It begins by discussing the conceptualization of SDOH as primary drivers of health inequities, underscoring that healthcare is only one piece of the larger puzzle in achieving overall well-being. The chapter highlights the importance of addressing various cultural, social, economic, and environmental factors that impact cognitive health, arguing that a comprehensive approach to health equity in neuropsychological research and practice must consider these broader conditions.

Introduction

Health equity is a global public health priority. Major institutions like the World Health Organization (WHO, 2010) and the US National Institute on Aging (Hill et al., 2015) have long emphasized the role of social, cultural, economic, and environmental factors in shaping health. For instance, while US life expectancy rose from 47 to 75 years in the twentieth century, these gains were uneven across racial

E. Tsoy (✉)
Department of Neurology, University of California, San Francisco, CA, USA
e-mail: elena.tsoy@ucsf.edu

Global Brain Health Institute, University of California, San Francisco, CA, USA

S. Franzen
Department of Neurology & Alzheimer Center, Erasmus MC University Medical Center, Rotterdam, The Netherlands
e-mail: s.franzen@erasmusmc.nl

M. Lanca and R. Fallows (eds.), *Advancing Neuropsychology Through Population Health*, https://doi.org/10.1007/978-3-032-22457-6_4

and economic groups (Woolf & Schoomaker, 2019). Life expectancy gaps have also widened between individuals with and without a college degree, and between those living in poverty vs. not (LaVeist et al., 2023; Woolf & Schoomaker, 2019). Health disparities impose a significant economic burden, with race-related disparities costing an estimated $421-$451 billion, and education-related disparities costing $940–$978 billion annually (LaVeist et al., 2023). These losses stem from premature deaths, reduced labor productivity, and increased healthcare costs, and they are likely to grow as the USA becomes a majority-minority population (LaVeist et al., 2023). Central to health equity is the concept of social determinants of health (SDOH)—the conditions in which people are born, grow, live, work, and age (Hill et al., 2015; WHO, 2010).

Social Drivers of Health and Healthcare Disparities

Early works on SDOH highlighted the limitations of focusing only on proximal risk factors for major diseases, such as health behaviors (e.g., smoking, diet) or biomarkers (e.g., cholesterol levels) (Link & Phelan, 1995; WHO, 2010). This narrow focus ignores the broader social conditions that serve as the "fundamental causes" of disease, putting certain individuals "at risk of risks" for poor health outcomes (Link & Phelan, 1995). Health is shaped by the complex interplay of cultural, social, economic, political, and environmental factors, affecting both individual and societal health outcomes. SDOH can thus be understood as structural conditions that influence health, reflecting policies, norms, and governance structures that lead to the inequitable distribution of power, resources, and opportunities (Adkins-Jackson et al., 2023). Additionally, while often used interchangeably, health and healthcare disparities are distinct concepts. Health disparities refer to differences in health outcomes—such as higher disease or disability burden—between groups (Alzheimer's Association, 2021; Hill et al., 2015). Healthcare disparities involve differences in access to care, insurance coverage, or care quality (Alzheimer's Association, 2021). Healthcare disparities often contribute to health disparities, but do not fully explain all differences in health outcomes.

SDOH Frameworks. Given the complexity of integrating numerous factors influencing health outcomes into effective policies, several SDOH conceptual frameworks have been developed. One model is the 2010 WHO Commission on Social Determinants of Health (CSDH) Conceptual Framework (WHO, 2010), which distinguishes between structural and intermediary SDOH. Structural factors, such as governance, macroeconomic policies, and cultural values, create social stratification. These factors are reflected in individual-level indicators like socioeconomic position, gender, race, ethnicity, education, occupation, and income. WHO suggests these structural factors affect health outcomes through intermediary determinants, including material circumstances (e.g., housing), behavioral and biological factors (e.g., smoking), and psychosocial variables (e.g., social support). Another model is the US National Institute on Aging (NIA) Health Disparities Research Framework (Hill et al., 2015). This framework organizes SDOH into analytical levels to inform aging policies, covering environmental, sociocultural, behavioral, and biological factors across the lifespan. The environmental level includes geographic/political, socioeconomic, and healthcare factors. Sociocultural factors encompass cultural, social, and psychological elements. The behavioral level includes coping strategies, psychosocial risk and resilience, and health behaviors. Biological factors include physiological indicators, genetic stability, and cellular function. Notably, the NIA framework highlights race, ethnicity, age, gender/sex identity, and disability status as key determinants of health disparities across all levels. The US National Institute on Minority Health and Health Disparities (NIMHD) recently developed a Health Disparities Research Framework, which represents a hybrid of the NIA framework and Bronfenbrenner's socioecological theory (Alvidrez et al., 2019). It expands on existing models by including the healthcare system as an additional level of analysis and categorizes individual SDOH factors into Bronfenbrenner's individual, interpersonal, community, and societal levels of influence (Bronfenbrenner, 1977). A comprehensive review of all existing SDOH frameworks is beyond the scope of this chapter, but it's important to note that no single universal theory exists. Nonetheless, these models are valuable for guiding efforts to reduce health inequities by providing a framework for generating research that informs policy changes and for designing person-centered clinical practices that improve care quality and patient outcomes.

Healthcare System as a SDOH. While healthcare access is a key determinant of health, SDOH create barriers that hinder people's ability to access and effectively use healthcare services. It's important to consider healthcare inequities within the context of different healthcare systems, as these systems provide distinct "backgrounds" for disparities. We review evidence on the role of SDOH in healthcare access in systems with and without universal healthcare coverage, using the US and European Union (EU) countries as examples. Our focus on systems is particularly relevant to neuropsychological services, which are often provided at secondary or tertiary levels and directly affected by healthcare resource distribution.

SDOH and Healthcare Access in the USA. In the USA, where universal healthcare coverage is not available to all, SDOH create complex barriers to access. Economic factors are particularly important, as economically disadvantaged individuals often cannot afford insurance premiums, co-pays, or out-of-pocket expenses, preventing timely care (Alzheimer's Association, 2021). Many unemployed or underemployed adults lack benefits like employer-provided insurance or paid sick leave, making medical costs prohibitive (Agency for Healthcare Research & Quality [AHRQ], 2019; Alzheimer's Association, 2021; Hinton et al., 2024). Additionally, limited health literacy, low English proficiency, and distrust of healthcare services can reduce healthcare access, leading to lower use of preventive services and poorer treatment adherence (AHRQ, 2019; Hinton et al., 2024). Systemic factors, rooted in historical inequities, further complicate access. These include shortages of culturally competent providers, insufficient healthcare resources in rural areas, and structural racism in medical practice (Adkins-Jackson et al., 2023; Alzheimer's Association, 2021;

AHRQ, 2019; Hinton et al., 2024; Airhihenbuwa & Liburd, 2006). Together, these factors create compounded barriers that affect health outcomes. For example, a study of 259 non-English-speaking stroke patients found that those without access to professional interpreters had worse post-stroke outcomes, even after adjusting for socioeconomic status and demographics (Luan Erfe et al., 2017). The relationship between SDOH and healthcare disparities in the USA is complex, but critical for understanding why the U.S. lags behind other high-income countries in healthcare performance. A recent report by the Commonwealth Fund found that the USA ranked last among 11 high-income countries on access, equity, and healthcare outcomes, despite having the highest healthcare spending (Schneider et al., 2021). While countries with universal healthcare perform better on these metrics, barriers related to SDOH persist, as discussed in the next section.

SDOH and Healthcare Access in Europe. Although most European countries offer near-universal coverage, significant variation exists within and between countries (Palm et al., 2021). In 2023, 3.8% of the EU population over 16 reported unmet medical needs (Eurostat, 2024). The reasons for these unmet needs vary—out-of-pocket expenses were the primary cause in Romania and Greece, while long waitlists were the main issue in Denmark and Slovenia. SDOH impact healthcare access in Europe in complex ways. Individuals with lower education levels are often the most affected, although poverty's effect on access is less consistent. Structural factors, such as the type of welfare model, also play a role. Health inequalities are lower in countries where social insurance is funded through contributions from employers, rather than general taxation or other means (Eikemo et al., 2008). While the general population in Europe generally has better care access compared to other countries, certain groups face challenges. Asylum seekers, irregular residents, people experiencing homelessness, and Roma populations may be partially or fully excluded from coverage or lack health insurance (Guerrero et al., 2024; Palm et al., 2021). These groups also face linguistic, financial, and informational barriers, along with racism, anti-migrant attitudes, and health-related prejudices when seeking care (Aljadeeah et al., 2024; Guerrero et al., 2024; Pattillo et al., 2023).

Social Determinants of Cognitive Health

Social determinants not only influence access to healthcare but also directly affect cognitive health outcomes. This section reviews evidence on the relationship between SDOH and cognitive abilities and decline, particularly in middle and late adulthood. Focusing on adulthood is important for two reasons. First, cognitive functioning follows a developmental trajectory, and studying adults who have experienced the cumulative effects of life course SDOH helps better understand these impacts. Second, examining mature populations helps identify SDOH that increase the risk of neurological disorders, as they bear the burden of these diseases. We organize this section around key factors, including education, economic well-being, employment, social and community context, and the physical and built environment. While these factors are among the most studied SDOH, they do not encompass all the variables that influence cognitive outcomes.

Education. Education is a key determinant of cognitive health. Across countries, there is a strong, stepwise relationship between educational attainment and life expectancy, with better-educated individuals living longer (Braveman & Gottlieb, 2014; Braveman et al., 2011). Education is one of the strongest predictors of cognitive performance as reflected in nearly all neuropsychological test norms. Studies worldwide consistently show that lower educational attainment increases the risk of dementia and other cognitive disorders, making it a promising prevention target (Lipnicki et al., 2019; Livingston et al., 2024). Education also influences brain development in adolescents (Judd et al., 2020) and gray matter volumes across the lifespan (Walhovd et al., 2022). Beyond attainment, the quality of education impacts cognitive abilities later in life (Crowe et al., 2013; Sisco et al., 2015), suggesting that the years of education alone don't fully explain cognitive health advantages or disadvantages. Additionally, low literacy has been shown to increase dementia risk, possibly more so than low education (Arce Rentería et al., 2019; Manly et al., 2003). Importantly, education not only stimulates cognitive engagement and reserve (Braveman & Gottlieb, 2014; Braveman et al., 2011; Livingston et al., 2024) but also provides the foundation for economic opportunities, social mobility, and the ability to navigate health information and make informed decisions. Inadequate education, conversely, perpetuates disadvantage, leading to poorer cognitive outcomes and limiting opportunities for cognitive enhancement.

Economic Well-being. The poverty-wealth dimension is another important SDOH for brain health. A WHO report from 21 countries estimated that up to 30% of poor brain health and disorders could be attributed to insufficient family income and adverse childhood experiences (Kessler et al., 2010). Children growing up in poverty are at higher risk for developmental delays, compromised brain organization, and lower cognitive function in adulthood (Chan et al., 2018; Hair et al., 2015). Early-life poverty also increases the risk of neurological diseases, including epilepsy, stroke, neuro-infections, and dementia (Maalouf et al., 2021; Wang et al., 2023). These long-term effects are likely related to economic constraints that limit access to education, nutrition, safe housing, and stimulating environments—critical components for healthy brain development. In adulthood, lower socioeconomic resources are linked to accelerated aging in physical, sensory, physiological, cognitive, and socioemotional domains (Steptoe & Zaninotto, 2020). Economic hardship is also strongly associated with chronic stress, a significant risk factor for impaired brain development and functioning (Evans & Schamberg, 2009). Chronic stress (allostatic load) leads to physiological changes affecting the nervous, endocrine, immune, cardiovascular, and metabolic systems, with overlap in brain function (McEwen & Gianaros, 2010). This stress-induced damage illustrates how social factors exert "under the skin" effects on health, highlighting the need to recognize these mechanisms in diagnosing and treating neurological disorders.

Employment. Employment as an SDOH encompasses factors related to intellectual stimulation and work conditions. Higher occupational complexity—jobs requiring greater cognitive engagement, critical thinking, or problem-solving—has been linked to better cognitive performance and a lower risk of cognitive decline and disorders (Almeida-Meza et al., 2021; Andel et al., 2005; Mayeda et al., 2020; Pool et al., 2016). Notably, most studies show that these relationships cannot be fully explained by educational background alone. The concept of occupational neuroplasticity suggests that highly professional workers have greater gray matter volumes compared to novices in areas relevant to job performance (Wu et al., 2020). Conversely, certain work conditions can negatively impact cognitive health. Jobs with high work-related stress and irregular hours (e.g., shift work) are associated with poorer cognitive outcomes (Andel et al., 2011; Bufano et al., 2024). Additionally, frequent work exposure to environmental chemical pollutants, such as pesticides, may increase the risk of neurological diseases and dementia (Elonheimo et al., 2021; Kulcsarova et al., 2023).

Social and Community Context. Social environments shape the developing brain and may impact cognitive trajectories into adulthood. Maltreatment, such as abuse, neglect, or manipulation, and other adverse childhood experiences (ACEs) can affect neurodevelopment and alter brain structure (Teicher & Samson, 2016). Emerging evidence also suggests that ACEs in general, and maltreatment in childhood specifically, are associated with dementia in late life (Abouelmagd et al., 2025). Conversely, strong social networks can reduce the risk of cognitive disorders. People who engage in frequent, high-quality social interactions tend to have better cognitive functioning in late life (Perry et al., 2022). Social connectedness contributes to cognitive reserve, highlighting that both cognitive and social enrichment are important for maintaining cognitive health throughout life (Peng et al., 2022). Conversely, loneliness, particularly among older adults, is linked to poorer cognitive health (Harrington et al., 2023), and individuals reporting more loneliness tend to belong to socially disadvantaged communities, such as low-income, low education, LGB + identity, or a migration background (Berlingieri et al., 2024). Additionally, neighborhood context plays a crucial role in access to social activities, food, safety, education, and health behaviors, independently affecting cognitive health (Kind & Buckingham, 2018). People in disadvantaged neighborhoods tend to have smaller cerebral and hippocampal volumes and greater Alzheimer's disease neuropathological changes at autopsy (Hunt et al., 2020; Powell et al., 2020). This issue is especially prominent in the USA, where the legacy of racial residential segregation continues to harm Black Americans and those living in poverty. Studies show that Black Americans often live in neighborhoods with fewer recreational facilities, health food stores, and higher crime rates, as well as greater exposure to environmental toxins and fewer high-quality healthcare facilities (Phelan & Link, 2015). Furthermore, housing instability, common in these neighborhoods, is associated with higher rates of cognitive dysfunction (Mullady et al., 2022).

Physical and Built Environment. Another key dimension of SDOH is the physical environment, which includes housing conditions, air quality, and access to green spaces. A Lancet Commission report found that environmental pollution contributes to 9 million deaths annually worldwide, with ambient air pollution and toxic chemical exposure increasing since 2000 (Fuller et al., 2022). Pollutants like fine particulate matter (PM2.5) have been linked to a higher risk of dementia and faster cognitive decline, particularly in urban areas with high industrialization and traffic (Weuve et al., 2021). Housing quality is directly tied to water and air quality and exposure to lead, mold, or dust—factors that impact health and well-being. Children exposed to lead in substandard housing exhibit lower cognitive skills, delayed physical development, and worse behavioral outcomes (Coley et al., 2013; Lidsky & Schneider, 2003). Additionally, studies show that neighborhood greenness is associated with better cognitive performance, larger cortical volumes, and a lower risk of cognitive impairment and dementia (Besser, 2021). Access to protected walking spaces encourages physical activity and mental stimulation, which are effective strategies for reducing the risks of neurological disorders and cognitive decline (Rovio et al., 2005; Stephen et al., 2017).

Disparities in Neuropsychological Care

The relationship between SDOH and cognitive health is especially relevant in the context of the current landscape of health equity in neuropsychology. This section highlights global disparities in access, quality, and outcomes of neuropsychological services.

Access to Care. In many regions, access to neuropsychological care is limited by financial and logistical barriers. In low- and middle-income countries, neuropsychology is an emerging field, and the shortage of trained specialists limits availability and access to services (Grote & Novitski, 2016). This gap is compounded by a resource-strained healthcare infrastructure and insufficient funding for sustainable provision of mental and cognitive care (Tsoy et al., 2021). In wealthier countries, disparities persist in underserved communities, particularly among people of color, those with low socioeconomic status, and rural residents (Saadi et al., 2017). While teleneuropsychology offers a potential solution to geographical barriers (Munro Cullum et al., 2014), its effectiveness is limited by digital literacy and technology access, especially in rural areas, communities of color, older adults, and those with low income and health literacy (Nouri et al., 2020).

Workforce. Cultural competence and representativeness in neuropsychology remain a significant challenge worldwide. In North America, only 9–13% of clinical neuropsychologists are from ethnic minority backgrounds (Elbulok-Charcape et al., 2014; Klipfel et al., 2023), creating a "chronic disconnect" between providers and an increasingly diverse patient population. This gap raises concerns about service availability, quality, and the profession's relevance, as noted in the American Academy of Clinical Neuropsychology's Relevance 2050 Initiative (Postal, 2018). Only about 15% of neuropsychologists in the USA and Canada provide services in languages other than English, despite projections that the minority of the US population will be monolingual English speakers by 2050 (Klipfel et al., 2023). Multicultural training is also inconsistent, with a third of neuropsychologists in North America receiving no such training (Elbulok-Charcape et al., 2014). In Europe, data on workforce diversity is lacking, but studies suggest underrepresentation of certain demographic groups in medicine as they advance in their careers (General Medical Council, 2023; Mulder et al., 2023). A Delphi study on European cross-cultural neuropsychology emphasized the need for better multicultural training, increased workforce diversity, and improvement in interpreter-mediated processes (Franzen et al., 2021), leading to the development of recommendations for interpreter-mediated assessment (Nielsen et al., 2024).

Research Methods. Most neuropsychological assessments are designed in 'Western,' English-speaking countries, and contain stimuli and procedures that may not be appropriate for individuals from diverse cultural and educational backgrounds (Ardila, 2005; Franzen et al., 2020; Fujii, 2023; Tsoy et al., 2021). Most normative data cohorts are also unrepresentative of populations at risk for social and health disadvantages. Disparities in behavioral science research, from which we draw conclusions about brain-behavior relationships, are staggering. While Western, Educated, Industrialized, Rich, and Democratic (WEIRD) populations make up 12% of the global population, they represent 96% of behavior science cohorts and 99% of developmental neuroscience cohorts (Fujii, 2023). While several approaches have been developed in the past to address these limitations in research studies, such as application of race-based neuropsychological norms in the USA, more progress is clearly needed to appropriately meet the needs of diverse patients seen in clinical practice.

Clinical Practice. Disparities in neuropsychological research contribute to a shortage of culturally appropriate neuropsychological measures and normative data, increasing the risk of misdiagnosis and missed interventions in culturally diverse patients (Daugherty et al., 2017; Tsoy et al., 2021). Studies also raise concerns about the cultural validity of using directly translated English-language tests or "language-free" measures (e.g., complex figure copy) in diverse communities, as factors related to test construction, procedures, and underlying constructs can affect the results (Nguyen et al., 2024). For translations and adaptations, proper guidelines, such as those by the International Test Commission, should be followed to ensure reliability and validity (Nguyen et al., 2024). In the USA, use of race-based norms for clinical decision making should be guided by person-centered considerations of the appropriateness of these norms to the patient's background and potential harms and benefits to the patient (e.g., false negative vs. false positive results). While a detailed discussion of the race-based adjustments is outside of the scope of this chapter, providers should be aware that this practice uses race as a crude proxy for lifelong social experiences, including many SDOH discussed in the previous section (Possin et al., 2021; Schneider et al., 2024).

Implementation Takeaway #1

Advancing cognitive health equity requires collaboration among policymakers, clinicians, and researchers to build a more inclusive and accessible system that meets the needs of all communities. Although systemic change is essential, individual clinicians can take concrete actions to address these barriers in their everyday practice. For example, clinicians may pursue cultural competence or cultural humility training to acquire more skills and knowledge about their patient populations and improve their ability to consider and reflect on one's own biases and implicit assumptions. Clinicians can also advocate for changes to processes within their organization, including purchasing or adopting freely available culturally sensitive tests and reducing access barriers—such as offering interpreter-supported assessments or telehealth options for patients living in remote regions. Both clinical and research neuropsychologists can also contribute dedicated efforts toward reducing barriers for entry for trainees and students from socioeconomically and culturally diverse backgrounds by engaging in pro bono mentorship activities and educational opportunities, which are frequently facilitated by professional organizations such as the International Neuropsychological Society.

Neuropsychology is increasingly recognized as essential in broader healthcare systems, yet it often remains siloed. The lack of interdisciplinary collaboration, such as coordination with primary care providers, limits the effectiveness of services. Integration of neuropsychological services within broader healthcare systems can facilitate greater access for underserved communities by easing the burden and complexity of navigating referrals and maximizing quality of care management (Brunette et al., 2022; Lanca, 2018). For example, in Europe, where neuropsychologists are fewer than other medical professionals (Kasten et al., 2021), some countries, like the Netherlands, offer specialized services such as multicultural memory clinics to improve access for underserved populations.

Advancing Health Equity in Neuropsychology

Neuropsychologists seek to understand brain-behavior relationships, and it is essential to consider the social, economic, and environmental factors influencing these relationships. SDOH not only affect cognitive health but also create systemic barriers to accessing neuropsychological care. Based on scientific evidence and ethical guidelines, we propose the following recommendations for advancing health equity in neuropsychology, organized by aspirational implementation goals for the next five (recommendations 1–4), ten (recommendations 5–8), and thirty (recommendations 9–10) years.

1. **Incorporate Comprehensive SDOH Assessments into Clinical Evaluations**

Neuropsychologists should routinely assess SDOH factors—such as social history, cultural beliefs, and barriers to care—and incorporate these into test selection, normative data use, and interpretation of results. Test conclusions should always be contextualized within the individual's cultural and socioeconomic background.

Rationale: A holistic approach to patient evaluations helps clinicians better understand cognitive difficulties, reducing the risk of misdiagnosis or over pathologizing culturally and socioeconomically driven differences.

2. **Tailor Cognitive Interventions to Address SDOH**

Neuropsychologists should tailor cognitive rehabilitation interventions to address social and environmental factors that may affect their effectiveness. For example, if physical activity is a part of the intervention plan, a provider should first ensure that a patient has access to safe environments in which these activities take place. Another example is development of a cognitive stimulation regimen for a patient with low educational attainment, where a provider should select or adapt evidence-based interventions to ensure that they are accessible and engaging for patients with different levels of literacy and numeracy. Neuropsychologists should also proactively collaborate with and refer patients to appropriate support services (e.g., social work) when SDOH such as poverty, housing insecurity, or social isolation are identified.

Rationale: Focusing solely on cognitive remediation without considering broader social factors may limit intervention effectiveness. Addressing social barriers can improve treatment adherence and enhance both short- and long-term outcomes.

3. **Implement Structured SDOH Data Collection in Cognitive Research**

Research neuropsychologists should develop structured tools to assess SDOH beyond basic demographics (e.g., educational attainment), incorporating factors that are key for cognitive health and show potential as future predictors. These tools should be standardized across cohorts nationally and internationally, capturing data from diverse cultural, geographic, and socioeconomic populations.

Rationale: Standardized SDOH data collection will allow researchers to test new hypotheses and address critical questions on social determinants of cognitive health. This evidence will support the development of targeted interventions and inform policy.

4. **Facilitate Global Brain Health Research Initiatives**

Neuropsychologists should enhance global brain health research to advance understanding of the epidemiology, progression, and treatment of cognitive disorders. By leveraging international consortia, neuropsychologists can improve the design, implementation, and evaluation of assessment methods, rehabilitation strategies, and reduce barriers to care. These initiatives will also support the development of culturally and socioeconomically fair measures, improving neuropsychological care worldwide.

Rationale: International research collaborations foster knowledge exchange, build capacity in regions with limited neuropsychological services, and improve care quality in high-resource nations.

5. **Strengthen Collaborative Care and Advocacy for Health Equity**

Neuropsychologists should collaborate with multidisciplinary teams, including primary care providers, medical specialists, social workers, and community organizations, to create comprehensive care plans that address both cognitive health and social stressors. This integrative model would require flexible diagnostic evaluations, improved provider consultations, and seamless integration of results into medical records. Several integrated memory clinics in the USA, for example, offer same-day multidisciplinary evaluations, including a neurology, neuropsychology, nursing, and social work visits, with results and recommendations shared with and implemented by primary care teams. This approach does not only reduce the potential for missed or overlooked clinical information but also minimizes the travel costs and time burden for patients and families.

Rationale: Many SDOH influencing cognitive health are beyond the purview of individual clinicians. Collaborative, multidisciplinary care models can maximize the impact of neuropsychology services and contribute to long-term solutions to reduce cognitive health disparities and improve access to care.

6. **Adopt Culturally Competent Practices in Assessment and Diagnosis**

Neuropsychologists should require cultural competence and diversity training in graduate programs and continuing education (Fujii, 2018). This training should cover the impact of systemic inequality, racism, and discrimination on cognitive health, as well as how social and cultural factors beyond language affect cognitive performance (Franzen et al., 2022; Fujii, 2018; Rivera Mindt et al., 2010).

Rationale: Cultural competence ensures that neuropsychologists are prepared to provide accurate diagnoses, effective treatment plans, and equitable care for diverse patient populations.

7. **Ensure Representativeness of Neuropsychology Workforce and Research Cohorts**

Neuropsychology graduate programs should prioritize recruiting candidates from underrepresented backgrounds and avoid selection processes that disadvantage diverse applicants (e.g., standardized test results) (Fujii, 2018). Researchers should also focus on recruiting racially, ethnically, culturally, and socioeconomically diverse populations for cognitive health studies, fostering community partnerships and collaborative research.

Rationale: A representative workforce is essential for quality, accessible, and relevant neuropsychological services. Neuropsychological research must involve diverse populations to ensure generalizability and meaningful impact.

8. **Expand Access to Neuropsychological Services for Underserved Populations**

Neuropsychologists should advocate for better access to care for underserved populations by supporting policy campaigns that expand neuropsychological coverage through government and private insurance (for additional discussion, please see Chapter 2). Research neuropsychologists should push for funding to increase services in rural and disadvantaged areas, utilizing low-cost technology and non-traditional service settings.

Rationale: Access to neuropsychological services is a critical issue, especially in low-income, rural, and minority communities. Promoting affordable access will help reduce cognitive health disparities and improve outcomes for all populations.

9. **Advocate for Policy Changes to Address Structural Inequities**

Neuropsychologists should advocate for policy changes that address structural SDOH causing health disparities. Professional organizations and providers should support policies that reduce educational disparities, increase employment opportunities, and alleviate poverty. Expanding public assistance, affordable housing, and social mobility are essential for optimal cognitive health.

Rationale: Neuropsychologists are well-positioned to advocate for systemic change, using evidence of the impact of cognitive health disparities on society and the economy to guide targeted policy interventions.

10. **Develop a Global Neuropsychological Infrastructure**

Neuropsychologists should contribute to global efforts to build neuropsychological services by engaging in educational, clinical, and research activities, collaborating with organizations like the WHO. Expanding global networks is imperative for improving care access, quality, and for ensuring longevity, relevance, and sustainability of our profession.

Rationale: Neuropsychology remains underrepresented worldwide. Supporting the training of local neuropsychologists ensures equitable access to services for all populations.

Implementation Takeaway #2

Systematic collection of SDOH data in both clinical and research settings is critical to advance person-centered practice of neuropsychology. Below are several examples of SDOH tools that have been developed to enhance clinical and research evaluations of patients' cognitive health.

1. National Alzheimer's Coordinating Center's Uniform Data Set Social Determinants of Health Form (Zuelsdorff et al., 2025)
2. Alzheimer's Association Social Determinants of Health and Dementia Risk Toolkit for Public Health Agencies (Alzheimer's Association, n.d.)
3. Brief Cultural Interview (Groen et al., 2017)
4. U.S. Centers for Medicare and Medicaid Services Accountable Health Communities Health-Related Social Needs Screening Tool (Centers for Medicare & Medicaid Services, n.d.)
5. American Academy of Family Physicians Social Needs Screening Tool (Billioux et al., 2017)

Conclusion

The interplay of various SDOH creates a complex web of factors that affect cognitive development, functioning, and decline. For example, children growing up in poverty may face cognitive delays and academic difficulties, which can impact their educational attainment, employment prospects, and psychological well-being. These early challenges can accumulate over time, leading to poorer outcomes in adulthood, such as financial strain, poor housing, limited healthcare access, high neighborhood disadvantage, and exposure to environmental pollutants. The cumulative effects of these interconnected SDOH can result in a higher burden of neurological diseases, accelerated aging, and early mortality.

The current state of health equity in neuropsychological services reveals persistent disparities in access, use, and quality worldwide. Although high-income countries have initiated efforts to address these inequities, gaps remain in cultural competence and workforce representativeness. Advancing cognitive health equity requires collaboration among policymakers, clinicians, and researchers to build a more inclusive and accessible system that meets the needs of all communities.

Neuropsychology can play a pivotal role in advancing global health equity by integrating SDOH into practice, addressing systemic health disparities, and ensuring culturally competent, interdisciplinary care globally.

Key Points in Review

Neuropsychology faces persistent disparities in access, quality, and use of its services. Neuropsychologists are uniquely positioned to promote brain health equity by incorporating evidence on social, economic, and environmental factors in cognitive health into its research and practice. For additional resources on addressing disparities in neuropsychological practice and research, please see:

- The ECLECTIC framework for incorporating the cultural context in neuropsychological evaluations (Fujii, 2018).
- The International Test Commission Guidelines for neuropsychological test translations and adaptations (Nguyen et al., 2024).
- European Consortium on Cross-Cultural Neuropsychology position statement on cross-cultural neuropsychological assessment (Franzen et al., 2022).

References

Abouelmagd, M. E., AbdelMeseh, M., Elrosasy, A., Eldeeb, H. A., & Nabil, Y. (2025). Adverse childhood experiences and risk of late-life dementia: A systematic review and meta-analysis. *Social Psychiatry and Psychiatric Epidemiology, 60*(5), 1087–1098. https://doi.org/10.1007/s00127-024-02676-4

Adkins-Jackson, P. B., George, K. M., Besser, L. M., Hyun, J., Lamar, M., Hill-Jarrett, T. G., Bubu, O. M., Flatt, J. D., Heyn, P. C., Cicero, E. C., Zarina Kraal, A., Pushpalata Zanwar, P.,

Peterson, R., Kim, B., Turner, R. W., 2nd, Viswanathan, J., Kulick, E. R., Zuelsdorff, M., Stites, S. D., … Babulal, G. (2023). The structural and social determinants of Alzheimer's disease–related dementias. *Alzheimer's & Dementia: The Journal of the Alzheimer's Association, 19*(7), 3171–3185. https://doi.org/10.1002/alz.13027

Agency for Healthcare Research and Quality. (2019). *2018 National Healthcare Quality and Disparities Report* (AHRQ Pub. No. 19-0070-EF). https://www.ahrq.gov/research/findings/nhqrdr/nhqdr18/index.html

Airhihenbuwa, C. O., & Liburd, L. (2006). Eliminating health disparities in the African American population: The interface of culture, gender, and power. *Health Education & Behavior: THe Official Publication of the Society for Public Health Education, 33*(4), 488–501. https://doi.org/10.1177/1090198106287731

Aljadeeah, S., Payedimarri, A. B., Kielmann, K., Michielsen, J., Wirtz, V. J., & Ravinetto, R. (2024). Access to medicines among asylum seekers, refugees and undocumented migrants across the migratory cycle in Europe: A scoping review. *BMJ Global Health, 9*(10), Article e015790. https://doi.org/10.1136/bmjgh-2024-015790

Almeida-Meza, P., Steptoe, A., & Cadar, D. (2021). Markers of cognitive reserve and dementia incidence in the English Longitudinal Study of Ageing. *The British Journal of Psychiatry: THe Journal of Mental Science, 218*(5), 243–251. https://doi.org/10.1192/bjp.2020.54

Alvidrez, J., Castille, D., Laude-Sharp, M., Rosario, A., & Tabor, D. (2019). The National Institute on Minority Health and Health Disparities Research Framework. *American Journal of Public Health, 109*(S1), S16–S20. https://doi.org/10.2105/AJPH.2018.304883

Alzheimer's Association. (2021). 2021 Alzheimer's disease facts and figures. *Alzheimer's & Dementia: The journal of the Alzheimer's Association, 17*(3), 327–406. https://doi.org/10.1002/alz.12328

Alzheimer's Association. (n.d.). *Social Determinants of Health Toolkit for Public Health Agencies.* https://www.alz.org/getmedia/1b7d00a3-dec3-47e5-9d14-00add522ae70/sdoh-toolkit-public-health-agencies_alzheimers-association.pdf

Andel, R., Crowe, M., Kåreholt, I., Wastesson, J., & Parker, M. G. (2011). Indicators of job strain at midlife and cognitive functioning in advanced old age. *The Journals of Gerontology: Series b, Psychological Sciences and Social Sciences, 66*(3), 287–291. https://doi.org/10.1093/geronb/gbq105

Andel, R., Crowe, M., Pedersen, N. L., Mortimer, J., Crimmins, E., Johansson, B., & Gatz, M. (2005). Complexity of work and risk of Alzheimer's disease: A population-based study of Swedish twins. *The Journals of Gerontology: Series B, Psychological Sciences and Social Sciences, 60*(5), P251–P258. https://doi.org/10.1093/geronb/60.5.p251

Arce Rentería, M., Vonk, J. M. J., Felix, G., Avila, J. F., Zahodne, L. B., Dalchand, E., Frazer, K. M., Martinez, M. N., Shouel, H. L., & Manly, J. J. (2019). Illiteracy, dementia risk, and cognitive trajectories among older adults with low education. *Neurology, 93*(24), e2247–e2256. https://doi.org/10.1212/WNL.0000000000008587

Ardila, A. (2005). Cultural values underlying psychometric cognitive testing. *Neuropsychology Review, 15*(4), 185–195. https://doi.org/10.1007/s11065-005-9180-y

Berlingieri, F., Barjaková, M., Garnero, A., & Mauri, C. (2024). Who feels lonely in the European Union? In S.V. Schnepf, B. d'Hombres, & C. Mauri. (Eds.), *Loneliness in Europe* (pp. 43–70). Population Economics. Springer. https://doi.org/10.1007/978-3-031-66582-0_3

Besser, L. (2021). Outdoor green space exposure and brain health measures related to Alzheimer's disease: A rapid review. *British Medical Journal Open, 11*(5), Article e043456. https://doi.org/10.1136/bmjopen-2020-043456

Billioux, A., Verlander, K., Anthony, S., & Alley, D. (2017). *Standardized screening for health-related social needs in clinical settings: The accountable health communities screening tool.* https://nam.edu/wp-content/uploads/2017/05/Standardized-Screening-for-Health-Related-Social-Needs-in-Clinical-Settings.pdf

Braveman, P., Egerter, S., & Williams, D. R. (2011). The social determinants of health: Coming of age. *Annual Review of Public Health, 32*, 381–398. https://doi.org/10.1146/annurev-publhealth-031210-101218

Braveman, P., & Gottlieb, L. (2014). The social determinants of health: It's time to consider the causes of the causes. *Public Health Reports (Washington, D.C.: 1974), 129*(Suppl 2), 19–31. https://doi.org/10.1177/00333549141291S206

Bronfenbrenner, U. (1977). Toward an experimental ecology of human development. *American Psychologist, 32*(7), 513–531.

Brunette, A. M., Rycroft, S. S., Colvin, L., Schwartz, A. W., Driver, J. A., Nothern, A., Harrington, M. B., & Jackson, C. E. (2022). Integrating neuropsychology into interprofessional geriatrics clinics. *Archives of Clinical Neuropsychology: THe Official Journal of the National Academy of Neuropsychologists, 37*(3), 545–552. https://doi.org/10.1093/arclin/acab084

Bufano, P., Di Tecco, C., Fattori, A., Barnini, T., Comotti, A., Ciocan, C., Ferrari, L., Mastorci, F., Laurino, M., & Bonzini, M. (2024). The effects of work on cognitive functions: A systematic review. *Frontiers in Psychology, 15*, 1351625. https://doi.org/10.3389/fpsyg.2024.1351625

Centers for Medicare & Medicaid Services, Innovation Center. (n.d.). *Accountable Health Communities (AHCM) health-related social needs screening tool.* https://www.cms.gov/priorities/innovation/files/worksheets/ahcm-screeningtool.pdf

Chan, M. Y., Na, J., Agres, P. F., Savalia, N. K., Park, D. C., & Wig, G. S. (2018). Socioeconomic status moderates age-related differences in the brain's functional network organization and anatomy across the adult lifespan. *Proceedings of the National Academy of Sciences of the United States of America, 115*(22), E5144–E5153. https://doi.org/10.1073/pnas.1714021115

Coley, R. L., Leventhal, T., Lynch, A. D., & Kull, M. (2013). Relations between housing characteristics and the well-being of low-income children and adolescents. *Developmental Psychology, 49*(9), 1775–1789. https://doi.org/10.1037/a0031033

Crowe, M., Clay, O. J., Martin, R. C., Howard, V. J., Wadley, V. G., Sawyer, P., & Allman, R. M. (2013). Indicators of childhood quality of education in relation to cognitive function in older adulthood. *The Journals of Gerontology: Series a, Biological Sciences and Medical Sciences, 68*(2), 198–204. https://doi.org/10.1093/gerona/gls122

Daugherty, J. C., Puente, A. E., Fasfous, A. F., Hidalgo-Ruzzante, N., & Pérez-Garcia, M. (2017). Diagnostic mistakes of culturally diverse individuals when using North American neuropsychological tests. *Applied Neuropsychology: Adult, 24*(1), 16–22. https://doi.org/10.1080/23279095.2015.1036992

Eikemo, T. A., Huisman, M., Bambra, C., & Kunst, A. E. (2008). Health inequalities according to educational level in different welfare regimes: A comparison of 23 European countries. *Sociology of Health & Illness, 30*(4), 565–582. https://doi.org/10.1111/j.1467-9566.2007.01073.x

Elbulok-Charcape, M. M., Rabin, L. A., Spadaccini, A. T., & Barr, W. B. (2014). Trends in the neuropsychological assessment of ethnic/racial minorities: A survey of clinical neuropsychologists in the United States and Canada. *Cultural Diversity & Ethnic Minority Psychology, 20*(3), 353–361. https://doi.org/10.1037/a0035023

Elonheimo, H. M., Andersen, H. R., Katsonouri, A., & Tolonen, H. (2021). Environmental substances associated with Alzheimer's disease—A scoping review. *International Journal of Environmental Research and Public Health, 18*(22), 11839. https://doi.org/10.3390/ijerph182211839

Eurostat. (2024). *Unmet Health Care Needs Statistics.* Web report. Retrieved March 2, 2025, from https://ec.europa.eu/eurostat/statistics-explained/index.php?title=Unmet_health_care_needs_statistics

Evans, G. W., & Schamberg, M. A. (2009). Childhood poverty, chronic stress, and adult working memory. *Proceedings of the National Academy of Sciences of the United States of America, 106*(16), 6545–6549. https://doi.org/10.1073/pnas.0811910106

Franzen, S., Papma, J. M., van den Berg, E., & Nielsen, T. R. (2021). Cross-cultural neuropsychological assessment in the European Union: A Delphi expert study. *Archives of Clinical*

Neuropsychology: THe Official Journal of the National Academy of Neuropsychologists, 36(5), 815–830. https://doi.org/10.1093/arclin/acaa083

Franzen, S., van den Berg, E., Goudsmit, M., Jurgens, C. K., van de Wiel, L., Kalkisim, Y., Uysal-Bozkir, Ö., Ayhan, Y., Nielsen, T. R., & Papma, J. M. (2020). A systematic review of neuropsychological tests for the assessment of dementia in non-Western, low-educated or illiterate populations. *Journal of the International Neuropsychological Society: JINS, 26*(3), 331–351. https://doi.org/10.1017/S1355617719000894

Franzen, S., Watermeyer, T. J., Pomati, S., Papma, J. M., Nielsen, T. R., Narme, P., Mukadam, N., Lozano-Ruiz, Á., Ibanez-Casas, I., Goudsmit, M., Fasfous, A., Daugherty, J. C., Canevelli, M., Calia, C., van den Berg, E., & Bekkhus-Wetterberg, P. (2022). Cross-cultural neuropsychological assessment in Europe: Position statement of the European Consortium on Cross-Cultural Neuropsychology (ECCroN). *The Clinical Neuropsychologist, 36*(3), 546–557. https://doi.org/10.1080/13854046.2021.1981456

Fujii, D. E. M. (2018). Developing a cultural context for conducting a neuropsychological evaluation with a culturally diverse client: The ECLECTIC framework. *The Clinical Neuropsychologist, 32*(8), 1356–1392. https://doi.org/10.1080/13854046.2018.1435826

Fujii, D. E. M. (2023). Incorporating intersectionality in neuropsychology: Moving the discipline forward. *Archives of Clinical Neuropsychology: THe Official Journal of the National Academy of Neuropsychologists, 38*(1), 154–167. https://doi.org/10.1093/arclin/acac075

Fuller, R., Landrigan, P. J., Balakrishnan, K., Bathan, G., Bose-O'Reilly, S., Brauer, M., Caravanos, J., Chiles, T., Cohen, A., Corra, L., Cropper, M., Ferraro, G., Hanna, J., Hanrahan, D., Hu, H., Hunter, D., Janata, G., Kupka, R., Lanphear, B., … Yan, C. (2022). Pollution and health: A progress update. *The Lancet Planetary Health, 6*(6), e535–e547. https://doi.org/10.1016/S2542-5196(22)00090-0

General Medical Council. (2023). *Tackling Disadvantage in Medical Education.* Web report. Retrieved March 2, 2025, from https://www.gmc-uk.org/-/media/documents/96887270_tackling-disadvantage-in-medical-education-020323.pdf

Grimmer, Y., Insensee, C., Becker, A., Banaschewski, T., Bokde, A. L. W., Quinlan, E. B., Desrivières, S., Flor, H., Grigis, A., Gowland, P., Heinz, A., Ittermann, B., Klingberg, T., et al. (2020). Cognitive and brain development is independently influenced by socioeconomic status and polygenic scores for educational attainment. *Proceedings of the National Academy of Sciences of the United States of America, 117*(22), 12411–12418. https://doi.org/10.1073/pnas.2001228117

Groen, S. P., Richters, A., Laban, C. J., & Devillé, W. L. (2017). Implementation of the cultural formulation through a newly developed brief cultural interview: Pilot data from the Netherlands. *Transcultural Psychiatry, 54*(1), 3–22. https://doi.org/10.1177/1363461516678342

Grote, C. L., & Novitski, J. I. (2016). International perspectives on education, training, and practice in clinical neuropsychology: Comparison across 14 countries around the world. *The Clinical Neuropsychologist, 30*(8), 1380–1388. https://doi.org/10.1080/13854046.2016.1235727

Guerrero, Z., Civišová, D., & Winkler, P. (2024). Mental health and access to care among the Roma population in Europe: A scoping review. *Transcultural Psychiatry, 61*(1), 118–130. https://doi.org/10.1177/13634615231200853

Hair, N. L., Hanson, J. L., Wolfe, B. L., & Pollak, S. D. (2015). Association of child poverty, brain development, and academic achievement. *JAMA Pediatrics, 169*(9), 822–829. https://doi.org/10.1001/jamapediatrics.2015.1475

Harrington, K. D., Vasan, S., Kang, J. E., Sliwinski, M. J., & Lim, M. H. (2023). Loneliness and cognitive function in older adults without dementia: A systematic review and meta-analysis. *Journal of Alzheimer's Disease: JAD, 91*(4), 1243–1259. https://doi.org/10.3233/JAD-220832

Hill, C. V., Pérez-Stable, E. J., Anderson, N. A., & Bernard, M. A. (2015). The National Institute on Aging Health Disparities Research Framework. *Ethnicity & Disease, 25*(3), 245–254. https://doi.org/10.18865/ed.25.3.245

Hinton, L., Tran, D., Peak, K., Meyer, O. L., & Quiñones, A. R. (2024). Mapping racial and ethnic healthcare disparities for persons living with dementia: A scoping review. *Alzheimer's &*

Dementia: The Journal of the Alzheimer's Association, 20(4), 3000–3020. https://doi.org/10.1002/alz.13612

Hunt, J. F. V., Buckingham, W., Kim, A. J., Oh, J., Vogt, N. M., Jonaitis, E. M., Hunt, T. K., Zuelsdorff, M., Powell, R., Norton, D., Rissman, R. A., Asthana, S., Okonkwo, O. C., Johnson, S. C., Kind, A. J. H., & Bendlin, B. B. (2020). Association of neighborhood-level disadvantage with cerebral and hippocampal volume. *JAMA Neurology, 77*(4), 451–460. https://doi.org/10.1001/jamaneurol.2019.4501

Kasten, E., Barbosa, F., Kosmidis, M. H., Persson, B. A., Constantinou, M., Baker, G. A., Lettner, S., Hokkanen, L., Ponchel, A., Mondini, S., Jonsdottir, M. K., Varako, N., Nikolai, T., Pranckeviciene, A., Harper, L., & Hessen, E. (2021). European clinical neuropsychology: Role in healthcare and access to neuropsychological services. *Healthcare (Basel, Switzerland), 9*(6), 734. https://doi.org/10.3390/healthcare9060734

Kessler, R. C., McLaughlin, K. A., Green, J. G., Gruber, M. J., Sampson, N. A., Zaslavsky, A. M., Aguilar-Gaxiola, S., Alhamzawi, A. O., Alonso, J., Angermeyer, M., Benjet, C., Bromet, E., Chatterji, S., de Girolamo, G., Demyttenaere, K., Fayyad, J., Florescu, S., Gal, G., Gureje, O., … Williams, D. R. (2010). Childhood adversities and adult psychopathology in the WHO World Mental Health Surveys. *The British Journal of Psychiatry: THe Journal of Mental Science, 197*(5), 378–385. https://doi.org/10.1192/bjp.bp.110.080499

Kind, A. J. H., & Buckingham, W. R. (2018). Making neighborhood-disadvantage metrics accessible—The Neighborhood Atlas. *The New England Journal of Medicine, 378*(26), 2456–2458. https://doi.org/10.1056/NEJMp1802313

Klipfel, K. M., Sweet, J. J., Nelson, N. W., & Moberg, P. J. (2023). Gender and ethnic/racial diversity in clinical neuropsychology: Updates from the AACN, NAN, SCN 2020 practice and "salary survey." *The Clinical Neuropsychologist, 37*(2), 231–285. https://doi.org/10.1080/13854046.2022.2054360

Kulcsarova, K., Bang, C., Berg, D., & Schaeffer, E. (2023). Pesticides and the microbiome-gut-brain axis: Convergent pathways in the pathogenesis of Parkinson's disease. *Journal of Parkinson's Disease, 13*(7), 1079–1106. https://doi.org/10.3233/JPD-230206

Lanca, M. (2018). Integration of neuropsychology in primary care. *Archives of Clinical Neuropsychology: THe Official Journal of the National Academy of Neuropsychologists, 33*(3), 269–279. https://doi.org/10.1093/arclin/acx135

LaVeist, T. A., Pérez-Stable, E. J., Richard, P., Anderson, A., Isaac, L. A., Santiago, R., Okoh, C., Breen, N., Farhat, T., Assenov, A., & Gaskin, D. J. (2023). The economic burden of racial, ethnic, and educational health inequities in the US. *JAMA, 329*(19), 1682–1692. https://doi.org/10.1001/jama.2023.5965

Lidsky, T. I., & Schneider, J. S. (2003). Lead neurotoxicity in children: Basic mechanisms and clinical correlates. *Brain: A Journal of Neurology, 126*(Pt 1), 5–19. https://doi.org/10.1093/brain/awg014

Link, B. G., & Phelan, J. (1995). Social conditions as fundamental causes of disease. *Journal of Health and Social Behavior*, *Spec No*, 80–94.

Lipnicki, D. M., Makkar, S. R., Crawford, J. D., Thalamuthu, A., Kochan, N. A., Lima-Costa, M. F., Castro-Costa, E., Ferri, C. P., Brayne, C., Stephan, B., Llibre-Rodriguez, J. J., Llibre-Guerra, J. J., Valhuerdi-Cepero, A. J., Lipton, R. B., Katz, M. J., Derby, C. A., Ritchie, K., Ancelin, M. L., Carrière, I., … for Cohort Studies of Memory in an International Consortium (COSMIC). (2019). Determinants of cognitive performance and decline in 20 diverse ethno-regional groups: A COSMIC collaboration cohort study. *PLoS Medicine, 16*(7), e1002853. https://doi.org/10.1371/journal.pmed.1002853

Livingston, G., Huntley, J., Liu, K. Y., Costafreda, S. G., Selbæk, G., Alladi, S., Ames, D., Banerjee, S., Burns, A., Brayne, C., Fox, N. C., Ferri, C. P., Gitlin, L. N., Howard, R., Kales, H. C., Kivimäki, M., Larson, E. B., Nakasujja, N., Rockwood, K., … Mukadam, N. (2024). Dementia prevention, intervention, and care: 2024 report of the Lancet standing Commission. *Lancet (London, England), 404*(10452), 572–628. https://doi.org/10.1016/S0140-6736(24)01296-0

Luan Erfe, B. M., Siddiqui, K. A., Schwamm, L. H., Kirwan, C., Nunes, A., & Mejia, N. I. (2017). Professional medical interpreters influence the quality of acute ischemic stroke care for patients who speak languages other than English. *Journal of the American Heart Association, 6*(9), Article e006175. https://doi.org/10.1161/JAHA.117.006175

Maalouf, M., Fearon, M., Lipa, M. C., Chow-Johnson, H., Tayeh, L., & Lipa, D. (2021). Neurologic complications of poverty: The associations between poverty as a social determinant of health and adverse neurologic outcomes. *Current Neurology and Neuroscience Reports, 21*(7), 29. https://doi.org/10.1007/s11910-021-01116-z

Manly, J. J., Touradji, P., Tang, M. X., & Stern, Y. (2003). Literacy and memory decline among ethnically diverse elders. *Journal of Clinical and Experimental Neuropsychology, 25*(5), 680–690. https://doi.org/10.1076/jcen.25.5.680.14579

Mayeda, E. R., Mobley, T. M., Weiss, R. E., Murchland, A. R., Berkman, L. F., & Sabbath, E. L. (2020). Association of work-family experience with mid- and late-life memory decline in US women. *Neurology, 95*(23), e3072–e3080. https://doi.org/10.1212/WNL.0000000000010989

McEwen, B. S., & Gianaros, P. J. (2010). Central role of the brain in stress and adaptation: Links to socioeconomic status, health, and disease. *Annals of the New York Academy of Sciences, 1186*, 190–222. https://doi.org/10.1111/j.1749-6632.2009.05331.x

Mulder, L., Wouters, A., Akwiwu, E. U., Koster, A. S., Ravesloot, J. H., Peerdeman, S. M., Salih, M., Croiset, G., & Kusurkar, R. A. (2023). Diversity in the pathway from medical student to specialist in the Netherlands: A retrospective cohort study. *The Lancet Regional Health. Europe, 35*, Article 100749. https://doi.org/10.1016/j.lanepe.2023.100749

Mullady, S. S., Castellanos, S., Lopez, L., Aguirre, G., Weeks, J., King, S., Valle, K., Goode, C., Tsoy, E., Possin, K., Miller, B., Kushel, M., & Lanata, S. (2022). Neurocognitive health of older adults experiencing homelessness in Oakland, California. *Frontiers in Neurology, 13*, Article 905779. https://doi.org/10.3389/fneur.2022.905779

Munro Cullum, C., Hynan, L. S., Grosch, M., Parikh, M., & Weiner, M. F. (2014). Teleneuropsychology: Evidence for video teleconference-based neuropsychological assessment. *Journal of the International Neuropsychological Society: JINS, 20*(10), 1028–1033. https://doi.org/10.1017/S1355617714000873

Nguyen, C. M., Rampa, S., Staios, M., Nielsen, T. R., Zapparoli, B., Zhou, X. E., Mbakile-Mahlanza, L., Colon, J., Hammond, A., Hendriks, M., Kgolo, T., Serrano, Y., Marquine, M. J., Dutt, A., Evans, J., & Judd, T. (2024). Neuropsychological application of the International Test Commission Guidelines for Translation and Adapting of Tests. *Journal of the International Neuropsychological Society: JINS, 30*(7), 621–634. https://doi.org/10.1017/S1355617724000286

Nielsen, T. R., Franzen, S., Watermeyer, T., Jiang, J., Calia, C., Kjærgaard, D., Bothe, S., & Mukadam, N. (2024). Interpreter-mediated neuropsychological assessment: Clinical considerations and recommendations from the European Consortium on Cross-Cultural Neuropsychology (ECCroN). *The Clinical Neuropsychologist, 38*(8), 1775–1805. https://doi.org/10.1080/13854046.2024.2335113

Nouri, S., Khoong, E. C., Lyles, C. R., & Karliner, L. (2020). Addressing equity in telemedicine for chronic disease management during the Covid-19 pandemic. *NEJM Catalyst Innovations in Care Delivery*. https://doi.org/10.1056/CAT.20.0123

Palm, W., Webb, E., Hernández-Quevedo, C., Scarpetti, G., Lessof, S., Siciliani, L., & van Ginneken, E. (2021). Gaps in coverage and access in the European Union. *Health Policy (Amsterdam, Netherlands), 125*(3), 341–350. https://doi.org/10.1016/j.healthpol.2020.12.011

Pattillo, M., Stieglitz, S., Angoumis, K., & Gottlieb, N. (2023). Racism against racialized migrants in healthcare in Europe: A scoping review. *International Journal for Equity in Health, 22*(1), 201. https://doi.org/10.1186/s12939-023-02014-1

Peng, S., Roth, A. R., Apostolova, L. G., Saykin, A. J., & Perry, B. L. (2022). Cognitively stimulating environments and cognitive reserve: The case of personal social networks. *Neurobiology of Aging, 112*, 197–203. https://doi.org/10.1016/j.neurobiolaging.2022.01.004

Perry, B. L., McConnell, W. R., Coleman, M. E., Roth, A. R., Peng, S., & Apostolova, L. G. (2022). Why the cognitive "fountain of youth" may be upstream: Pathways to dementia risk and resilience through social connectedness. *Alzheimer's & Dementia: The Journal of the Alzheimer's Association, 18*(5), 934–941. https://doi.org/10.1002/alz.12443

Phelan, J. C., & Link, B. G. (2015). Is racism a fundamental cause of inequalities in health? *Annual Review of Sociology, 41*, 311–330. https://doi.org/10.1146/annurev-soc-073014-112305

Pool, L. R., Weuve, J., Wilson, R. S., Bültmann, U., Evans, D. A., & Mendes de Leon, C. F. (2016). Occupational cognitive requirements and late-life cognitive aging. *Neurology, 86*(15), 1386–1392. https://doi.org/10.1212/WNL.0000000000002569

Possin, K. L., Tsoy, E., & Windon, C. C. (2021). Perils of race-based norms in cognitive testing: The case of former NFL players. *JAMA Neurology, 78*(4), 377–378. https://doi.org/10.1001/jamaneurol.2020.4763

Postal, K. (2018). President's Annual State of the Academy Report. *The Clinical Neuropsychologist, 32*(1), 1–9. https://doi.org/10.1080/13854046.2017.1406993

Powell, W. R., Buckingham, W. R., Larson, J. L., Vilen, L., Yu, M., Salamat, M. S., Bendlin, B. B., Rissman, R. A., & Kind, A. J. H. (2020). Association of neighborhood-level disadvantage with Alzheimer disease neuropathology. *JAMA Network Open, 3*(6), Article e207559. https://doi.org/10.1001/jamanetworkopen.2020.7559

Rivera Mindt, M., Byrd, D., Saez, P., & Manly, J. (2010). Increasing culturally competent neuropsychological services for ethnic minority populations: A call to action. *The Clinical Neuropsychologist, 24*(3), 429–453. https://doi.org/10.1080/13854040903058960

Rovio, S., Kåreholt, I., Helkala, E. L., Viitanen, M., Winblad, B., Tuomilehto, J., Soininen, H., Nissinen, A., & Kivipelto, M. (2005). Leisure-time physical activity at midlife and the risk of dementia and Alzheimer's disease. *The Lancet Neurology, 4*(11), 705–711. https://doi.org/10.1016/S1474-4422(05)70198-8

Saadi, A., Himmelstein, D. U., Woolhandler, S., & Mejia, N. I. (2017). Racial disparities in neurologic health care access and utilization in the United States. *Neurology, 88*(24), 2268–2275. https://doi.org/10.1212/WNL.0000000000004025

Schneider, A. L. C., Reyes, A., Henegan, J. A., Kamath, V., Wruck, L., Pike, J. R., Gross, A., Walker, K., Kucharska-Newton, A., Coresh, J., Mosley, T. H., Gottesman, R. F., & Griswold, M. (2024). Evaluating social determinants of health-based alternatives to race-based cognitive normative models. *Neurology, 103*(11), Article e210030. https://doi.org/10.1212/WNL.0000000000210030

Schneider, E.C., Shah, A., Doty, M.M., Tikkanen, R., Fields, K., & Williams II, R.D. (2021). *Mirror, mirror 2021. Reflecting poorly: Health care in the U.S. compared to other high-income countries* (The Commonwealth Fund report). https://www.commonwealthfund.org/publications/fund-reports/2021/aug/mirror-mirror-2021-reflecting-poorly

Sisco, S., Gross, A. L., Shih, R. A., Sachs, B. C., Glymour, M. M., Bangen, K. J., Benitez, A., Skinner, J., Schneider, B. C., & Manly, J. J. (2015). The role of early-life educational quality and literacy in explaining racial disparities in cognition in late life. *The Journals of Gerontology: Series b, Psychological Sciences and Social Sciences, 70*(4), 557–567. https://doi.org/10.1093/geronb/gbt133

Stephen, R., Hongisto, K., Solomon, A., & Lönnroos, E. (2017). Physical activity and Alzheimer's disease: A systematic review. *The Journals of Gerontology: Series a, Biological Sciences and Medical Sciences, 72*(6), 733–739. https://doi.org/10.1093/gerona/glw251

Steptoe, A., & Zaninotto, P. (2020). Lower socioeconomic status and the acceleration of aging: An outcome-wide analysis. *Proceedings of the National Academy of Sciences of the United States of America, 117*(26), 14911–14917. https://doi.org/10.1073/pnas.1915741117

Teicher, M. H., & Samson, J. A. (2016). Annual Research Review: Enduring neurobiological effects of childhood abuse and neglect. *Journal of Child Psychology and Psychiatry, and Allied Disciplines, 57*(3), 241–266. https://doi.org/10.1111/jcpp.12507

Tsoy, E., Sideman, A. B., Piña Escudero, S. D., Pintado-Caipa, M., Kanjanapong, S., Al-Rousan, T., Mbakile-Mahlanza, L., de Oliveira, M. O., De la Cruz Puebla, M., Zygouris, S., Mohamed, A. A.,

Ibrahim, H., Goode, C. A., Miller, B. L., Valcour, V., & Possin, K. L. (2021). Global perspectives on brief cognitive assessments for dementia diagnosis. *Journal of Alzheimer's Disease: JAD, 82*(3), 1001–1013. https://doi.org/10.3233/JAD-201403

Walhovd, K. B., Fjell, A. M., Wang, Y., Amlien, I. K., Mowinckel, A. M., Lindenberger, U., Düzel, S., Bartrés-Faz, D., Ebmeier, K. P., Drevon, C. A., Baaré, W. F. C., Ghisletta, P., Johansen, L. B., Kievit, R. A., Henson, R. N., Madsen, K. S., Nyberg, L., R Harris, J., Solé-Padullés, C., … Brandmaier, A. M. (2022). Education and income show heterogeneous relationships to lifespan brain and cognitive differences across European and US cohorts. *Cerebral Cortex, 32*(4), 839–854. https://doi.org/10.1093/cercor/bhab248

Wang, A. Y., Hu, H. Y., Ou, Y. N., Wang, Z. T., Ma, Y. H., Tan, L., & Yu, J. T. (2023). Socioeconomic status and risks of cognitive impairment and dementia: A systematic review and meta-analysis of 39 prospective studies. *The Journal of Prevention of Alzheimer's Disease, 10*(1), 83–94. https://doi.org/10.14283/jpad.2022.81

Weuve, J., Bennett, E. E., Ranker, L., Gianattasio, K. Z., Pedde, M., Adar, S. D., Yanosky, J. D., & Power, M. C. (2021). Exposure to air pollution in relation to risk of dementia and related outcomes: An updated systematic review of the epidemiological literature. *Environmental Health Perspectives, 129*(9), Article 096001. https://doi.org/10.1289/EHP8716

Woolf, S. H., & Schoomaker, H. (2019). Life expectancy and mortality rates in the United States, 1959–2017. *JAMA, 322*(20), 1996–2016. https://doi.org/10.1001/jama.2019.16932

World Health Organization. (2010). *A Conceptual Framework for Action on the Social Determinants of Health* (Commission on Social Determinants of Health discussion paper). https://www.who.int/publications/i/item/9789241500852

Wu, H., Yan, H., Yang, Y., Xu, M., Shi, Y., Zeng, W., Li, J., Zhang, J., Chang, C., & Wang, N. (2020). Occupational neuroplasticity in the human brain: A critical review and meta-analysis of neuroimaging studies. *Frontiers in Human Neuroscience, 14*, 215. https://doi.org/10.3389/fnhum.2020.00215

Zuelsdorff, M., Abner, E. L., Balls-Berry, J. E., Jicha, G. A., Lanata, S., Maestre, G. E., Rosselli, M., Stites, S. D., Whitmer, R. A., Wilkins, C. H., & Barnes, L. L. (2025). Introducing social determinants of health to the Alzheimer's Disease Research Center network: Development and implementation in the Uniform Data Set. *Alzheimer's & Dementia: The Journal of the Alzheimer's Association, 21*(5), Article e70279. https://doi.org/10.1002/alz.70279

Part II
Neuropsychological Applications in Population Health at the Organizational and Community Level

Chapter 5
Advancing Access to Neuropsychological Services for Children and Adolescents

Molly Colvin and Trevor A. Hall

Executive Summary
Although pediatric neuropsychology is integrated into standard clinical care guidelines for multiple pediatric conditions, there is still a large unmet need for services. This chapter builds a case for adopting population health strategies to develop new practice models that expand timely access to care. We describe triage strategies and provide examples of how screening and brief evaluations can be applied to inpatient and outpatient pediatric neuropsychological practices. We also review the literature demonstrating the impact of these methods and outline opportunities for further research. Collectively, these techniques may improve efficient, equitable, and expanded access to pediatric neuropsychological services.

M. Colvin (✉)
Neuropsychology Division, Massachusetts General Hospital, Boston, MA, USA
e-mail: mcolvin@mgh.harvard.edu

AMC Department of Psychiatry, Mass General Brigham, Boston, MA, USA

Department of Psychiatry, Harvard Medical School, Boston, MA, USA

T. A. Hall
Divisions of Pediatric Psychology & Pediatric Critical Care, Pediatric Critical Care & Neurotrauma Recovery Program, Portland, OR, USA
e-mail: halltr@ohsu.edu

Oregon Health & Science University, Portland, OR, USA

Doernbecher Children's Hospital, Portland, OR, USA

M. Lanca and R. Fallows (eds.), *Advancing Neuropsychology Through Population Health*, https://doi.org/10.1007/978-3-032-22457-6_5

Pediatric Neuropsychology Through a Population Health Lens

Pediatric neuropsychologists are asked to evaluate children and adolescents who have neurobehavioral or neurocognitive symptoms. Evaluations provide information about the developing brain (that may be following an atypical trajectory) to provide intervention and accommodation recommendations aimed at improving functional outcomes. The essential role of pediatric neuropsychology has been recognized by its inclusion in standard clinical care guidelines for multiple pediatric conditions, including but not limited to childhood cancer (Baum et al., 2017), epilepsy (Wilson et al., 2015), multiple sclerosis (Foley & Portnoy, 2018), Turner syndrome (Gravholt et al., 2024), Duchenne muscular dystrophy (Birnkrant et al., 2018), and spina bifida (Jordan et al., 2025).

From a population health model perspective, traditional pediatric neuropsychological evaluations are *secondary* services, as evaluations happen after symptom onset and are designed to limit the impact of the condition being evaluated. Pediatric neuropsychologists working within a rehabilitation setting to mitigate the impact of a condition on long-term functioning provide *tertiary* services (Hardy et al., 2017). In these roles, the neuropsychologist identifies gaps between a child's current functioning and their environmental expectations, making treatment and educational recommendations that aim to reduce or minimize the size of that gap (Cassidy & Neumann, 2023). Increased awareness of the heightened risk of neuropsychological deficits in chronic conditions (e.g., sickle cell disease, epilepsy, cancer, brain injury) has also led to recommendations for surveillance screening (e.g., Baum et al., 2017; Gragert & Ris, 2011). As such, pediatric neuropsychology plays an increasing role in providing *primary* services that aim for earlier identification or even prevention of later cognitive or behavioral concerns (Cassidy & Neumann, 2023; Hardy et al., 2017).

Considering the epidemiology of neurodevelopmental and neurological disorders in pediatric patients, the effective integration of neuropsychological services into *primary*, *secondary*, and *tertiary* care will require a fundamental shift in current standard practice models. Moreover, it is imperative for the field to find ways to leverage technological advances to improve access (e.g., telehealth platforms), ecological validity of test results (e.g., computerized assessment tools), throughput and efficiency (e.g., artificial intelligence), and tracking of patient outcomes (e.g., integrated data management systems) to name a few. In addition, compared to adult-oriented practitioners, pediatric neuropsychologists are uniquely positioned to understand the influence of social determinants of health (e.g., poverty, housing instability, food insecurity, access to early education and healthcare) and adverse childhood experiences on brain development and functioning; this position should be leveraged in the enhancement of pediatric care models.

Expanding the roles of pediatric neuropsychologists within healthcare systems may improve patient quality of life and reduce long-term healthcare expenditures (Fisher et al., 2022; Glen et al., 2019). However, expansion also places additional demands on limited resources at a time when pediatric neuropsychology services already face high demand and long waitlists. In a recent survey of neuropsychologists about their practice, pediatric providers reported spending an average of 13.5 h (SD = 4.4) performing a clinical evaluation. This is considerably longer than reported for those performing adult evaluations (M = 8.9 h, SD = 3.2) (Sweet et al., 2020), and slightly longer than reported by pediatric neuropsychologists several years earlier (M = 12.5 h, SD = 3.9; Sweet et al., 2015). Given the length of existing waiting lists and the size of the potential population of children and adolescents who would benefit from neuropsychological services, there is a need to move practices away from exclusive reliance on lengthy comprehensive evaluations. As such, there is a need to enhance models of care to allow for improved screening, triage, and follow-up to ensure that the resources within neuropsychological practices are being optimally allocated and are financially viable. Additionally, longitudinal tracking and reporting of neuropsychological health outcomes to demonstrate the importance of timely and equitable access to pediatric neuropsychology is important.

Building Scalable Pediatric Neuropsychological Services

Although first conceptualized as a research paradigm, Hardy and et al., (2017) applied a population health perspective to describe a three-tiered system of neuropsychological assessment that recommends more intensive services for patients in pediatric medical settings. At the first level, there is universal monitoring for neuropsychological dysfunction. All at-risk children within a population would be regularly screened using measures that could be easily administered and interpreted by a trained member of the child's healthcare team (e.g., questionnaire, brief computerized assessment, etc.). Patients who show deficits move on to targeted screening, which includes a brief neuropsychological assessment (2–3 h), along with additional symptom questionnaires for the caregiver and sometimes education professionals. Comprehensive neuropsychological evaluations are reserved for patients at high risk of neurocognitive difficulties, either because of treatment or direct effects of a medical condition (e.g., brain tumor) or because they demonstrate significant difficulties on targeted screening (Hardy et al., 2017).

Baum et al. (2017) proposed a similar model for neuropsychologists to follow in caring for pediatric oncology patients, recommending that clinical surveillance (via a mixture of clinical interviews, screening questionnaires, and record review) be performed by the medical team before involving the neuropsychologist, who may provide different levels of service depending on the patient's needs. In their model, there are also targeted and comprehensive neuropsychological evaluations, as well as consultations and screening assessments. Consultations are provided by the neuropsychologists but do not involve testing. Rather, the consultations focus on providing guidance and psychoeducation, as well as gathering information to determine whether testing is necessary. Consultations can also occur at any point in time (e.g., prior to screening assessment or before/after evaluations).

Expanding the role of the neuropsychologist to include different types of evaluations tailored to the needs of patients and referring providers would represent a significant change for many. However, it would also potentially fill the service gaps created by pediatric neuropsychology's overreliance on traditional *secondary* service models. This is particularly important in a pediatric population given that the brain is developing and thus the system-based limits related to accessing timely interventions can have destructive downstream impacts on health-related outcomes (Dodd et al., 2018; Hall et al., 2022; Hall, Greene et al., 2022; Williams et al., 2023).

Bridging Inpatient and Outpatient Care Example

Critical neurologic injuries and illnesses that are first treated inpatient are often associated with long-term neuropsychological morbidities, and are thus, from a population health perspective, also well suited for *tertiary* and *primary* models of care. These conditions include traumatic brain injury (TBI)/trauma (e.g., motor vehicle accident, fall, non-accidental trauma), infectious/inflammatory conditions (e.g., meningitis, encephalitis), hypoxic-ischemic injury (e.g., cardiac arrest, heart defects, strangulation, near drowning), stroke (e.g., hemorrhagic, ischemic), and other critical illnesses (e.g., sepsis, severe pneumonia) (Williams et al., 2018). Unfortunately, despite the high morbidities associated with many neurocritical injuries and illnesses (Pollack et al., 2014) because of limited programs and scant available resources (Williams et al., 2022), few children receive inpatient rehabilitation or systematic outpatient follow-up services, which includes access to neuropsychological monitoring, assessment, and intervention (Greene et al., 2014; Keenan et al., 2013).

The Pediatric Critical Care and Neurotrauma Recovery Program (PCCNRP; TH is the Associate Director) at Oregon Health & Science University (OHSU) is a clinical program that utilizes a timely and integrated approach to bridge service gaps between inpatient admissions to longitudinal outpatient support. The PCCNRP has evolved to include a highly integrated model of care that starts in the inpatient setting and continues with recurrent outpatient follow-up visits (as needed) throughout a patient's recovery. The multiprofessional team proactively identifies and treats post-neurocritical care issues in physical, cognitive, emotional, and psychosocial/family health domains that historically often went undetected by utilizing a combination of school and medical record review, focused interviewing, direct objective assessment/evaluation, and questionnaires reported by the patient and family. It was clear from the start that the PCCNRP needed to adopt both a *tertiary* and a *primary* model of care (see Fig. 5.1) that could be adapted over time to meet the needs of children in a timely, equitable, and efficient manner; a model that could bidirectionally generate and answer research questions aimed at improving health outcomes in this vulnerable population. The PCCNRP uses a combination of approaches mentioned above—Hardy et al., (2017) and Baum et al. (2017).

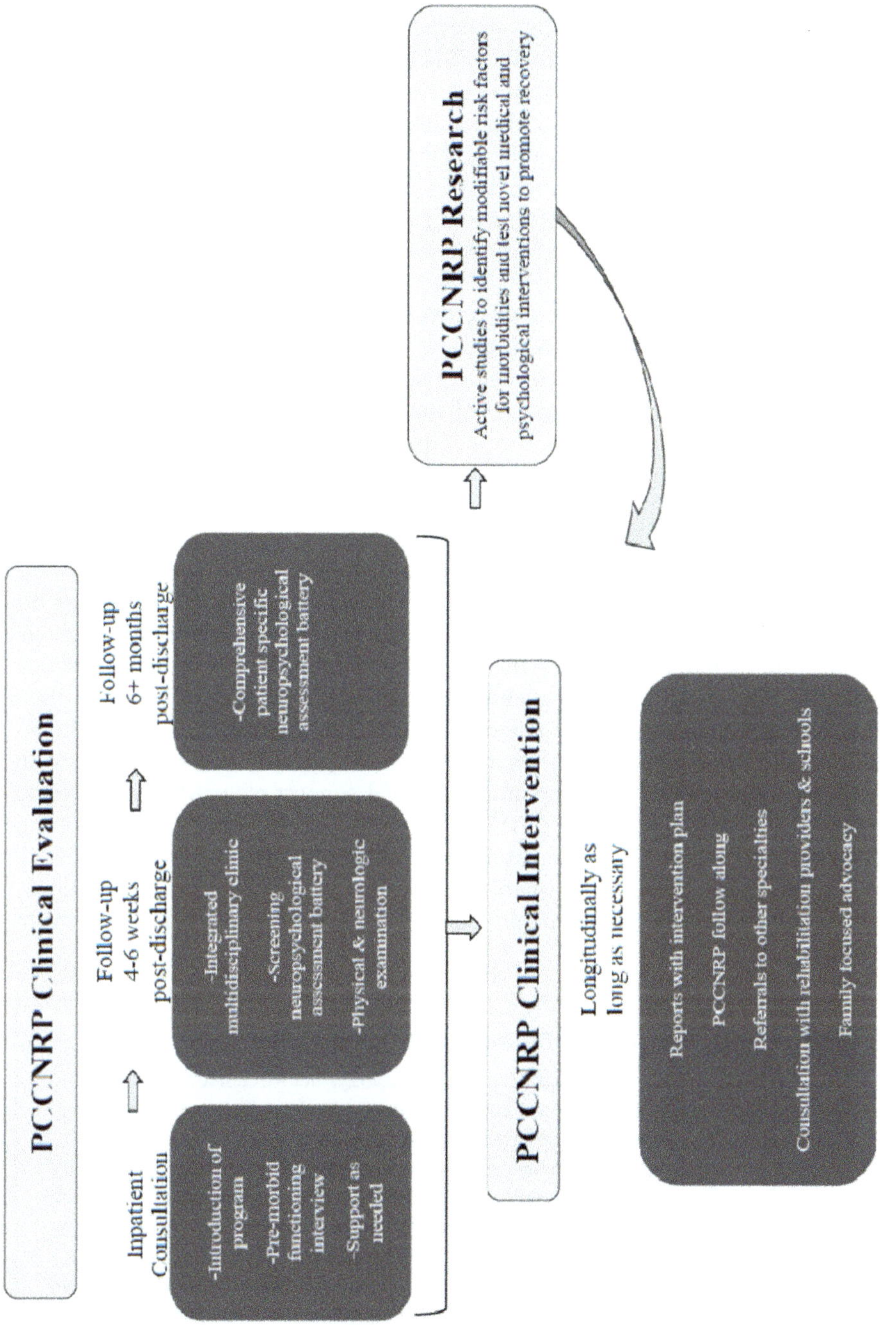

Fig. 5.1 The pediatric critical care and neurotrauma recovery program (PCCNRP) model of care

First, the PCCNRP team works to connect with every eligible child and their family when they are acutely hospitalized to: (1) establish care by introducing the family to the program; (2) address any acute recovery needs related to hospital adjustment that the inpatient medical team identifies as potential issues; and (3) conduct an interview focused on pre-hospitalization levels of functioning, which often includes gaining permission to access information from the school setting (when applicable) that is utilized clinically while developing plans of care. At discharge, the medical team then orders follow-up in the PCCNRP early recovery phase clinic. Staff within the PCCNRP utilize the information gained from the inpatient admission in concert with the medical discharge orders to secure any needed preauthorization for neuropsychological services.

Appointments for the early recovery clinic ideally occur four to six weeks after being home from the hospital, and the annual show rates to the clinic hover around 75%, which is ~15–20% higher in comparison to other co-located clinics in the children's hospital. The critical care physician on the team completes both a physical and neurological exam, while the neuropsychologist completes a targeted and abbreviated neurocognitive assessment focused mostly on attentional regulation, cognitive efficiency, and aspects of executive function given the common impact observed in these areas in the acute recovery phase—as well as an assessment of emotional functioning within the child and family (Table 5.1). Five integrated evaluations are typically scheduled; this approach has drastically improved access to pediatric neuropsychology for these high-need children and families (from four available appointments each month to 20). After the first appointment, it is common practice for the PCCNRP team to refer patients with identified struggles to relevant, often within the same health system, treatment providers (e.g., pediatric psychology, physical/occupational/speech-language therapies, neurology, etc.) and to connect with schools to collaboratively develop an educational support plan. After considering factors described by Baum et al. (2017), around 40 to 50% of the children seen in the acute phase clinic are identified as needing additional follow-up in the PCCNRP long-term recovery phase clinic where more traditional individualized comprehensive neurocognitive assessments are provided 10 to 12 months after being home from the hospital.

Implementation Takeaway #1: Developing Multiprofessional Teams

- Research shows that the integration of psychology, neuroscience, and medicine enhances patient/family-centered care, optimizes recovery outcomes in pediatric populations, and enhances accessible and equitable care.
- Pediatric neuropsychology teams often include primary care providers, specialty physicians (from various specialties depending on patient population), physical therapists, occupational therapists, speech-language pathologists, and education professionals. Also, in many care models, parents/caregivers are part of the team.
- Differences in training, clinical priority variation, schedule alignment, delays in referrals, insurance authorization problems, geographical constraints, and various

Table 5.1 Targeted/abbreviated neuropsychological exam by age ranges

Domain	3 m–35 m	3 years	4 Years	5 years	6–7 years	8–16 years	17+
Estimate of premorbid cognition	N/A	N/A	N/A	**WRAT-5** Word Reading	**WRAT-5** Word Reading	**WRAT-5** Word Reading	**WRAT-5** Word Reading
Executive functioning	N/A	**WPPSI-IV** Bug Search Cancellation	**WPPSI-IV** Bug Search Cancellation Picture Span Zoo Locations	**CMS** Numbers **WPPSI-IV** Bug Search Cancellation	**CMS** Numbers **WISC-V** Coding Symbol Search	**CMS** Numbers **WISC-V** Coding Symbol Search **D-KEFS** Trails	**WAIS-IV** Digit Span Coding Symbol Search **D-KEFS** Trails
Memory & learning	N/A	N/A	N/A	**ChAMP** Lists (Im, Delayed, Recall)	**ChAMP** Lists (Im, Delayed, Recall)	**ChAMP** Lists (Im, Delayed, Recall)	**ChAMP** Lists (Im, Delayed, Recall)
Language verbal	N/A	**WPPSI-IV** Receptive Vocabulary Picture Naming Information	**WPPSI-IV** Receptive Vocabulary Picture Naming Information Similarities	**NEPSY-II** Word Generation	**NEPSY-II** Word Generation	**D-KEFS** Verbal Fluency	**D-KEFS** Verbal Fluency
Visual-spatial nonverbal	N/A	**WPPSI-IV** Block Design Object Assembly	**WPPSI-IV** Block Design Object Assembly Matrix Reasoning	**As Indicated**	**As Indicated**	**As Indicated**	**As Indicated**
Fine motor dexterity	N/A	**Purdue Pegboard**	**Purdue Pegboard**	**Grooved Pegboard**	**Grooved Pegboard**	**Grooved Pegboard**	**Grooved Pegboard**

(continued)

Table 5.1 (continued)

Domain	3 m–35 m	3 years	4 Years	5 years	6–7 years	8–16 years	17+
Developmental screening	**Bayley-4**	N/A	N/A	N/A	N/A	N/A	N/A
Parent completed measures	ABAS-3 (Ages 3 months to 4 years) BRIEF-P (Age 3 years to 5 years) or BRIEF-2 (Ages 6 years and over) PedsQL Family Impact (1 month version); Core (1 month version); Fatigue (1 month version) Sleep Disturbance Scale for Children PROMIS Pain Intensity; Pain Behavior; Cognitive; Anxiety; Depression PTSD PC screen						

administration priorities are among the challenges often experienced while building a multiprofessional care team.
- Addressing these challenges requires a proactive and relational approach supported by data to demonstrate effectiveness and value.
- Creating something new takes time and dedication, so find your initial collaborators and share your vision. Then start tracking data related to access and outcomes to make the case for program enhancement/expansion.
- Be ready to adapt and grow as the system demands flex and the refinement of your model occurs.

Diversifying Outpatient Neuropsychological Services

In addition to the bridges built between care settings as described above, opportunities exist to expand access to outpatient neuropsychological services to improve the care of children and adolescents who have medical and neurodevelopmental conditions. Scientific advances allow for early identification of conditions that are known to be associated with cognitive, psychiatric, and/or psychosocial difficulties, even prior to symptom onset (e.g., in utero detection of genetic disorders or neurological disorders). Early screening programs focus on detection of neurodevelopmental disorders, recognizing the importance of early intervention in optimizing long-term outcomes (e.g., autism spectrum disorder). Children and adolescents may also be more likely to live longer and have more fulfilling lives with chronic or progressive neurological conditions. As with inpatient care, outpatient neuropsychological services can be integrated at the levels of *primary*, *secondary*, and *tertiary* care.

To meet these integration needs, there needs to be fundamental shifts in many practice models. Many practices already have long waitlists, potentially contributing to delayed diagnosis and treatment, provider and caregiver dissatisfaction, and increasing no-show rates (Cass et al., 2020). At a time when technology that allows for quantification of human behavior is being rapidly adopted (e.g., wearable devices that monitor sleep patterns and heart rates), provider and patient frustration with neuropsychology access may push them toward other opportunities that assess cognitive functioning. To maintain viability, neuropsychological practices need to focus on appropriate scaling and timing of evaluation procedures to minimize unnecessary evaluations and increase efficiency.

The COVID-19 pandemic was a catalyst for change in that many pediatric neuropsychology practices had to rapidly adjust their methods to continue to provide patient care under vastly different circumstances. Remote testing by telehealth became more common, as did the integration of telehealth for clinical interviews and parent feedback sessions. Research on assessment using telehealth expanded, and there are ongoing efforts to improve it and to permanently codify insurance reimbursement for teleneuropsychological services (Sperling et al., 2024). Additional insurance codes will likely be needed to allow for easy adoption and expansion of the targeted neuropsychological services described below, but this will likely first require more research demonstrating their efficacy and benefit. Below, we describe the current landscape of pediatric neuropsychology generally, identifying promising research in expanding access through innovative practice models, while also identifying current gaps in care.

Triage

For pediatric neuropsychology clinics, which often face high demand for services, the importance of effective triage cannot be understated. At a minimum, triage should identify those who may not need an evaluation, either because there is no significant evidence of cognitive impairment or because ongoing treatment methods are sufficient and effective. However, making this determination is challenging. A combination of tailored referral forms and targeted discussions with referring providers about the potential role of neuropsychology may be needed (e.g., Cass et al., 2020; Mietchen et al., 2025). It is important to note that practitioners (both neuropsychologists and referral sources) are often overcommitted and have little available time for targeted discussions; nonetheless, when establishing a triage system for a specific population of patients, building these connections (and developing stakeholder buy in) is a vital component that ideally becomes less of a time burden as the model is utilized. Additional factors to consider include patient characteristics, as well as clinic resources, particularly the availability of stratified neuropsychological services (e.g., whether a targeted evaluation can be performed if that is more appropriate than a comprehensive evaluation).

Clinical urgency, or the potential risk of delaying access to care, is the second major factor to consider in triage. This is also often a multifactorial decision that involves integrating knowledge of the clinical condition and patient characteristics. Baum et al. (2017) described four factors that can be considered over the course of development to predict the need for neuropsychological assessment in pediatric oncology patients, although these can be more broadly applied: (1) pre-existing child factors (e.g., age at diagnosis, premorbid functioning), (2) environmental/family factors (e.g., distance to care, access to resources), (3) developmental factors (e.g., cognitive or neurological developmental factors, schooling), and (4) medical/treatment variables (e.g., extent of central nervous system involvement and nature of treatment).

From a population health perspective, several of these factors relate to social determinants of health (e.g., access to education, access to resources). In the wake of psychosocial disruption during the COVID-19 pandemic, which had disproportionate negative impacts on children and adolescents for those already impacted by social and economic disparities, Colvin et al. (2024) argued for the adoption of risk-based assessment models, which prioritize screening and evaluation of youth at high risk for neurodevelopmental disorders who also may not have had access to diagnosis and intervention due to racial or economic disparities. To appropriately determine risk, caregiver questionnaires about developmental history and functioning (adaptive, attentional, learning, affective, and behavioral) may add critical information to classify the type and severity of concerns (Zabel et al., 2021).

Patient/Caregiver Consultations

Neuropsychological consultations are brief interventions, typically between the neuropsychologist and the patient and/or their caregiver, that do not involve testing. The child may not always need to be present for these consultations, depending on the reason for the consultation and/or data available. Referrals for consultations can be generated via the use of triaging systems as described above. They can also emerge programmatically within new service lines of care in specialty populations such as described by Baum et al. (2017) and demonstrated in the PCCNRP example earlier in this chapter. Although testing may not be performed, consultations still require the neuropsychologist to apply specialized knowledge. During a consultation, the neuropsychologist may integrate prior testing with a clinical interview and medical records review to offer diagnostic impressions and treatment recommendations. From a conceptual standpoint, consultations are closely aligned with feedback sessions in that they require the neuropsychologist to rely on therapeutic principles and specialized knowledge of brain-behavior relationships to provide a direct intervention. Below, we discuss several clinical scenarios where consultations may be particularly effective in expanding access to care and minimizing unnecessary evaluations.

Triage and Treatment Planning. In cases when there is insufficient information from the referral data to determine the need for neuropsychological evaluation, consultations may be particularly useful in assisting triage, while also providing psychoeducation to the family. The Baum et al. (2017) and PCCNRP examples discussed earlier highlight this. Taking it a step further, in the outpatient setting, consultations may be especially useful for triaging cases that present with non-specific developmental concerns. In these cases, the differential diagnosis is often broad (e.g., idiopathic neurodevelopmental disorder, psychiatric disorder, normal developmental variability), and testing may not always be appropriate. There may also be prior testing available from school evaluations that determine eligibility for special education services. Colvin et al. (2022) described a consultation model of leveraging these school records data to quickly identify children who have learning or attentional disorders, which became particularly important following educational disruption during the COVID-19 pandemic. Mietchen et al. (2025) used a similar process with patients who had non-specific concerns about learning, attention, and/or behavior, and found that 25% did not need an evaluation.

Early Identification and Prevention. The integration of neuropsychological consultation into primary prevention models may allow for earlier identification of challenges in high-risk patients (e.g., congenital heart disease) (Cassidy & Neumann, 2023). Consultations have also been shown to help prevent complications and unnecessary interventions. For example, neuropsychological consultations have been shown to reduce the severity of post-concussive symptoms in pediatric patients (Kirkwood et al., 2016; Patricios et al., 2023). Importantly, parents indicated high satisfaction with these visits (Kirkwood et al., 2017). This model could be extended to other patient populations, such as functional neurological disorders, where delays in diagnosis and care may complicate presentations (Silverberg & Rush, 2023; Van Patten et al., 2024). Similarly, one might hypothesize that consultations resulting in faster re-routing of those who do not need neuropsychological services to appropriate treatment providers (e.g., psychiatry) may prevent the worsening of symptoms.

Family Psychoeducation and Follow-Up. Consultations also allow neuropsychologists to communicate with patients and families as circumstances change, without necessarily performing additional testing. Gragert and Ris (2011) and Baum et al. (2017) proposed that consultations could be helpful for pediatric oncology patients as they continue in their recovery process, providing targeted advice as patients reach new developmental stages. Applying this model to a wide range of patient populations could potentially extend the time between re-evaluations, expanding access to evaluations while strengthening the relationship between the neuropsychologist and the patient/family through more regular contact.

Screening Assessments: Challenges and Opportunities

A 2014 American Psychological Association (APA) work group described several key characteristics differentiating screening tools from psychological assessment measures. Briefly, screening tools are intended to indicate the risk or likelihood of a condition or to monitor treatment progress, outcomes, or changes in symptoms over time. They are brief, narrow in scope, and are not definitively diagnostic (APA, 2014; Roebuck-Spencer et al., 2017). Many are designed to favor false positives over false negatives so that cases are not prematurely excluded from needed evaluations. Sensitivity and reliability may be further impacted by different administration techniques (e.g., by clinicians, support staff, electronic devices, or by patients themselves) (Bauer et al., 2012; Roebuck-Spencer et al., 2017).

Cognitive screening is common in geriatric populations to determine whether there is evidence of cognitive impairment warranting neuropsychological evaluation (Roebuck-Spencer et al., 2017). Some of these screening measures have been shown to correlate strongly with neuropsychological test performance (e.g., Zarrella et al., 2023) and to be more sensitive to cognitive impairment than a physician's standard clinical exam (Roebuck-Spencer et al., 2017). Implementation of similar screening methods for pediatric services may eliminate unnecessary evaluations while improving access to those who need them.

Unfortunately, there are relatively few well-validated cognitive screening measures for children and adolescents, at least in part because normative expectations rapidly and continuously shift during neurodevelopment (Bryce et al., 2021). For example, a brief cognitive screening measure for a 6-year-old is unlikely to be as sensitive as for a 14-year-old, especially if the measure needs to broadly assess cognitive functions and permit tracking of developmental progress over time. Consistent with this, a recent review of cognitive screening measures that have been used in adolescence or early adulthood (ages 12–25) found that none of the measures could be recommended (Bryce et al., 2021). However, a more recent study found that screening using subtests of the NIH Toolbox had significant predictive value for cognitive impairment in pediatric epilepsy patients (Patrick et al., 2025), but larger studies across patient populations are still needed. Such measures would allow neuropsychology to be more easily integrated into primary prevention, or universal monitoring of at-risk patient populations (Hardy et al., 2017).

In the absence of well-validated objective cognitive screening measures, most pediatric screening methods have relied on caregiver report questionnaires. Indeed, some practices paired a clinical interview with caregiver questionnaires to detect neuropsychological difficulties during the initial phases of the COVID-19 pandemic, when there were limitations on in-person care (Loman et al., 2020). However, effective interpretation of caregiver questionnaires also needs to consider potential threats to validity, as well as the potential influence of linguistic and cultural factors on the interpretation of questions. These factors may partially account for mixed findings on the ability of caregiver report questionnaires to predict who will show clinical difficulties on neuropsychological testing. While Wolfe et al., (2022) showed that caregiver questionnaires could be effective in predicting intellectual and academic test performance in oncology patients, conflicting results were found in similar studies of pediatric patients with multiple sclerosis (Nguyen-Martinez et al., 2024) and traumatic brain injury (Larson et al., 2023).

In a recent study, Williams and et al., (2025) paired screening questionnaires with parent consultation to determine whether patients referred from the neonatal neurodevelopmental follow-up program needed in-person evaluations. Of the 85 patients who were seen for consultation, 50 proceeded to testing due to the presence of neurocognitive concerns, 18 were determined not to need testing, and the others were deferred and/or referred for family support. Importantly, high scores on the parent screening questionnaires were predictive of who was ultimately referred for evaluation.

Altogether, there is a need to develop sensitive screening methods to identify and monitor pediatric patients who have neurocognitive difficulties. Existing research suggests that the efficacy of these tools may be enhanced when caregiver reports and patient characteristics are considered, but considerable research needs to be done to develop effective protocols that can be used at scale. This has led some to explore the possibility of fully automated cognitive screening, although more work is needed within clinical populations (e.g., Singh et al., 2021; see Chapter 10).

Weighing Risks and Benefits of Targeted Neuropsychological Services

Research within specific patient populations has shown that brief and targeted neuropsychological evaluations can significantly improve access to care. For example, pediatric patients with a concussion may not need full neuropsychological evaluations but evaluations may be uniquely helpful in post-concussion management of children who have unusual symptom trajectories (e.g., persistent symptoms or prolonged recovery), those at risk for long-term cognitive or behavioral difficulties, and those who have other neurological or developmental concerns (Patricios et al., 2023).

Neuropsychologists have also explored whether targeted evaluations may help expand access to services for pediatric epilepsy patients. Nussbaum et al. (2021) describe a triage model that starts by prioritizing patients who need evaluations for pre-surgical planning and then leveraging telehealth for assessment when there are appropriate patient characteristics. Even brief evaluations may be critical in identifying patients with epilepsy who have cognitive difficulties. A recent study compared performances on a brief cognitive evaluation between pediatric patients with epilepsy who were and who were not referred for evaluation and found similar rates of cognitive impairment. This suggests that a significant portion of pediatric epilepsy patients who are not referred for testing may have cognitive difficulties that could be identified by brief evaluations (Patrick et al., 2025).

Similarly, brief or targeted neuropsychological evaluations have been used to identify patients who may have autism spectrum disorder (ASD). Such primary prevention models have been developed using telehealth applications of autism screening measures, including the TELE-ASD-PEDS (Corona, et al., 2020) for children who are at higher risk of neurodevelopmental disorders given their birth histories (Raches et al., 2024). In the Massachusetts General Hospital (MGH; MC is the Director) clinic, we have been using this methodology to identify young patients who need further neuropsychological evaluation related to a possible ASD diagnosis so that they may be appropriately and quickly routed to needed interventions. The first step of these evaluations is completed via telehealth. A clinical interview, the TELE-ASD-PEDS, and standardized questionnaires are administered to determine whether there is clear evidence of the presence or absence of ASD. If so, then the clinical decision is rendered at this visit. If not, then the patient is scheduled for an in-person follow-up evaluation, which may include assessing relevant aspects of cognitive functioning.

A common assumption is that targeted outpatient neuropsychological services are of lesser quality than full-length evaluation. Yet there is little research to support a full-length neuropsychological evaluation as the gold standard for every patient. Because consultations and targeted evaluations allow neuropsychologists to provide the right service at the right time, they prevent unnecessary evaluations and build greater flexibility into scheduling, potentially reducing waitlists. Shorter waitlists potentially alleviate the pressure for neuropsychologists to be overly comprehensive for fear that it may take months or even years for a patient to get another appointment.

If a referring provider or family has access to a neuropsychologist when needed, even for consultation, then this may increase, rather than decrease, provider and patient satisfaction with targeted and briefer neuropsychological services.

Implementation Takeaway #2: Putting Triage into Practice

- In addition to offering traditional full-length evaluations, outpatient neuropsychology practices should consider adding consultations and targeted evaluations. Potential benefits include: improving access to care, reducing wait lists, eliminating unnecessary evaluations, and ensuring that the right care at the right time.
  - Neuropsychology consultations are brief interventions with patients and/or their caregivers that do not involve testing and can assist with: 1) triage and treatment planning, 2) early identification and prevention, and 3) family psychoeducation and follow-up.
  - Screening measures need to continue to be developed, which can be integrated with consultations or implemented as part of brief evaluations. These may be helpful in determining which patients need full evaluations.
  - Targeted evaluations, either in person or telehealth, may be helpful in homing in on specific areas of concern, determining who may require additional testing, and expanding access to patients who may not have otherwise received any neuropsychological services.
- Effective triage is a critical component of building a diversified outpatient practice. Two key questions need to be answered during triage: 1) What kind of evaluation does the patient need, if any? and 2) Is the evaluation urgent? Multiple factors will contribute to decision-making, and should include patient variables related to social determinants of health. Building a good triage system may require an investment in creating tailored referral forms and fostering conversations with referring providers about neuropsychology's role and range of services.

Conclusion

The models described above provide a description of how screening and brief evaluations can be applied to both inpatient and outpatient pediatric neuropsychological practice to improve access to care and monitor developmental progress or recovery in response to interventions, while also effectively allocating scarce resources. These innovations are needed to maintain relevance within a rapidly evolving healthcare system. Neuropsychology is already recognized as critical in clinical care guidelines for many patient populations and has the potential to play an even larger role in prevention (primary care) and recovery (tertiary care).

Meeting this need will require adopting new models of care, including consultations, targeted evaluations, and better triage models. It will be important to continue the momentum from the COVID-19 pandemic to leverage telehealth and technological advances to reach more patients, especially those in rural areas, to screen and intervene for high-risk children and adolescents. It will be especially important to consider how neuropsychology can be integrated with mobile devices that measure biometric data or use artificial intelligence (AI) to screen for different conditions. Such advances have the potential to inform education and health policy to address inequities and the promotion of brain health across the lifespan. As new innovative models informed by population health models are implemented, it will be critical to document their value and outcomes to maintain and grown neuropsychology's role in the evolving healthcare system.

Key Points in Review

- Pediatric neuropsychological services can be developed to provide primary, secondary, and tertiary interventions within both inpatient and outpatient environments that allow for expanded access to timely, equitable, and appropriate evaluations and interventions.
- Innovative practice models that are informed by population health models and technological advances will improve care for pediatric patients who have medical, neurodevelopmental, and/or psychiatric conditions, while also solidifying the neuropsychologists' critical role on multidisciplinary teams.
- Effective triage methods balance patient characteristics, specialized knowledge of medical conditions and developmental trajectories, and presenting concerns. Diversified outpatient neuropsychological services may include patient/caregiver consultation, screening or targeted evaluations, and comprehensive evaluations.
- Challenges in building a diversified outpatient neuropsychology service include building flexible systems to support administrative and financial success. There is also a need to combat an unvalidated assumption that more testing is better care, including within our profession. As health care professionals, neuropsychologists are qualified to make the best determination about the timing and scope of an intervention and should communicate this clearly with parents and referring providers who may be used to "ordering testing." Integration of briefer and targeted services allows neuropsychologists to provide the right service at the right time, increasing both provider and patient satisfaction.

References

American Psychological Association Practice Organization. (2014, December). *Distinguishing between screening and assessment for mental and behavioral health problems: A statement from an American Psychological Association Practice Organization work group on screening and psychological assessment.* http://www.apapracticecentral.org/reimbursement/billing/assessment-screening.aspx

Bauer, R. M., Iverson, G. L., Cernich, A. N., Binder, L. M., Ruff, R. M., & Naugle, R. I. (2012). Computerized neuropsychological assessment devices: Joint position paper of the American Academy of Clinical Neuropsychology and the National Academy of Neuropsychology. *Archives of Clinical Neuropsychology, 27*(3), 362–373. https://doi.org/10.1093/arclin/acs027

Baum, K. T., Powell, S. K., Jacobson, L. A., Gragert, M. N., Janzen, L. A., Paltin, I., Rey-Casserly, C. M., & Wilkening, G. N. (2017). Implementing guidelines: Proposed definitions of neuropsychology services in pediatric oncology. *Pediatric Blood & Cancer, 64*(8), Article e26446. https://doi.org/10.1002/pbc.26446

Birnkrant, D. J., Bushby, K., Bann, C. M., Apkon, S. D., Blackwell, A., Colvin, M. K., Cripe, L., Herron, A. R., Kennedy, A., Kinnett, K., Naprawa, J., Noritz, G., Poysky, J., Street, N., Trout, C. J., Weber, D. R., & Ward, L. M. (2018). Diagnosis and management of Duchenne muscular dystrophy, part 3: Primary care, emergency management, psychosocial care, and transitions of care across the lifespan. *The Lancet Neurology, 17*(5), 445–455. https://doi.org/10.1016/S1474-4422(18)30026-7

Bryce, S. D., Bowden, S. C., Wood, S. J., & Allott, K. (2021). Brief, performance-based cognitive screening in youth aged 12–25: A systematic review. *Journal of the International Neuropsychological Society, 27*(8), 835–854. https://doi.org/10.1017/S1355617720001241

Cass, J., Fristad, M. A., Valleru, J., Gallup, J., & Butter, E. (2020). Improving wait times for pediatric neuropsychology services. *Evidence-Based Practice in Child and Adolescent Mental Health, 5*(2), 128–138. https://doi.org/10.1080/23794925.2020.1784057

Cassidy, A. R., & Neumann, A. A. (2023). Optimizing neurodevelopmental outcomes following fetal diagnosis of congenital heart disease: A call for primary prevention neuropsychology. *Child Neuropsychology, 29*(7), 1155–1177. https://doi.org/10.1080/09297049.2023.2190966. PMID: 36942716.

Colvin, M. K., Forchelli, G. A., Reese, K. L., Capawana, M. R., Beery, C. S., Murphy, J., & Braaten, E. B. (2022). Neuropsychology consultation to identify learning disorders in children and adolescents: A proposal based on lessons learned during the COVID-19 pandemic. *Child Neuropsychology, 28*(5), 671–688. https://doi.org/10.1080/09297049.2021.2006839

Colvin, M. K., Reesman, J., & Glen, T. (2024). Altered trajectories: Considering the long-term impact of educational disruption during the COVID-19 pandemic on neurodevelopment and a call to action for neuropsychology. *Archives of Clinical Neuropsychology, 39*(3), 305–312. https://doi.org/10.1093/arclin/acae021

Corona, L., Hine, J., Nicholson, A., Stone, C., Swanson, A., Wade, J., Wagner, L., Weitlauf, A., & Warren, Z. (2020). *TELE-ASD-PEDS: A telemedicine-based ASD evaluation tool for toddlers and young children.* Vanderbilt University Medical Center. https://vkc.vumc.org/vkc/triad/tele-asd-peds

Dodd, J. N., Hall, T. A., Guilliams, K., Guerriero, R. M., Wagner, A., Malone, S., Williams, C. N., Hartman, M. E., & Piantino, J. (2018). Optimizing neurocritical care follow-up through the integration of neuropsychology. *Pediatric Neurology, 89*, 58–62. https://doi.org/10.1016/j.pediatrneurol.2018.09.007

Fisher, E. L., Zimak, E., Sherwood, A. R., & Elias, J. (2022). Outcomes of pediatric neuropsychological services: A systematic review. *The Clinical Neuropsychologist, 36*(6), 1265–1289. https://doi.org/10.1080/13854046.2020.1853812

Foley, F. W., & Portnoy, J. G. (2018). Neuropsychology in the integrated MS care setting. *Archives of Clinical Neuropsychology, 33*(3), 330–338. https://doi.org/10.1093/arclin/acy003

Glen, E. T., Hostetter, G., Ruff, R. M., Roebuck-Spencer, T. M., Denney, R. L., Perry, W., Fazio, R. L., Garmoe, W. S., Bianchini, K. J., & Scott, J. G. (2019). Integrative care models in neuropsychology: A National Academy of Neuropsychology education paper. *Archives of Clinical Neuropsychology, 34*(2), 141–151. https://doi.org/10.1093/arclin/acy092

Gravholt, C. H., Andersen, N. H., Christin-Maitre, S., Davis, S. M., Duijnhouwer, A., Gawlik, A., Maciel-Guerra, A. T., Gutmark-Little, I., Fleischer, K., Hong, D., Klein, K. O., Prakash, S. K., Shankar, R. K., Sandberg, D. E., Sas, T. C. J., Skakkebæk, A., Stochholm, K., & van der Velden, J. A., International Turner Syndrome Consensus Group, & Backeljauw, P. F. (2024). Clinical practice guidelines for the care of girls and women with Turner syndrome. *European Journal of Endocrinology, 190*(6), G53–G151. https://doi.org/10.1093/ejendo/lvae050

Gragert, M. N., & Ris, M. D. (2011). Neuropsychological late effects and rehabilitation following pediatric brain tumor. *Journal of Pediatric Rehabilitation Medicine, 4*

Greene, N. H., Kernic, M. A., Vavilala, M. S., & Rivara, F. P. (2014). Variation in pediatric traumatic brain injury outcomes in the United States. *Archives of Physical Medicine and Rehabilitation, 95*(6), 1148–1155. https://doi.org/10.1016/j.apmr.2014.02.020

Hall, T. A., Greene, R. K., Lee, J. B., Leonard, S., Bradbury, K. R., Drury, K., Recht, G., Randall, J., Norr, M. E., & Williams, C. N. (2022). Post-intensive care syndrome in a cohort of school-aged children and adolescent ICU survivors: The importance of follow-up in the acute recovery phase. *Journal of Pediatric Intensive Care*. Advance online publication. https://doi.org/10.1055/s-0042-1747935

Hall, T. A., Leonard, S., Bradbury, K., Holding, E., Lee, J., Wagner, A., Duvall, S., & Williams, C. N. (2022b). Post-intensive care syndrome in a cohort of infants and young children receiving integrated care via a pediatric critical care and neurotrauma recovery program: A pilot investigation. *The Clinical Neuropsychologist, 36*(3), 639–663. https://doi.org/10.1080/13854046.2020.1797176

Hardy, K. K., Olson, K., Cox, S. M., Kennedy, T., & Walsh, K. S. (2017). Systematic review: A prevention-based model of neuropsychological assessment for children with medical illness. *Journal of Pediatric Psychology, 42*(8), 815–822. https://doi.org/10.1093/jpepsy/jsx060

Jordan, L. L., Costello, R., MacDonald, B., Heffelfinger, A., Jones, E. F., Zabel, T. A., & Queally, J. T. (2025). Evaluating access to neuropsychological services for individuals with spina bifida: Insights from the 2022 provider survey. *Topics in Spinal Cord Injury Rehabilitation*. Advance online publication. https://doi.org/10.46292/sci24-00023

Keenan, H. T., Murphy, N. A., Staheli, R., & Savitz, L. A. (2013). Healthcare utilization in the first year after pediatric traumatic brain injury in an insured population. *The Journal of Head Trauma Rehabilitation, 28*(6), 426–433. https://doi.org/10.1097/HTR.0b013e31825935b8

Kirkwood, M. W., Peterson, R. L., Connery, A. K., Baker, D. A., & Forster, J. (2016). A pilot study investigating neuropsychological consultation as an intervention for persistent postconcussive symptoms in a pediatric sample. *The Journal of Pediatrics, 169*, 244–249. https://doi.org/10.1016/j.jpeds.2015.10.086

Kirkwood, M. W., Peterson, R. L., Baker, D. A., & Connery, A. K. (2017). Parent satisfaction with neuropsychological consultation after pediatric mild traumatic brain injury. *Child Neuropsychology, 23*(3), 273–283. https://doi.org/10.1080/09297049.2015.1105809

Larson, K. R., Demers, L. A., Holding, E. Z., Williams, C. N., & Hall, T. A. (2023). Variability across caregiver and performance-based measures of executive functioning in an acute pediatric neurocritical care population. *Neurotrauma Reports, 4*(1), 97–106. https://doi.org/10.1089/neur.2022.0083

Loman, M., Vogt, E., Miller, L., Landsman, R., Duong, P., Kasten, J., Heffelfinger, A., et al. (2020). "How to" operate a pediatric neuropsychology practice during the COVID-19 pandemic: Real tips from one practice's experience. *Child Neuropsychology, 27*(2), 251–279. https://doi.org/10.1080/09297049.2020.1830962

Mietchen, J. J., Cieminski, T. M., & Kessler-Jones, A. M. (2025). Your clinical interview is data: The benefit of telehealth appointments to triage referrals made to pediatric neuropsychology. *The Clinical Neuropsychologist*, 1–20. Advance online publication. https://doi.org/10.1080/13854046.2025.2456160

Nguyen-Martinez, A., Weigand, B., Wolfe, K., Kammeyer, R., Schreiner, T., & Hutaff-Lee, C. (2024). Clinical utility of brief screening measures during neuropsychological consultation for pediatric onset multiple sclerosis. *Journal of the International Neuropsychological Society, 30*(10), 977–984. https://doi.org/10.1017/S1355617724000419

Nussbaum, N. L., Young, S. R., DeLeon, R. C., Engelmann, M. L., & Schraegle, W. A. (2021). The future is now: Pediatric neuropsychological presurgical epilepsy evaluation in the age of COVID-19. *Epileptic Disorders, 23*(2), 274–280. https://doi.org/10.1684/epd.2021.1274

Patricios, J. S., Schneider, K. J., Dvorak, J., Ahmed, O. H., Blauwet, C., Cantu, R. C., Davis, G. A., Echemendia, R. J., Makdissi, M., McNamee, M., Broglio, S., Emery, C. A., Feddermann-Demont, N., Fuller, G. W., Giza, C. C., Guskiewicz, K. M., Hainline, B., Iverson, G. L., Kutcher,

J. S., … Meeuwisse, W. (2023). Consensus statement on concussion in sport: The 6th International Conference on Concussion in Sport–Amsterdam, October 2022. *British Journal of Sports Medicine, 57*(11), 695–711. https://doi.org/10.1136/bjsports-2023-106898

Patrick, K. E., Shields, A. N., Dustin, H. A., Patel, A. D., & McNally, K. (2025). *Cognitive screening informs referrals for neuropsychological evaluation in children with epilepsy*. Advance online publication. https://doi.org/10.1111/epi.18421

Pollack, M. M., Holubkov, R., Funai, T., Clark, A., Berger, J. T., Meert, K., Newth, C. J. L., Shanley, T., Moler, F., Carcillo, J., Berg, R. A., Dalton, H., Wessel, D. L., Harrison, R. E., Doctor, A., Dean, J. M., Jenkins, T. L., & Network, C. P. C. C. (2014). Pediatric intensive care outcomes: Development of new morbidities during pediatric critical care. *Pediatric Critical Care Medicine, 15*(9), 821–827. https://doi.org/10.1097/PCC.0000000000000250

Raches, C. M., Hines, E. N., Hines, A. C., & Scott, E. K. (2024). Identifying autism spectrum disorder in a high-risk follow-up program through quality improvement methodology. *Pediatric Quality & Safety, 9*(2), Article e717. https://doi.org/10.1097/pq9.0000000000000717. PMID: 38576888.

Roebuck-Spencer, T. M., Glen, T., Puente, A. E., Denney, R. L., Ruff, R. M., Hostetter, G., & Bianchini, K. J. (2017). Cognitive screening tests versus comprehensive neuropsychological test batteries: A National Academy of Neuropsychology education paper. *Archives of Clinical Neuropsychology, 32*(4), 491–498. https://doi.org/10.1093/arclin/acx021

Silverberg, N. D., & Rush, B. K. (2023). Neuropsychological evaluation of functional cognitive disorder: A narrative review. *The Clinical Neuropsychologist, 38*(2), 302–325. https://doi.org/10.1080/13854046.2023.2228527

Singh, S., Strong, R. W., Jung, L., Li, F. H., Grinspoon, L., Scheuer, L. S., Passell, E. J., Martini, P., Chaytor, N., Soble, J. R., & Germine, L. (2021). The TestMyBrain Digital Neuropsychology Toolkit: Development and psychometric characteristics. *Journal of Clinical and Experimental Neuropsychology, 43*(8), 786–795. https://doi.org/10.1080/13803395.2021.2002269. PMID: 34907842.

Sperling, S. A., Acheson, S. K., Fox-Fuller, J., Colvin, M. K., Harder, L., Cullum, C. M., Randolph, J. J., Carter, K. R., Espe-Pfeifer, P., Lacritz, L. H., Arnett, P. A., & Gillaspy, S. R. (2024). Teleneuropsychology: From science to policy to practice. *Archives of Clinical Neuropsychology, 39*(2), 227–248. https://doi.org/10.1093/arclin/acad066

Sweet, J. J., Benson, L. M., Nelson, N. W., & Moberg, P. J. (2015). The American Academy of Clinical Neuropsychology, National Academy of Neuropsychology, and Society for Clinical Neuropsychology (APA Division 40) 2015 TCN professional practice and 'salary survey': Professional practices, beliefs, and incomes of U.S. neuropsychologists. *The Clinical Neuropsychologist, 29*(8), 1069–1162. https://doi.org/10.1080/13854046.2016.1140228

Sweet, J. J., Klipfel, K. M., Nelson, N. W., & Moberg, P. J. (2020). Professional practices, beliefs, and incomes of U.S. neuropsychologists: The AACN, NAN, SCN 2020 practice and "salary survey." *The Clinical Neuropsychologist, 35*(1), 7–80. https://doi.org/10.1080/13854046.2020.1849803

Van Patten, R., Mordecai, K., & LaFrance, W. C. (2024). The role of neuropsychology in the care of patients with functional neurological symptom disorder. *Journal of the International Neuropsychological Society, 30*(7), 710–717. https://doi.org/10.1017/S1355617724000249

Williams, C. N., Piantino, J., McEvoy, C., Fino, N., & Eriksson, C. O. (2018). The burden of pediatric neurocritical care in the United States. *Pediatric Neurology, 89*, 31–38. https://doi.org/10.1016/j.pediatrneurol.2018.07.013

Williams, C. N., Hall, T. A., Francoeur, C., Kurz, J., Rasmussen, L., Hartman, M. E., O'Meara, A. I., Ferguson, N. M., Fink, E. L., Walker, T., Drury, K., Carpenter, J. L., Erklauer, J., Press, C., Wainwright, M. S., Lovett, M., Dapul, H., Murphy, S., Risen, S., … Pediatric Neurocritical Care Research Group (PNCRG). (2022). Continuing care for critically ill children beyond hospital discharge: Current state of follow-up. *Hospital Pediatrics, 12*(4), 359–393. https://doi.org/10.1542/hpeds.2021-006464

Williams, C. N., Hall, T. A., Baker, V. A., Chertow, D. J., Vanderlind, W. M., Bosworth, C. C., & Hartman, M. E. (2023). Follow-up after PICU discharge for patients with acquired brain injury: The role of an abbreviated neuropsychological evaluation and a return-to-school program. *Pediatric Critical Care Medicine, 24*(10), 807–817. https://doi.org/10.1097/pcc.0000000000003303

Williams, T. S., Taylor, M. M., Green, R. R., Lyon R., Bondi, B. C., Desire, N. (2025). Development of a neuropsychological service pathway for school-aged neonatal follow up: A feasibility pilot. *Archives of Clinical Neuropsychology*, acaf061.

Wilson, S. J., Baxendale, S., Barr, W., Hamed, S., Langfitt, J., Samson, S., Watanabe, M., Baker, G. A., Helmstaedter, C., Hermann, B. P., & Smith, M.-L. (2015). Indications and expectations for neuropsychological assessment in routine epilepsy care: Report of the ILAE Neuropsychology Task Force, Diagnostic Methods Commission, 2013–2017. *Epilepsia, 56*(5), 674–681. https://doi.org/10.1111/epi.12962

Wolfe, K. R., Hutaff-Lee, C., & Wilkening, G. (2022). Neuropsychological screening in pediatric multidisciplinary clinics: Group characteristics and predictive utility. *Archives of Clinical Neuropsychology, 37*(4), 789–797. https://doi.org/10.1093/arclin/acab090

Zabel, T. A., Jacobson, L. A., Pritchard, A. E., Mahone, E. M., & Kalb, L. (2021). Pre-appointment online assessment of patient complexity: Towards a personalized model of neuropsychological assessment. *Child Neuropsychology, 27*(2), 232–250. https://doi.org/10.1080/09297049.2020.1822310

Zarrella, G. V., Kay, C. D., Gettens, K., Sherman, J. C., & Colvin, M. K. (2023). Addenbrooke's Cognitive Examination-Third Edition predicts neuropsychological test performance. *The Journal of Neuropsychiatry and Clinical Neurosciences, 35*(2), 178–183. https://doi.org/10.1176/appi.neuropsych.21080196

Chapter 6
Modifying Neuropsychological Practice to Promote Early Detection and Intervention of Cognitive Disorders

Robert Fallows and Caleb Pearson

Executive Summary
This chapter provides a brief overview of the critical importance of early detection and intervention in managing cognitive disorders within the framework of population health. By intervening at the earliest stages of cognitive decline, healthcare providers can prevent the progression to more severe conditions or potentially limit burden (secondary prevention), thereby enhancing patients' quality of life. The chapter then advocates for increasing the role of neuropsychology within primary care settings to facilitate the early identification of cognitive issues, allowing for timely and targeted interventions. This approach not only helps in detecting cognitive disorders early but also supports the overall goal of population health by making neuropsychological services more accessible to a broader population. A model to adapt similar population health approaches to specialized clinics, using an epilepsy program as a model is then discussed.

R. Fallows (✉)
Samaritan Health Services, Samaritan Medical Group, Corvallis, OR, USA
e-mail: rfallows@samhealth.org

C. Pearson
University of Kansas Medical Center, Departments of Neurosurgery, Neurology, and Psychiatry, Kansas City, KS, USA
e-mail: cpearson2@kumc.edu

M. Lanca and R. Fallows (eds.), *Advancing Neuropsychology Through Population Health*, https://doi.org/10.1007/978-3-032-22457-6_6

Early Detection: A Case for Neuropsychology Embracing Population Health

Primordial and primary interventions, covered in Chap. 2, represent valuable opportunities for neuropsychologists to have significant population level impact, but are not often readily adaptable to the clinical roles in which these providers already operate. Secondary prevention is more readily applicable to standard clinical practice, and includes screening, early diagnosis and treatment, which has shown improved outcomes for neurological populations. For example, when early intervention is offered for individuals with multiple sclerosis (MS), there is a significant reduction in disability status years later (Landfeldt et al., 2018). In fact, the effects of early intervention have been so promising that calls for collaboration between insurance, pharmaceutical companies, and clinical researchers have been advanced in acknowledgment that "time matters" (Cerqueira et al., 2018) with efforts to improve stepped care intervention policies with this population. While early identification of MS often relies on non-neuropsychological methods such as lumbar puncture and magnetic resonance imaging, the disease itself often has heterogeneous manifestations ranging from physical to emotional and cognitive. The role of the neuropsychologist in identifying those at risk of cognitive and emotional impact and offering early, non-pharmaceutical intervention should not be overlooked. Specifically, individuals with MS have shown cognitive and emotional improvement from increased exercise (Li et al., 2023), engagement with mindfulness and acceptance-based interventions (Han, 2022), and cognitive rehabilitation (Chen et al., 2021).

Early diagnosis is central to secondary prevention, and neuropsychology's role is pivotal for many cognitive disorders. Specifically, at a time when there is increased interest in advancing neuroimaging techniques, spinal fluid, and blood biomarkers for early detection of dementia, groups such as the American Geriatrics Society have raised concerns that there is not sufficient evidence yet for early treatment intervention of biomarker positive, but cognitively normal patients (2023). Neuropsychology is often overlooked as a 'biomarker' in determining when/if these patients will develop mild cognitive impairment and/or dementia. Similarly overlooked are the non-pharmaceutical interventions. One must start to ask how much of that tendency to overlook neuropsychology and non-pharmaceutical interventions is driven by problems with access and time. Specifically, there is a clear access difference between a blood draw and a comprehensive neuropsychological evaluation and a time and access difference between taking a pill versus attending educational skill-building classes. Models for improving neuropsychology access must be explored as a blood test will never be able to reveal how a person's memory is functioning or how their level of executive dysfunction does or does not impact their daily functional abilities. Further, reducing barriers to engagement for non-pharmaceutical interventions (e.g., placing rehabilitation and psychoeducation in highly accessible service lines, such as primary care) and building continued research that demonstrates response to intervention is needed. For example, research examining multi-modal health intervention programs that promote secondary prevention in mild cognitive impairment and early stage dementia is very encouraging (Chandler et al., 2019; Smith et al., 2017). Notably, these programs do not necessarily need to target primary central nervous system disorders, and the rehabilitation care does not need to be delivered by psychologists in order to be effective, as one study examining nurse-lead rehabilitation in diabetes demonstrated (Cuevas et al., 2019). However, these programs need increased specificity to benefit all members of a population, as the success of these interventions within culturally diverse communities is often lacking (Azar et al., 2024).

Ultimately, the ability to access these interventions can be dependent on access, for which triage discussed in Chap. 2 holds significant promise. The following two sections of this chapter elaborate on this concept with two practice models which implemented triage-based approaches to care and focus on team integration of the neuropsychologists. While triaged based models are newer to the practice of psychology in general, their importance in driving population health outcomes cannot be understated and many barriers (e.g., provider education, patient acceptance/interest) can be more easily overcome while others (e.g., reimbursement) will require continued advocacy (Lucy et al, 2025). Critically, better triaging increases access to care, which in turn can promote earlier identification of cognitive disruption and earlier intervention. While the goal remains improved patient outcomes, these models also keep neuropsychology at the forefront of clinical practice as an accessible service and not a luxury for the fortunate few.

Primary Care as the Central Hub for Population Health Management

In 2019, there were over 1 billion physician office visits in the United States with more than 50% of those occurring in primary care (Santo & Kang, 2019). The chronic care model emphasizes the importance of primary care, and studies show that high-quality, regular primary care access improves outcomes and reduces costs (Rose et al., 2019). Health and clinical psychologists have been co-located in primary care for decades (McDaniel & deGruy, 2014) and have demonstrated significant benefit in driving forward the chronic care model (see Chap. 8), reducing total cost of care while improving healthcare outcomes. While the integration of neuropsychologists into this space is relatively new (Fallows, 2019; Lanca, 2018), it is clear that the demand has risen with primary care physicians becoming one of the more common referral sources to neuropsychologists (Sweet et al., 2020). Moreover, the benefits of having neuropsychologists co-located in primary care are significant. For example, in evaluation of a single practice, Fallows (2019) was able to demonstrate that patients were 3.2 times more likely to complete a cognitive evaluation by a neuropsychologist simply by being located in the primary care clinic. If the patient was able to have a brief introduction to the provider prior to the referral being formally made, (also known as a "warm hand-off"), the odds of evaluation completion jumped to 5.7 times that of the traditional route.

Neuropsychologists working in primary care have specialized competencies and their practices are adapted to meet the needs of primary care settings. McDaniel et al. (2014) outlined six core competency clusters with essential components that psychologists possess and sample behavioral anchors for consideration. Of these, neuropsychologists/psychologists must clearly possess the knowledge of the biological, cognitive, and affective components of health and illness as well as knowledge of how sociocultural and economic factors interact with health and illness. Although some of these core competencies are already familiar to the average neuropsychologist, acquiring skills in *rapid* assessment of the patient's needs, engaging in longitudinal monitoring of patients, balancing the multiple ethical standards across a multidisciplinary team, and applying principles of population-based care may be newer competencies for primary care neuropsychologists to develop. In another publication on this topic, the APA Services, Inc.'s (2018) resolution on psychologists practicing in primary care and specialty health care settings details some of the ongoing challenges to co-located or coordinated care, the benefit that psychologists offer to these settings, and the need for continued advocacy on reimbursement within these settings.

For neuropsychologists working in a primary care setting, there are several shifts in typical neuropsychological practice that are critical. First, neuropsychologists must acknowledge that they are on the front lines of healthcare and that the range of referral questions are going to be broader. Patients want to know many different things about their cognitive health and may be interested in everything from risk of attention-deficit/hyperactivity disorder (ADHD) and autism spectrum disorder (ASD) to what their new diagnosis of Moya-Moya means for their future. The neuropsychologist who becomes an integral member of the care team is prepared to assist the primary care providers in providing education, supporting brief rehabilitation efforts, conducting cognitive screening, and carrying out brief to slightly more comprehensive evaluations. The primary care neuropsychologist must have a clear sense of their boundaries of competence and have developed referral resources when patient care needs exceed those boundaries. An almost certain way to fail in the primary care setting is to not be available for a "curbside" consultation when needed, to decline a warm hand-off, or to tell a primary care provider "no, I don't see those patients". Taking the "yes, and…" approach and providing solutions to the patient and their care team quickly builds trust and rapport, making the neuropsychologist an indispensable care team member.

In her 2018 paper on integrating neuropsychology services into primary care, Lanca proposed a stepped care model akin to how primary care manages many other conditions. Specifically, the patient that comes in and complains of some stomach tightness and pain after eating is not immediately referred to gastroenterology. Rather, the primary care provider completes an initial examination and may order laboratory tests or imaging studies to rule out more common conditions. There may be some trial of medication or other therapies based on early results and, if the patient does not respond or there is indication of other need, a referral to a specialty care provider for consultation may be initiated. Similarly, neuropsychologists can take a triaged

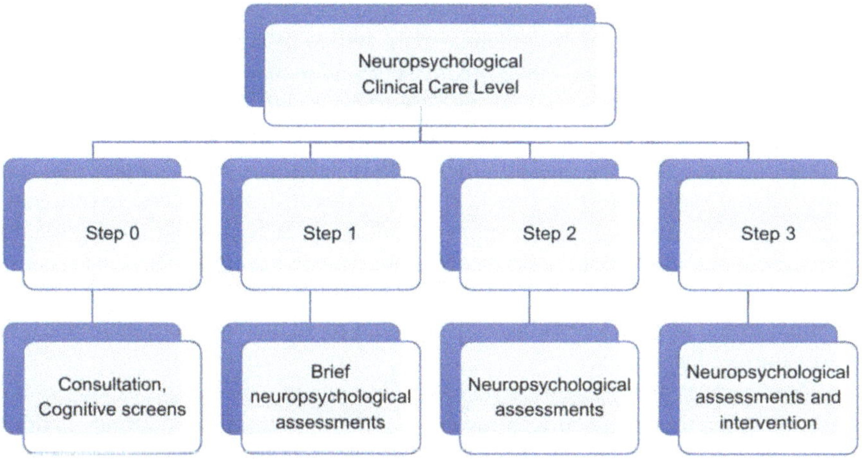

Fig. 6.1 Stepped care model for neuropsychology

approach to care (see Fig. 6.1) that ranges from conducting a cognitive screen (Step 0) to taking on the full range of care needs for a patient, including interventional care (Step 3). Neuropsychologists may also consider what elements of care they need to be fully involved in versus those that they tap on their care team (e.g., psychometry or the physician/advanced practitioner's medical assistant (MA) or clinic nurse) to manage. For example, using an MA to complete a risk stratification tool (e.g., Mini-Cog) (Hilsabeck et al., 2024) to determine what patients need screening by the clinic nurse with a more robust screening tool (e.g., SLUMS) as part of their annual wellness visit may make incoming caseload more manageable for the neuropsychologist, depending on the size of the clinic. Further, longitudinal screening in some cases may provide diagnostic answers allowing the neuropsychologist to shorten their battery or repurpose their time with the patient and their family toward education and support.

When results of care are completed, the neuropsychologist makes sure to discuss these with the care team. Here, there are numerous benefits to the patient. For example, the neuropsychologist who sees the 90-year-old patient with a chronic history of hypothyroidism may be curious about a thyroid-stimulating hormone lab that was marked as elevated by the electronic medical record's (EMR) automated system. However, in discussing the case "curbside" with the physician, the neuropsychologist is informed that the lab value is actually within an empirically safe range for older adults based on emerging research, not taken into consideration by the automated reporting system in the EMR, creating more diagnostic clarity.

Another significant modification or shift in typical neuropsychology practice is that neuropsychological reports need to be significantly streamlined and presented in a manner that is helpful for the stakeholder. As noted by Postal et al (2018), stakeholders typically regard neuropsychological reports as too long and riddled with jargon. In a primary care setting, asking oneself: does a primary care physician know what a WAIS-5 is and what the potential pros and cons of using that measure vs a Stanford-Binet are? Does the nurse practitioner understand why the neuropsychologist reported scaled scores vs T-scores to present results, and what the mean and standard deviation for those scales are? The answer is almost certainly "no" and, with that in mind, one must question the utility of lengthy tables that describe such scores in detail to the referring provider or the patient. Instead, neuropsychologist may consider the use of graphs or other visual aids which uses common cognitive descriptors to quickly 'paint the picture' for the referring provider. Beyond communication to the referring provider, these may also serve as a conversational aid with the patient in the feedback session, helping them to visualize where their strengths and weaknesses lie.

In summary, expanding neuropsychology into primary care requires attention to integration rather than mere co-location in order to be successful. Adopting historical neuropsychology outpatient operating procedures into the neuropsychology primary care clinic are likely to result in barriers, and neuropsychologists should consider how to triage care, simplify reports, and meet the needs of patients and providers through the facilitation of warm hand-offs and curbside consultations. Doing so has demonstrated better likelihood of completing evaluations, which creates opportunities for earlier identification to start early intervention in order to reduce the risk of downstream consequences.

Implementation Takeaway #1

Moving into the primary care setting requires a shift in practice. Providers need to:

1. Understand the core competencies required to operate as a member of an interdisciplinary team as well as some of the regulatory/financial challenges
2. Adapt their care model to be responsive to the needs of the patients in the care setting, considering a triaged care model approach
3. Be flexible, available, and resourceful—saying "no" or "not right now" to a primary care physician seeing 20–25 patients a day is a quick path toward losing the care team's trust.

Adapting Lessons Learned in Primary Care to an Epilepsy Clinic

A Primer on the Neuropsychology of Epilepsy

A primary care model of neuropsychology can also be adapted to neuropsychology specialty practices, such as those involving large scale epilepsy programs. While epilepsy neuropsychologists often focus on surgical treatment planning, there are other aspects of the disease that can benefit from neuropsychological expertise.

Epilepsy is a chronic disease of the brain characterized by unpredictable and recurrent seizures. Seizures are defined by the International League Against Epilepsy (ILAE) as, "transient occurrence of signs and/or symptoms due to abnormal excessive synchronous neuronal activity of the brain" (Fisher et al., 2005). These transient abnormal neuronal discharges not only impact our patients from a neurophysiological perspective, but also cognitively and psychologically. Indeed, both the ILAE and International Bureau for Epilepsy (IBE) specifically point out the impact that epilepsy has on an individual's cognitive, psychological, and social well-being in their updated definition of seizures and epilepsy (Fisher et al., 2005). Given this, clinical psychologists and neuropsychologists, are often asked to evaluate and treat patients with epilepsy and their work with these patients can demonstrate the power of secondary and tertiary prevention in the chronic care model.

To better understand how a chronic care model applies to epilepsy, it is important to briefly address the epidemiology and course of the disease. Epilepsy affects men and women of all ages worldwide with only a slightly higher prevalence in men compared to women (Beghi, 2020). The age of onset is bimodal with younger and older individuals having their first seizure more commonly than those in middle adulthood (Engel & Moshé, 2024). Nevertheless, seizures can arise at any point in the lifespan. Epilepsy can be subdivided into two categories, focal epilepsies, which arise from a specific location within the brain and generalized epilepsies that begin and spread throughout the whole brain (Engel & Moshé, 2024). Both types of epilepsies impact cognitive functioning; however, focal epilepsies can have a greater impact on specific subregions of the brain, which in turn tend to impact circumscribed cognitive abilities at a greater level (Elger et al., 2004). Generalized epilepsies tend to cause global cognitive dysfunction and are primarily characterized by a frontostriatal pattern of impairment seen on tests of processing speed, attention, and executive functioning (Engel & Moshé, 2024). The depth of the impact on cognitive functioning from both generalized and focal epilepsies can range from non-existent or subtle to severe and profound.

To better understand how a neuropsychologist can treat those with epilepsy, it is important to understand the impact that epilepsy can have on the natural history of both cognitive developments early in life, and cognitive aging later in the lifespan. As neuropsychologists, we understand that cognition is not a group of static abilities, but a set of dynamic attributes that change over the course of one's life. Factors like age, social and societal pressures, adverse childhood events, mental health, education, and chronic diseases such as epilepsy can have a large impact on these abilities both in terms of development early in life and the natural trajectory of decline as an individual ages. These factors amount to what is often termed "cognitive reserve" (Kremen et al., 2022). There is evidence that those who eventually develop epilepsy have deficits on neuropsychological examination even prior to their first seizure occurrence (Jackson-Tarlton et al., 2020). In addition to this, those with epilepsy, particularly drug-resistant epilepsies, often age cognitively at a greater rate than their peers—a concept known as accentuated aging (Bernas et al., 2020). Figure 6.2 shows the theoretical impact of both development and normal age-related decline in individuals with epilepsy. While it is thought that better seizure control can alter

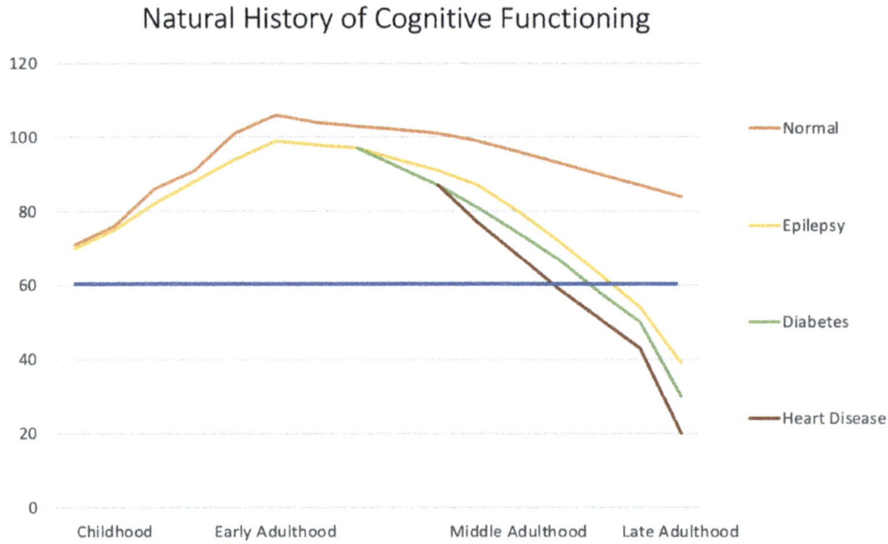

Fig. 6.2 Typical and abnormal development and aging in those with and without epilepsy (This figure represents normal cognitive development and aging (orange), as well as the typical cognitive development and aging of those with epilepsy (yellow). The blue line represents a theoretical loss of functional ability whereas individuals who fall below this line are no longer independent. The green and brown lines show the potential cumulative impact of cognitive decline with various chronic conditions such as diabetes and heart disease. By utilizing psychoeducation and lifestyle interventions early on, it is possible to nullify the added cognitive decline caused by these diseases (secondary prevention))

these trajectories that is not always the case. For this reason, it is important to counsel patients on epilepsy's impact on cognitive health.

In addition to epilepsy, there are many other potentially comorbid chronic conditions that can also alter cognitive development and aging in our patients. For example, diseases that impact metabolic functioning, liver or kidney functioning, as well as conditions such as heart disease, and cerebrovascular disease also adversely impact cognition. These conditions can have a cumulative effect on cognitive aging (Fig. 6.2) and by preventing or reducing the impact of these diseases on a patient's overall health, we preserve cognitive functioning and reduce the chance of premature functional loss (secondary prevention). In other words, we can attenuate cognitive aging in our patients with epilepsy by engaging in secondary and tertiary prevention strategies. This process of intervention to prevent the development of comorbid conditions or inhibit their effect is part of the chronic care model. Indeed, one of the first points of education and intervention in the second author's (CP) practice as a neuropsychologist is to aid patients in understanding the impact of and provide interventions to mitigate other more preventable forms of chronic illness (secondary prevention). In this way, we do not necessarily impact the effect of epilepsy on our patients' cognitive development or aging, but we provide the type of patient education and lifestyle interventions that prevent other diseases from further eroding cognitive health.

Comorbid Conditions as Targets for Intervention in Epilepsy

In addition to the impact that comorbid diseases can have on those with epilepsy, the cognitive functioning of individuals with epilepsy can also be impacted by other external factors. It is important to understand and consider these factors and how they interact to adversely impact cognition. For instance, the medication taken to control seizures often influences cognitive performance in those with epilepsy (Park & Kwon, 2008). Many patients, especially older individuals, also take medications that have anticholinergic side effects. These medications in particular have been shown to impact cognitive performance, fall risk, and even elevate the risk of death in older adults (Broder et al., 2022; Myint et al., 2015). There is also mounting evidence that anticholinergic medications can impact the cognitive performance of younger individuals as well (Cebron Lipovec et al., 2020). Although medications are often necessary for the health of the individual, psychoeducation on the impact of these medications on cognition is often useful to help patients understand their symptoms. It can also be useful to make referrals to a pharmacist, if available, who specializes in polypharmacy. At the very least, communication with the patient's treating provider about concerns of cognitive impairment related to medication use and the risks and benefits of such medications can be discussed.

Epilepsy can also affect sleep performance. Individuals can have nocturnal seizures that arise out of sleep, which can significantly disrupt the normal sleep patterns of those with epilepsy (Engel & Moshé, 2024). Obstructive sleep apnea (OSA) is another common issue that is often present in those with epilepsy (Goyal et al., 2023). Although not a direct cause of epilepsy, obstructive sleep apnea has been shown to worsen seizure frequency in those with epilepsy (Jaseja et al., 2021) and has been linked to a higher risk of the sudden unexpected death in epilepsy (SUDEP) (Soontornpun et al., 2024). OSA can also impact cognitive performance in and of itself (Gnoni et al., 2023) and these individuals carry a greater risk of cerebrovascular diseases including stroke (Yaggi et al., 2005). Finally, OSA has been linked to various metabolic diseases such as obesity, diabetes, and cardiovascular disease, which can also impact cognitive functioning, overall health, and quality of life in patients with epilepsy (Framnes & Arble, 2018; Moheet et al., 2015).

Psychiatric disorders effect approximately one third of individuals with epilepsy due to both the physiological impact of epilepsy on the brain and various psychosocial factors that are more common in individuals with epilepsy (Mula et al., 2021). Psychological conditions typically seen in those with epilepsy are often mood and anxiety disorders but can also include other less common conditions such as psychotic disorders. Individuals with epilepsy who have comorbid psychiatric conditions can also have additional cognitive deficits related to the treatment of their psychiatric conditions or the psychiatric condition themselves. Psychosis, mood disorders, impulse control disorders, and anxiety disorders have all been linked to cognitive dysfunction. Unipolar and bipolar depression for instance often impact abilities such as attention, executive functioning and memory (Marvel & Paradiso, 2004). Executive functioning and non-verbal memory deficits have been identified as common cognitive deficits suffered by individuals with obsessive compulsive disorder (Suhas & Rao, 2019), and those with psychosis often experience generalized cognitive impairment (Sheffield et al., 2018). Given the high level of comorbidity and the potential cognitive and health related consequences of psychiatric disorders in those with epilepsy, individuals should be routinely screened and treated when necessary.

Finally, there are several social factors that must be considered when treating patients with epilepsy. These factors often complicate treatment and impact cognitive health and overall quality of life. Factors such as under- or unemployment due to epilepsy, lack of transportation due to driving limitations and social isolation can all impact a patient's mental and cognitive health. There is evidence that those with epilepsy have higher rates of obesity than the general population (Janousek et al., 2013) likely owing, in part, to the social and physical isolation that often accompanies individuals with this disease, as well as the side effects of many antiseizure medications. Social and physical isolation not only impact the mental health of those with epilepsy, but there is some evidence that it can also impact cognitive health (Cardona & Andrés, 2023). Obesity too can impact cognitive health due to higher rates of metabolic diseases, inflammation, and vascular changes (Nguyen et al., 2014). It is often useful to screen patients for barriers that may impact social and physical isolation and make referrals to social work to aid with transportation, employment opportunities, or disability applications. Counseling on weight loss and the impact that this can have on physical, cognitive, and mental health are also important interventions.

The Neuropsychologist in the Epilepsy Clinic

Neuropsychologists strive to aid in the assessment and treatment of cognitive complaints seen in those with epilepsy. Indeed, a special report of the International League Against Epilepsy Neuropsychology Task Force (Wilson et al., 2015), endorsed routine screening of cognition, mood, and behavior in all individuals with new-onset epilepsy, as well as existing patients with epilepsy who have cognitive complaints. The task force also endorsed routine provision of feedback to patients, their families, and their treating providers about the implications of neuropsychological assessment results. Having neuropsychologists involved in all aspects of epilepsy care maximizes early identification of cognitive dysfunction and allows intervention early in the disease course.

In the second author's (CP) clinic, neuropsychologists are tasked with performing approximately two neuropsychological evaluations daily. Neuropsychological evaluations are conducted using a psychometrician, which allows the neuropsychologist ample time to perform clinical interviews, give feedback, and write reports. Given the reports in our interdisciplinary clinic are brief and focused, and that much of the history and workup has been done by a neurologist or other provider prior to the neuropsychologist seeing the patient, the neuropsychologist also has time to perform what we term, "Brain Health Consultations." To this end, each new patient is given a set of three questions prior to their initial appointment with their epileptologist: Are you having memory concerns, is there impact of cognitive functioning on your work or schooling, and/or are you prescribed two or more anti-epileptic drugs (AEDs) (Fig. 6.3). Two or more "yes" answers to these questions prompt a warm hand-off to our neuropsychologists following the patient's consultation with their primary epilepsy provider. The primary provider will explain to the patient the reason for the additional 15-to-30-min appointment with the neuropsychologist and an introduction is made prior to the primary provider excusing themselves from the visit. At this point, the neuropsychologist conducts a brief assessment that consists of either a neurobehavioral status examination or a more formalized computer assessment using the NIH Toolbox (Fox et al., 2022). The purpose of this examination is twofold. First, it is important to understand the patient's cognitive functioning to provide appropriate feedback and education on the cause of their potential cognitive dysfunction. For instance, language complaints that can be attributed to inattention or poor executive functioning rather than a dysfunctional language system. This has implications for the etiology of the cognitive symptom as non-specific attention and executive deficits are more likely attributable to medication side effects, sleep dysfunction, or depression compared to a more focal finding of naming deficits or verbal memory dysfunction, which is often seen in a dominant temporal lobe epilepsy (Zhao et al., 2014).

When neuropsychological screening suggests focal dysfunction that points to lateralized or localized cognitive deficits, a full neuropsychological examination is then ordered. When findings are non-focal, other potential sources of cognitive dysfunction such as those described above are considered. For instance, if a patient has several anticholinergic medications, it is briefly mentioned to the patient as a potential contributing factor and discussed with their provider. Occasionally a referral to a pharmacist may be made for more patient/provider education or adjustment of their medication. When depression appears to be a significant factor, a referral to one of the clinic's health psychologists for brief treatment and further workup is considered. The goal of the brain health consultation is not to treat the patient for every possible source of cognitive impairment, but to collaborate with the patient and their treating provider to find possible sources of poor cognitive health and offer treatments (Fig. 6.3). Indeed, by incorporating behavioral health interventions targeting lifestyle changes, psychoeducation, and providing appropriate referrals, neuropsychologists can make a profound impact on the health of our patients.

Implementation Takeaway #2

The goal of these consultations is not to find exact answers for patients, but to generate ideas in a collaborative effort with both the patient and their provider. These ideas can lead to lifestyle interventions (increased physical activity, smoking cessation), referrals to other providers for treatment of comorbid conditions that are often missed (i.e.,

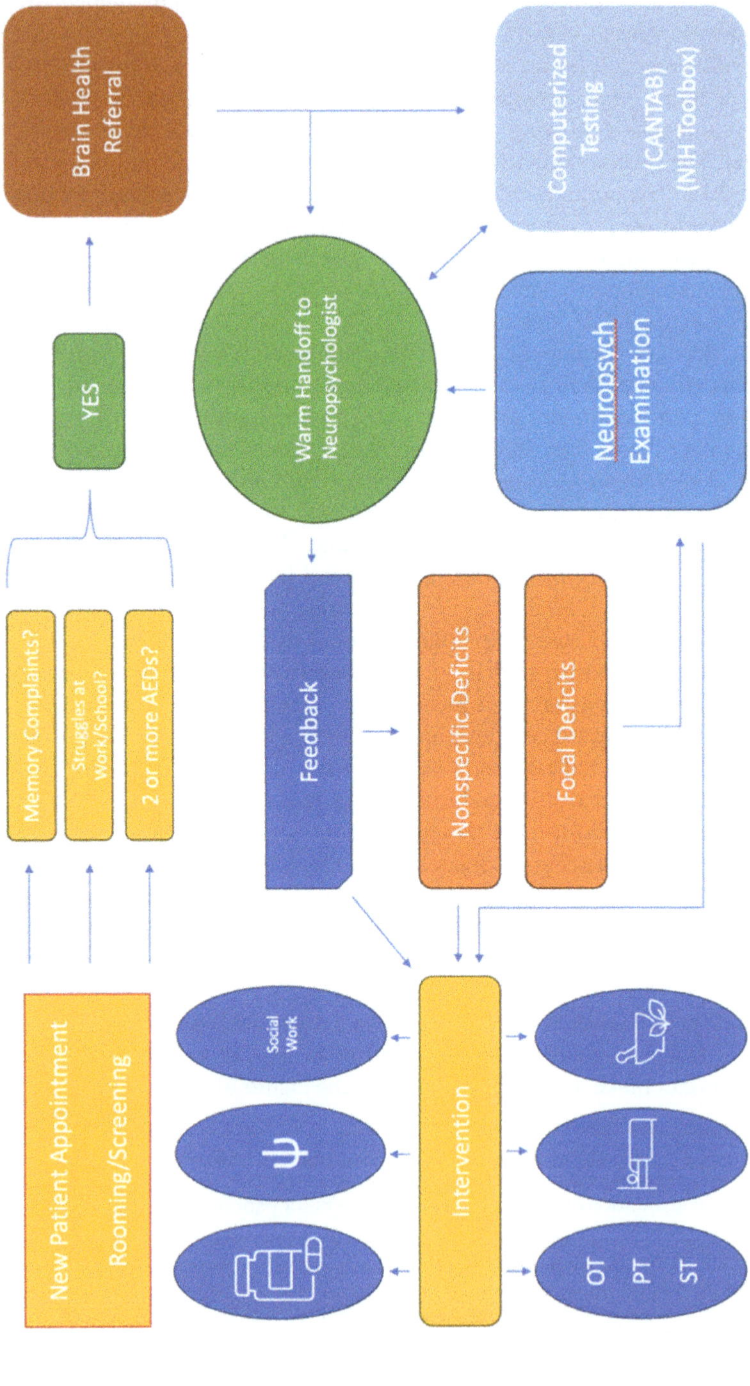

Fig. 6.3 Brain health consultation care model (This figure represents the model of brain health consultations utilized in the care of the second author's (CP) patients with epilepsy. Each new patient is screened by nursing staff prior to their appointment with their primary provider. If the patient answers yes to two or more of these questions, they are provided a consultation with a neuropsychologist. Note the interventions on this figure. Pharmacy, psychology/psychiatry, social work, medication consultation with their provider, and physical, occupational, and speech therapy consults are often utilized to help treat comorbid conditions or disorders)

obstructive sleep apnea or mood disorders), or potential medication changes (reducing anticholinergic medications, reduced reliance on diphenhydramine for sleep, etc.).

Conclusion

The integration of neuropsychologists into care teams has important implications in realizing the true intent of the biopsychosocial model and improving population health through increasing early identification and intervention of cognitive health. Regardless of care setting and population, adapting neuropsychological practices to include triaging of care and collaboration with both the care team and patient are essential. Within primary care, especially in consideration of the aging population, the focus may be on dementia screening and longitudinal tracking, early interventions for secondary prevention, and general promotion of cognitive health. However, the primary care neuropsychologist in this setting should also adapt their practice to meet the needs of a diverse range of individuals and consider different competencies required and tools (e.g., warm hand-offs) that are essential to population health management. Within an epilepsy clinic, providers appreciate that these patients may have a myriad of social, psychological, and cognitive comorbidities that impact cognitive and psychological functioning. These comorbidities warrant treatment and are often amenable to behavioral health or lifestyle interventions. The goal of the neuropsychologist is to work collaboratively with the patient and their provider to maximize cognitive and behavioral health.

Considering the quadruple aim's focus and rising care costs within the US healthcare system, future research on integration of neuropsychologists into specialty and primary care clinics will need to focus on the cost effectiveness of neuropsychological intervention and its impact on overall quality of life in these care settings. Early identification and intervention are just one component of population health though—neuropsychologists must also keep an eye toward other factors such as primary and primordial interventions which have the potential to significantly reduce the prevalence and/or burden of neurological disorders. Intentional focus on diverse populations in terms of both access to these services as well as tailored approaches to drive similar outcomes is essential. Being integrated in either a primary care or epilepsy setting hold potential promises here, and the likelihood of reaching diverse groups within these multidisciplinary care settings versus a stand-alone practice is worthy of future investigation. From an administrative/sustainability perspective, research should also focus on the impact of overall productivity of those neuropsychologists engaged in similar clinic models compared to more traditional models of neuropsychological care.

Key Points in Review

1. Early detection of cognitive disorders is essential in reducing the burden of these disorders on patients and their stakeholders.
2. Neuropsychologists must evolve their practices to meet the needs of the population they serve and integration of providers with subsequent logistical adaptations provides promise in realizing the benefits of population health.
3. Within a specialty clinic setting, individuals with epilepsy often suffer from physical, psychological, cognitive, and social comorbidities that impact health and overall quality of life. Neuropsychological interventions should be multi-faceted and include interventions focused on reducing the risk of comorbid conditions such as obesity, heart disease, and other metabolic disorders.
4. Neuropsychologists should embrace the care team and refer to multidisciplinary team members when able to better treat cognitive or psychiatric conditions related to sleep, polypharmacy, psychiatric illness, etc.
5. Similar to dementia screening models within primary care, neuropsychologists should screen all patients with epilepsy even if the patient does not have active complaints of cognitive or psychiatric dysfunction

References

American Geriatrics Society. (2023, August). Draft NIA-AA revised clinical criteria for Alzheimer's disease. https://www.americangeriatrics.org/sites/default/files/inline-files/AGS%20Comments%20on%20Draft%20NIA-AA%20Revised%20Clinical%20Criteria%20for%20Alzheimer's%20Disease%20(8%2016%2023)%20FINAL_0.pdf

APA Services, Inc. (2018, September). Resolution on psychologists in integrated primary care and specialty health care settings. https://www.apaservices.org/about/resolution-integrated-care.pdf

Azar, M., Stelmokas, J., Stringer, A., & Arias, F. (2024). Nonpharmacological treatment for older adults with mild cognitive impairment: Considerations for culturally informed clinical practice and research. *Neuropsychology, 38*(7), 609–621. https://doi.org/10.1037/neu0000965

Beghi, E. (2020). The epidemiology of epilepsy. *Neuroepidemiology, 54*(2), 185–191.

Bernas, A., Breuer, L. E. M., Lamerichs, R., de Louw, A. J. A., Aldenkamp, A. P., & Zinger, S. (2020). Accelerated cognitive ageing in epilepsy: Exploring the effective connectivity between resting-state networks and its relation to cognitive decline. *Heliyon, 6*(6), Article e03951. https://doi.org/10.1016/j.heliyon.2020.e03951

Broder, J. C., Ryan, J., Shah, R. C., Lockery, J. E., Orchard, S. G., Gilmartin-Thomas, J. F., Fravel, M. A., Owen, A. J., Woods, R. L., Wolfe, R., Storey, E., Murray, A. M., & Ernst, M. E. (2022). Anticholinergic medication burden and cognitive function in participants of the ASPREE study. *Pharmacotherapy, 42*(2), 134–144. https://doi.org/10.1002/phar.2652

Cardona, M., & Andrés, P. (2023). Are social isolation and loneliness associated with cognitive decline in ageing? *Frontiers in Aging Neuroscience, 15*, 1075563. https://doi.org/10.3389/fnagi.2023.1075563

Cerqueira, J. J., Compston, D. A. S., Geraldes, R., Rosa, M. M., Schmierer, K., Thompson, A., Tinelli, M., & Palace, J. (2018). Time matters in multiple sclerosis: Can early treatment and long-term follow-up ensure everyone benefits from the latest advances in multiple sclerosis? *Journal of neurology, neurosurgery, and psychiatry, 89*(8), 844–850. https://doi.org/10.1136/jnnp-2017-317509

Cebron Lipovec, N., Jazbar, J. & Kos, M. (2020). Anticholinergic burden in children, adults and older adults in Slovenia: A nationwide database study. *Sci Rep, 10*, 9337. https://doi.org/10.1038/s41598-020-65989-9

Chandler, M. J., Locke, D. E., Crook, J. E., Fields, J. A., Ball, C. T., Phatak, V. S., Dean, P. M., Morris, M., & Smith, G. E. (2019). Comparative effectiveness of behavioral interventions on quality of life for older adults with mild cognitive impairment: A randomized clinical trial. *JAMA network open, 2*(5), e193016. https://doi.org/10.1001/jamanetworkopen.2019.3016

Chen, M. H., Chiaravalloti, N. D., & DeLuca, J. (2021). Neurological update: Cognitive rehabilitation in multiple sclerosis. *Journal of neurology, 268*(12), 4908–4914. https://doi.org/10.1007/s00415-021-10618-2

Cuevas, H. E., Stuifbergen, A. K., Brown, S. A., & Ward, C. (2019). A nurse-led cognitive training intervention for individuals with type 2 diabetes. *Research in gerontological nursing, 12*(4), 203–212. https://doi.org/10.3928/19404921-20190612-01

Elger, C. E., Helmstaedter, C., & Kurthen, M. (2004). Chronic epilepsy and cognition. *The Lancet. Neurology, 3*(11), 663–672. https://doi.org/10.1016/S1474-4422(04)00906-8

Engel, J., & Moshé, S. L. (Eds.). (2024). Epilepsy: a comprehensive textbook (3rd ed.). Wolters Kluwer.

Fallows, R. (2019). Integration of neuropsychology into primary care: A retrospective analysis of outcomes and lessons learned from a single provider practice. *Professional Psychology: Research and Practice, 50*(6), 419-426.

Fisher, R. S., van Emde Boas, W., Blume, W., Elger, C., Genton, P., Lee, P., & Engel, J., Jr. (2005). Epileptic seizures and epilepsy: Definitions proposed by the International League Against Epilepsy (ILAE) and the International Bureau for Epilepsy (IBE). *Epilepsia, 46*(4), 470–472.

Framnes, S. N., & Arble, D. M. (2018). The bidirectional relationship between obstructive sleep Apnea and metabolic disease. *Frontiers in Endocrinology, 9*, 440. https://doi.org/10.3389/fendo.2018.00440

Fox, R. S., Zhang, M., Amagai, S., Bassard, A., Dworak, E. M., Han, Y. C., Kassanits, J., Miller, C. H., Nowinski, C. J., Giella, A. K., Stoeger, J. N., Swantek, K., Hook, J. N., & Gershon, R. C. (2022). Uses of the NIH toolbox® in clinical samples: A scoping review. *Neurology. Clinical Practice, 12*(4), 307–319. https://doi.org/10.1212/CPJ.0000000000200060

Goyal, M., Mishra, P., & Jaseja, H. (2023). Obstructive sleep apnea and epilepsy: Understanding the pathophysiology of the comorbidity. *International Journal of Physiology, Pathophysiology and Pharmacology, 15*(4), 105–114.

Gnoni, V., Mesquita, M., O'Regan, D., Delogu, A., Chakalov, I., Antal, A., Young, A. H., Bucks, R. S., Jackson, M. L., & Rosenzweig, I. (2023). Distinct cognitive changes in male patients with obstructive sleep apnoea without co-morbidities. *Frontiers in Sleep, 2*, 1097946. https://doi.org/10.3389/frsle.2023.1097946

Han, A. (2022). Effects of mindfulness-and acceptance-based interventions on quality of life, coping, cognition, and mindfulness of people with multiple sclerosis: A systematic review and meta-analysis. *Psychology, health & medicine, 27*(7), 1514–1531. https://doi.org/10.1080/13548506.2021.1894345

Hilsabeck, R. C., Perry, W., Lacritz, L., Arnett, P. A., Shah, R. C., Borson, S., Galvin, J. E., Roaten, K., Daven, M., Hwang, U., Ivey, L., Joshi, P., Parish, A. L., Wood, J., Woodhouse, J., Tsai, J., Sorweid, M., & Subramanian, U. (2024). Improving early detection of cognitive impairment in older adults in primary care clinics: Recommendations from an interdisciplinary geriatrics summit. *Annals of family medicine, 22*(6), 543–549. https://doi.org/10.1370/afm.3174

Jackson-Tarlton, C. S., Whatley, B. P., Kasheke, G. D. S., Pohlmann-Eden, B., & Omisade, A. (2020). A prospective pilot study of cognitive impairment and mood in adults with first seizure, new-onset epilepsy, and newly diagnosed epilepsy at time of initial seizure presentation. *Epilepsy & Behavior : E&b, 112*, Article 107359. https://doi.org/10.1016/j.yebeh.2020.107359

Janousek, J., Barber, A., Goldman, L., & Klein, P. (2013). Obesity in adults with epilepsy. *Epilepsy & Behavior : e&b, 28*(3), 391–394. https://doi.org/10.1016/j.yebeh.2013.05.012

Jaseja, H., Goyal, M., & Mishra, P. (2021). Drug-Resistant epilepsy and obstructive sleep apnea: Exploring a link between the two. *World Neurosurgery, 146*, 210–214. https://doi.org/10.1016/j.wneu.2020.11.099

Kremen, W. S., Elman, J. A., Panizzon, M. S., Eglit, G. M. L., Sanderson-Cimino, M., Williams, M. E., Lyons, M. J., & Franz, C. E. (2022). Cognitive reserve and related constructs: A unified framework across cognitive and brain dimensions of aging. *Frontiers in Aging Neuroscience, 14*, Article 834765. https://doi.org/10.3389/fnagi.2022.834765

Lanca, M. (2018). Integration of neuropsychology in primary care. *Archives of Clinical Neuropsychology, 33*(3), 269–279. https://doi.org/10.1093/arclin/acx135

Landfeldt, E., Castelo-Branco, A., Svedbom, A., Löfroth, E., Kavaliunas, A., & Hillert, J. (2018). The long-term impact of early treatment of multiple sclerosis on the risk of disability pension. *Journal of neurology, 265*(3), 701–707. https://doi.org/10.1007/s00415-018-8764-4

Li, G., You, Q., Hou, X., Zhang, S., Du, L., Lv, Y., & Yu, L. (2023). The effect of exercise on cognitive function in people with multiple sclerosis: A systematic review and meta-analysis of randomized controlled trials. *Journal of neurology, 270*(6), 2908–2923. https://doi.org/10.1007/s00415-023-11649-7

Lucy, C. A., Orkopoulou, E., Arble, E., Waltz, T. J., & Maragakis, A. (2025). Stepping in the right direction? Exploring mental health providers' beliefs about, training in, and use of stepped-care practices. *Professional Psychology: Research and Practice, 56*(4), 324–335. Advance online publication. https://doi.org/10.1037/pro0000627

Marvel, C. L., & Paradiso, S. (2004). Cognitive and neurological impairment in mood disorders. *The Psychiatric clinics of North America, 27*(1), 19–viii. https://doi.org/10.1016/S0193-953X(03)00106-0

McDaniel, S. H., & deGruy, F. V. III. (2014). An introduction to primary care and psychology. *American Psychologist, 69*(4), 325–331. https://doi.org/10.1037/a0036222

McDaniel, S. H., Grus, C. L., Cubic, B. A., Hunter, C. L., Kearney, L. K., Schuman, C. C., Karel, M. J., Kessler, R. S., Larkin, K. T., McCutcheon, S., Miller, B. F., Nash, J., Qualls, S. H., Connolly, K. S., Stancin, T., Stanton, A. L., Sturm, L. A., & Johnson, S. B. (2014). Competencies for psychology practice in primary care. *The American psychologist, 69*(4), 409–429. https://doi.org/10.1037/a0036072

Moheet, A., Mangia, S., & Seaquist, E. R. (2015). Impact of diabetes on cognitive function and brain structure. *Annals of the New York Academy of Sciences, 1353*, 60–71. https://doi.org/10.1111/nyas.12807

Mula, M., Kanner, A. M., Jetté, N., & Sander, J. W. (2021). Psychiatric comorbidities in people with epilepsy. *Neurology. Clinical Practice, 11*(2), e112–e120. https://doi.org/10.1212/CPJ.0000000000000874

Myint, P. K., Fox, C., Kwok, C. S., Luben, R. N., Wareham, N. J., & Khaw, K. T. (2015). Total anticholinergic burden and risk of mortality and cardiovascular disease over 10 years in 21,636 middle-aged and older men and women of EPIC-Norfolk prospective population study. *Age and Ageing, 44*(2), 219–225. https://doi.org/10.1093/ageing/afu185

Nguyen, J. C., Killcross, A. S., & Jenkins, T. A. (2014). Obesity and cognitive decline: Role of inflammation and vascular changes. *Frontiers in Neuroscience, 8*, 375. https://doi.org/10.3389/fnins.2014.00375

Park, S. P., & Kwon, S. H. (2008). Cognitive effects of antiepileptic drugs. *Journal of Clinical Neurology (Seoul, Korea), 4*(3), 99–106. https://doi.org/10.3988/jcn.2008.4.3.99

Postal, K., Chow, C., Jung, S., Erickson-Moreo, K., Geier, F., & Lanca, M. (2018). The stakeholders' project in neuropsychological report writing: A survey of neuropsychologists' and referral sources' views of neuropsychological reports. *The Clinical Neuropsychologist, 32*(3), 326–344. https://doi.org/10.1080/13854046.2017.1373859

Rose, A. J., Timbie, J. W., Setodji, C., Friedberg, M. W., Malsberger, R., & Kahn, K. L. (2019). Primary care visit regularity and patient outcomes: An observational study. *Journal of general internal medicine, 34*(1), 82–89. https://doi.org/10.1007/s11606-018-4718-x

Santo, L., & Kang, K. (2019). National ambulatory medical care survey: 2019 national summary tables. https://doi.org/10.15620/cdc:123251

Sheffield, J. M., Karcher, N. R., & Barch, D. M. (2018). Cognitive deficits in psychotic disorders: A lifespan perspective. *Neuropsychology Review, 28*(4), 509–533. https://doi.org/10.1007/s11065-018-9388-2

Smith, G., Chandler, M., Locke, D. E., Fields, J., Phatak, V., Crook, J., Hanna, S., Lunde, A., Morris, M., Graff-Radford, M., Hughes, C. A., Lepore, S., Cuc, A., Caselli, M., Hurst, D., Wethe, J., Francone, A., Eilertsen, J., Lucas, P.,… Cochran, D. (2017). Behavioral interventions to prevent or delay dementia: Protocol for a randomized comparative effectiveness study. *JMIR research protocols, 6*(11), e223. https://doi.org/10.2196/resprot.8103

Soontornpun, A., Mouchati, C., Andrews, N. D., Bena, J., Grigg-Damberger, M. M., & Foldvary-Schaefer, N. (2024). Obstructive sleep apnea is associated with risk for Sudden Unexpected Death in Epilepsy (SUDEP) using rSUDEP-7. *Epilepsy & Behavior : E&b, 161*, Article 110121. https://doi.org/10.1016/j.yebeh.2024.110121

Suhas, S., & Rao, N. P. (2019). Neurocognitive deficits in obsessive-compulsive disorder: A selective review. *Indian Journal of Psychiatry, 61*(Suppl 1), S30–S36. https://doi.org/10.4103/psychiatry.IndianJPsychiatry_517_18

Sweet, J. J., Klipfel, K. M., Nelson, N. W., & Moberg, P. J. (2020). Professional practices, beliefs, and incomes of U.S. neuropsychologists: The AACN, NAN, SCN 2020 practice and "salary survey." *The Clinical Neuropsychologist, 35*(1), 7–80. https://doi.org/10.1080/13854046.2020.1849803

Wilson, S. J., Baxendale, S., Barr, W., Hamed, S., Langfitt, J., Samson, S., Watanabe, M., Baker, G. A., Helmstaedter, C., Hermann, B. P., & Smith, M. L. (2015). Indications and expectations for neuropsychological assessment in routine epilepsy care: Report of the ILAE neuropsychology task force, diagnostic methods commission, 2013–2017. *Epilepsia, 56*(5), 674–681.

Yaggi, H. K., Concato, J., Kernan, W. N., Lichtman, J. H., Brass, L. M., & Mohsenin, V. (2005). Obstructive sleep apnea as a risk factor for stroke and death. *The New England Journal of Medicine, 353*(19), 2034–2041. https://doi.org/10.1056/NEJMoa043104

Zhao, F., Kang, H., You, L., Rastogi, P., Venkatesh, D., & Chandra, M. (2014). Neuropsychological deficits in temporal lobe epilepsy: A comprehensive review. *Annals of Indian Academy of Neurology, 17*(4), 374–382. https://doi.org/10.4103/0972-2327.144003

Chapter 7
The Community Context and Cognitive Health of Older Adults: Understanding Mechanisms and Pathways to Intervention

Abbey M. Hamlin, Victoria Leyva, and Alexandra L. Clark

Executive Summary
The community context encompasses a broad array of economic, social, built, healthcare, and educational factors that have been increasingly recognized for their role in shaping cognitive health outcomes. In this chapter, we (1) introduce a framework that emphasizes the community is an essential area of study, (2) detail ways researchers have measured community-level factors and discuss links to cognitive health disparities, (3) identify the biosocial mechanisms by which the community context may operate to impact cognition, and (4) highlight community-level interventions and make assessment recommendations for neuropsychologists to leverage that promote cognitive health.

Introduction

An estimated 416 million people worldwide are currently impacted by Alzheimer's disease (AD), and this number is projected to rapidly rise in coming decades as the population ages (Gustavsson et al., 2023). Effective disease-modifying treatments are presently limited and there is an urgent need to identify modifiable targets that

A. M. Hamlin · V. Leyva · A. L. Clark (✉)
Department of Psychology, The University of Texas at Austin, Austin, TX, USA
e-mail: alexandra.clark@austin.utexas.edu

A. M. Hamlin
e-mail: amh8767@my.utexas.edu

V. Leyva
e-mail: victoria.leyva@austin.utexas.edu

M. Lanca and R. Fallows (eds.), *Advancing Neuropsychology Through Population Health*, https://doi.org/10.1007/978-3-032-22457-6_7

may prevent or delay the onset of AD and AD-related dementias (AD/ADRD). Most research efforts have centered on identifying modifiable individual-level risk and resilience factors (e.g., physical activity, diet), which have been shown to account for approximately 40% of the risk of developing AD/ADRD (Livingston et al., 2020). While this illustrates the potential power of taking proactive preventative measures, interventions that target individual-level factors alone may be insufficient for effectively managing AD/ADRD at the population level.

A growing body of research has demonstrated that community characteristics fundamentally shape health outcomes (Besser et al., 2017; Clay et al., 2022; Yen et al., 2009). Researchers have drawn on public and private data sources (e.g., census records, geospatial mapping) to identify key community-level features (Diez Roux & Mair, 2010), revealing that the availability of economic resources, green space, and social infrastructure is associated with both levels and rates of cognitive decline in older adults (Besser et al., 2017; Michael et al., 2024). However, at present, there is no consensus as to what contextual features are most strongly associated with AD/ADRD and may therefore be ideal intervention targets (Diez Roux & Mair, 2010; Michael et al., 2024). There is also a need to better understand the mechanisms by which contextual exposures may "get under the skin" to indirectly shape late-life cognitive and brain health outcomes (Finlay et al., 2022). Finally, there is a paucity of research on the implementation of community-level interventions, which is problematic given that the distribution of community-level resources may also play an important role in racial/ethnic disparities of AD/ADRD (Clark et al., 2022; Hamlin et al., 2025).

The Link Between the Community Context and AD/ADRD Outcomes

The relationship between the community context and AD/ADRD outcomes involves: (1) direct pathways, in which environmental conditions influence cognitive, brain, and everyday functioning outcomes, and (2) indirect pathways, in which the environment shapes individual-level factors (e.g., biological processes, psychosocial functioning, and health behaviors) that are directly linked to cognitive aging and neurodegeneration. Figure 7.1 provides an overview of these relationships and is the theoretical model that directs our own research investigations. The direct and indirect pathways depicted can be moderated by individual-level characteristics (e.g., race/ethnicity, gender, socioeconomic status) and should be examined across the life course (e.g., early-, mid-, and late-life). The life course perspective is a key piece of the model, as the impact of community-level exposures is often cumulative (Clarke et al., 2014), or there may be sensitive or critical periods when environmental exposures exert particularly strong effects (George et al., 2020).

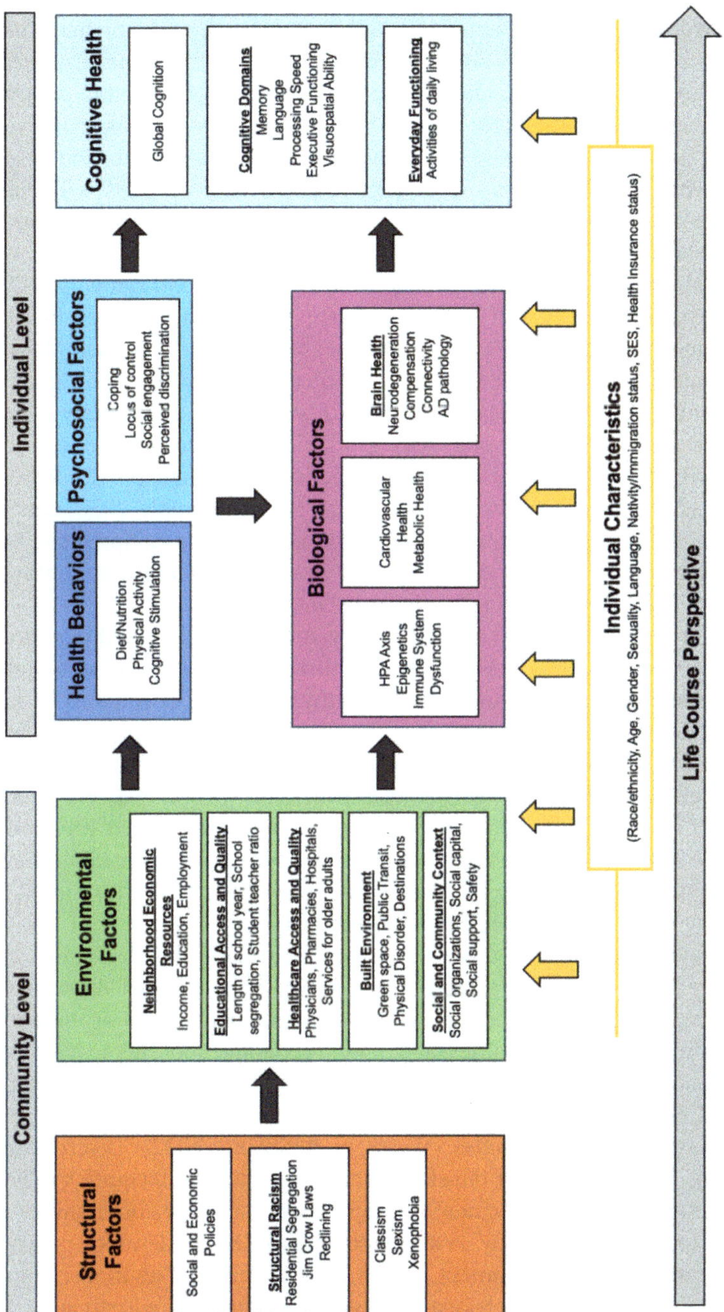

Fig. 7.1 Conceptual model of links between community context and cognitive health

Informed by Bronfenbrenner's ecological systems theory, our model emphasizes that health outcomes are the byproduct of dynamic interactions between individuals and the larger ecological systems in which they exist (Bronfenbrenner, 1977). These systems span from macro-level structural policies to micro-level neighborhood factors that are delineated under the "community-level" box within the framework. While the community shapes individual-level health outcomes, individual characteristics and needs will also affect how people engage with and respond to community-based interventions. The most effective interventions will operate across multiple socio-ecological levels—addressing both environmental constraints and individual-level factors.

The model also borrows content from the Healthy People 2030 campaign (Office of Disease Prevention and Health Promotion, n.d.), which has identified that there are five community-level features relevant to health outcomes: (1) neighborhood economic resources, (2) education access and quality, (3) healthcare access and quality, (4) built environment features, and (5) social and community context. However, there are alternative frameworks available, and there has been no clear consensus on which features should be prioritized in research studies (Finlay et al., 2022; Griffith et al., 2023; Hill et al., 2015). The Healthy People 2030 campaign conceptualization has been adopted into our work, as it offers a comprehensive and policy-relevant categorization of environmental domains that are measurable and hypothesized to indirectly and directly impact AD/ADRD risk.

Structural forces—including economic policy, urban planning, and institutional practices—have fundamentally shaped the distribution and quality of community-level features that represent each of the five Healthy People 2030 domains (Adkins-Jackson et al., 2023). These structural forces have systematically constrained access to important environmental resources for racially/ethnically minoritized older adults due to interlocking systems of racism, classism, and xenophobia. As a result, racially/ethnically minoritized and socioeconomically disadvantaged groups have often borne the brunt of disinvestment and exclusionary policies, leading them to reside in communities with unequal concentrations of both health-promoting and health-depleting resources (Williams & Collins, 2001).

Neighborhood economic resources have been shaped by discriminatory mortgage lending practices (known as redlining), urban renewal, and disinvestment (Swope & Hernández, 2019). These policies have restricted wealth accumulation, reduced homeownership opportunities, and limited economic mobility in historically marginalized communities. Educational access and quality factors are intimately tied to racially and economically segregated school systems and perpetuated by local property tax-based funding formulas (Weathers & Sosina, 2022). Discriminatory health planning, underinvestment in safety-net institutions, and inequities in health insurance coverage and reimbursement practices have left many communities with limited access to healthcare. Lastly, investments in built (e.g., sidewalks, parks, and safe housing) and social environment resources (e.g., civic institutions, community organizations) have disproportionately favored wealthier, predominately Non-Hispanic White neighborhoods via discriminatory zoning laws and urban planning (Finlay et al., 2022). Ultimately, today's community context reflects the cumulative impact of upstream structural forces that have operated over decades. Researchers studying the role of the community context on AD/ADRD outcomes must consider these structural and historical dynamics, as they have implications for study design, measurement decisions, and the interpretation of findings.

Direct Links Between the Community Context and AD/ADRD Outcomes

Studies linking contextual features to AD/ADRD outcomes have occasionally yielded mixed results. These inconsistencies may partially stem from critical differences in sample characteristics (e.g., racial/ethnic demographics) and contextual settings (e.g., urban vs. rural). However, the lack of standardization in how contextual features are measured also limits comparability across studies, making it more difficult to draw conclusions about the role of contextual features in shaping cognitive health (Besser et al., 2017). In the section that follows, we concentrate on a set of commonly utilized objective and subjective measures to operationalize these domains and discuss measurement issues to address in future research investigations.

Neighborhood Economic Resources

Neighborhood economic resources represent the extent to which a community context is characterized by economic stability and access to economic opportunities. Neighborhood economic resources are typically measured as a composite of multiple objective socioeconomic indicators (e.g., income, education, employment, poverty) assessed at the community level (e.g., area deprivation index [ADI], neighborhood disadvantage). These measures can be calculated at multiple geographic levels (e.g., block group, census tract), as well as across different time points (e.g., 2000, 2010) using census data (Clarke et al., 2012; Kind & Buckingham, 2018).

A recent systematic review of 15 studies suggested that there is moderately strong evidence for the association between neighborhood economic resources and cognitive outcomes (Besser et al., 2017). The majority of studies demonstrate that lower neighborhood economic resources characterized by higher ADI or individual indicators (e.g., proportion below the poverty line) are associated with worse cognition, greater AD/ADRD pathology (Powell et al., 2020), smaller total and hippocampal brain volume (Hunt et al., 2020), and alterations in functional connectivity (Rakesh et al., 2021). However, evidence for the effects of neighborhood economic resources on rates of cognitive decline has been inconclusive, with some studies finding that lower neighborhood economic resources are associated with faster rates of cognitive decline (Hunt et al., 2021; Vassilaki et al., 2023), while others have found no significant association (Meyer et al., 2017; Zeki Al Hazzouri et al., 2011). One study showed that the effects of neighborhood economic resources varied by race such that living in a community with fewer economic resources was associated with faster rates of decline in cognitive and functional outcomes among Black, but not non-Hispanic White adults (Clark et al., 2022; Hamlin et al., 2025). Black older adults may experience the double disadvantage of living in an economically deprived community without the personal financial resources to help cope, increasing their susceptibility to the negative impacts of low economic resources on cognitive health outcomes compared to non-Hispanic White older adults.

Despite the growing use of neighborhood economic resource measures in AD/ADRD research, there remain several challenges to effectively measuring this construct. Research has demonstrated that the ADI is not stable across place and time, which makes it problematic to compare neighborhood economic resources between neighborhoods or use the same indicator variables today that were used in past decades (Berg et al., 2021). For example, median gross rent was shown to be a stronger indicator of neighborhood financial strength in the state of New York compared to Minnesota (Berg et al., 2021). In terms of neighborhood economic resources over time, National Neighborhood Data Archive (NaNDA) measures of neighborhood disadvantage from 2000 to 2016 included the proportion of female-headed families and the proportion of residents identifying as non-Hispanic Black, but these variables no longer reflect concentrated economic disadvantage in the recent 2016–2020 American Community Survey (ACS) data (Clarke & Melendez, 2023). This change represents how the link between certain social characteristics and neighborhood economic resources has weakened over time. Researchers should consider identifying which socioeconomic indicators are most relevant to their sample and are most stably related to economic resources over time.

Educational Access and Quality

Educational access and quality refer to the availability of educational opportunities, levels of educational attainment, as well as the conditions within schools that may affect the quality of education. The accessibility of educational opportunities may be measured by utilizing public establishment data to examine the spatial distribution and availability of K-12 schools, community colleges, university campuses, and trade or technical schools within neighborhoods. Neighborhood-level educational attainment has been examined using census data to quantify the proportion of residents with higher levels of education (e.g., bachelor's degree or higher) within a census tract (Meyer et al., 2017). Educational quality can also be measured by leveraging public education data that characterizes the level of school funding per student, curriculum, length of school year, student–teacher ratios, literacy levels, urban versus rural location, and school segregation levels (Crowe et al., 2013; Seblova et al., 2023; Sisco et al., 2015).

While individual-level educational attainment has been extensively studied as a protective factor for cognitive health, community-level measures of educational quality have received less attention (Glymour & Manly, 2008). Studies have found that increases in mandatory years of schooling and attending school in a county with higher student–teacher ratios were associated with higher levels of cognitive functioning (Crowe et al., 2013; Glymour et al., 2008). The use of school-based longitudinal cohorts (e.g., Project Talent Aging Study) has allowed researchers to obtain more granular measures of school quality (e.g., dropout rates, teacher education levels, school size) and they found that attending a high school with a higher number of teachers with graduate training was most consistently associated with better late-life cognitive functioning (Seblova et al., 2023). Evidence for the effects of school-based segregation on cognitive outcomes is mixed; several studies have found that attending a segregated school is associated with worse cognitive outcomes in late life (Gutierrez et al., 2024; Mantri et al., 2019), while other studies have reported worse cognitive and physical performance among Black older adults who attended desegregated schools (Lamar et al., 2020; Wolinsky et al., 2012). The experience of school desegregation likely had both positive and negative consequences for Black older adults who may have gained access to schools with higher quality resources but were subsequently exposed to interpersonal discrimination from non-Hispanic White students and teachers.

Although measures of educational quality and resources have been increasingly incorporated into longitudinal cohorts, this research has largely relied on retrospective reports that ask participants to answer questions pertaining to select time periods (e.g., elementary school, age 10). These retrospective reports are subject to measurement error and do not allow researchers to examine whether exposures to features of educational contexts during different epochs (e.g., elementary school, high school, college) are more strongly related to cognitive outcomes. Future prospective studies should consider collecting educational histories, which would allow researchers to better quantify the length of exposure to different educational contexts and integrate measures of educational quality from public archival data at a more granular level.

Healthcare Access and Quality

Healthcare access and quality refer to the availability of healthcare services (e.g., primary care, outpatient clinics) and establishments (e.g., pharmacies), as well as perceived access to those services (Burstin et al., 2016). Living in a community with fewer healthcare establishments has been associated with lower levels of cognition (Clay et al., 2022) and higher odds of cognitive impairment (Mullins et al., 2021). However, other studies have found that higher access to healthcare was associated with faster rates of memory and reasoning decline, particularly among White participants, and a higher risk of ADRD diagnosis (Hamlin et al., 2025; Rebok et al., 2023). These findings suggest that individuals who have greater healthcare access start out with higher baseline levels of cognitive function and cognitive reserve in mid-life and may therefore have further to fall when cognitive health begins deteriorating in later life.

Disparate patterns of findings may also be related to variability across studies in terms of accounting for important individual-level variables (e.g., health insurance) that determine healthcare access and utilization (Kirby & Kaneda, 2005). For example, urban environments may have greater availability of healthcare facilities that are adjacent to communities of color (Small & McDermott, 2006). However, racially/ethnically minoritized adults often have more limited health insurance coverage, which can reduce their ability to access these resources (Hargraves & Hadley, 2003). Examining which types of health insurance (e.g., Medicare, Medicaid) are adopted by these hospital systems and the number of low-income patients treated in these facilities may be important ways to better understand the availability of healthcare resources and who can access them. Future research incorporating healthcare quality measures, including the racial/ethnic diversity of medical providers, patterns of hospital segregation, and disparities in treatment outcomes, may be especially important for understanding AD/ADRD risk (Nelson, 2002).

Built Environment

The built environment encompasses the physical infrastructure of the community context including the streets, parks, buildings, public transit, and land use. Greater access to green space (Besser et al., 2023), public transit (Chan et al., 2023), and neighborhood amenities (e.g., physical/recreational facilities, retail destinations, eating places; Besser et al., 2018; Finlay et al., 2021a) have been associated with better cognitive outcomes. Positive associations between green space and MRI measures (e.g., cortical thickness, volumes) have also been observed (Besser, 2021). However, some studies have shown that living in a context with greater urban density had no effect or was negatively associated with cognition, and effects on cognitive outcomes have differed across racial/ethnic groups (Besser et al., 2018; Clarke et al., 2012). One qualitative study revealed that although Black individuals were more likely to live in neighborhoods with denser museums and cultural institutions, fewer Black participants reported visiting these institutions likely due to the fact that these institutions have historically excluded them (Finlay et al., 2021b).

It may also be the case that perceptions of the physical environment are more directly related to cognitive health than objective measures. Subjective assessments of neighborhood physical disorder (e.g., vandalism, vacant homes) may reflect the lived experiences of community members and better capture how individuals psychologically and behaviorally respond to their community context (Weden et al., 2008). Prior research has shown that perceiving higher levels of physical disorder was associated with worse levels of cognition and mediated the relationship between objective measures of the built environment and cognitive outcomes (Lee & Waite, 2018). Additional work is needed to further characterize both objective and subjective aspects of the built environment to determine their relative influences on cognitive health.

Social and Community Context

The social and community context is characterized by the social features of the environment including social connections between community members, social capital, levels of safety/social disorder, and norms. While social measures usually consist of these non-physical aspects of the community context, some researchers have also considered social infrastructure (e.g., social services, social destinations, religious institutions) as important features of the social and community context given that physical places dedicated to social engagement can directly facilitate social behaviors (Clay et al., 2022; Diez Roux & Mair, 2010; Yen et al., 2009). Objective measures, including the density of civic and social organizations, and subjective measures, such as perceived social cohesion, have been linked to better cognitive outcomes (Finlay et al., 2022; Zaheed et al., 2019). However, other studies have observed negative associations between social environment measures (e.g., social destinations, social cohesion) and cognitive outcomes (Besser et al., 2018; Estrella et al., 2020). The lack of culturally specific measures may partially explain mixed evidence given that measures of social environment may not always capture the social aspects that are most relevant to Black and Latino older adults, leading to an underestimation of the unique sources of psychosocial resiliency. For example, our previous work has shown that greater participation in social activities was associated with better cognitive performance among non-Hispanic White, but not Black older adults (Hamlin et al., 2022). The measure of social activity did not include participation in religious/spiritual groups, which may be a particularly salient form of social engagement among Black older adults (Kraal et al., 2019). Developing better measures of sociocultural factors (e.g., Black social capital, religiosity, familismo) is especially needed to help clarify which factors may underly the "barrio advantage" in which minoritized older adults residing in segregated communities largely surrounded by their peers exhibit better cognitive health outcomes despite experiencing socioeconomic disadvantages (Padeiro et al., 2022).

Indirect Pathways Between the Community Context and AD/ADRD Outcomes

Community-level factors can also influence individual cognitive health outcomes indirectly through biological, behavioral, and psychosocial mechanisms. However, studies that directly examine mediational models of these pathways are limited (Clarke & Nieuwenhuijsen, 2009).

Biological Mechanisms

Research has consistently shown that living in a community context with few economic resources, deteriorating physical infrastructure, and higher crime is associated with chronic stress (Barrington et al., 2014; Sharifian et al., 2020). Chronic stress disrupts multiple biological systems and causes "wear and tear" on the body that can be characterized by overactivation of the hypothalamic–pituitary–adrenal (HPA) axis, immune system dysfunction (e.g., dampened or overactive immune response), and poor metabolic and cardiovascular health (Kuo et al., 2019; Lupien et al., 2018). Allostatic load refers to the cumulative burden of prolonged stress exposure across multiple biological systems and has been directly linked to poor consequences for cognitive and brain health outcomes (Juster et al., 2010). Moreover, extrinsic factors, such as exposure to air pollution, have been associated with alterations in gene expression (e.g., DNA methylation) and accelerated rates of biological aging (Yannatos et al., 2023).

Behavioral and Psychosocial Mechanisms

Health behaviors that are strongly linked to cognitive function—such as physical activity, eating nutritious foods, and cognitive stimulation—are often shaped by the community context. For example, the presence of recreational facilities and grocery stores has been associated with higher levels of physical activity and better access to healthy foods (Frank et al., 2022; McCormack & Shiell, 2011). In contrast, safety concerns, limited walkability, or the presence of polluting sites may discourage health-promoting behaviors (Yu et al., 2023). Features of the community context may also facilitate cognitively stimulating behaviors that maintain brain structure and connectivity. For example, the availability of cultural and learning institutions (e.g., museums, libraries) may provide opportunities for intellectually stimulating activities (Besser et al., 2018; Finlay et al., 2021b).

Psychosocial mechanisms (e.g., social engagement, adaptive coping, locus of control) may be especially important sources of cognitive resilience within marginalized communities experiencing resource deprivation. Communities characterized by high levels of social cohesion and collective efficacy (e.g., ethnic enclaves) may foster positive psychosocial factors (e.g., higher internal locus of control) within individuals that help protect cognitive functioning (Clark et al., 2024; Hamlin et al., 2025). At the same time, some communities may have historical and cultural features (e.g., legacy of Jim Crow, residential segregation) that increase the likelihood of experiencing racial discrimination, which has been associated with worse cognitive function among racially/ethnically minoritized older adults (Barnes et al., 2012).

Important Limitations and Future Directions

Quantifying aspects of the community context can be incredibly difficult, as is apparent from our brief review of measurement strategies in the current literature. While novices may have to invest a considerable amount of time into coding in order to integrate public geographic data into research studies, open science initiatives centered on the sharing of code from seasoned researchers can help ease the task at hand and enhance reproducibility. Given that the effects of community context are often small in magnitude, it can be difficult to parse out any indirect effects of individual health mechanisms when examining AD/ADRD outcomes. Large cohort studies such as Health and Aging Brain: Health Disparities Study—which includes a large, diverse sample of Black, Hispanic, and Non-Hispanic White individuals, along with robust biomarker plasma and neuroimaging biomarker data—hold incredible promise for providing important insight in the coming years (Petersen et al., 2025). Relatedly, merely living near a resourced area does not guarantee access to benefits—engagement may be shaped by a range of individual-level, interpersonal, and systemic barriers. The use of wearable activity trackers that collect geospatial data can help us to better understand the link between environmental exposures and actual health behaviors (e.g., walking, sleep). Ultimately, knowing which specific mechanisms are most relevant to the individual and the context they live within can inform precision medicine approaches.

Most studies of community context have measured environmental features cross-sectionally, but communities can experience gradual or rapid changes in physical and social features and individuals are usually exposed to different community contexts throughout their life course. Changing administrative boundaries for census tracts and block groups make it more challenging to estimate community exposures across time. However, public databases have harmonized census tract boundaries between census years to improve estimation of the true effect of community-level changes (Logan et al., 2014). Residential histories can also allow researchers to link existing cohort data to geocoded, time-concordant measures of community context. This improves estimation of the effects of cumulative exposures to environmental features and allows researchers to determine how changes in community context impact AD/ADRD risk.

Implementation Takeaway #1

While existing studies have examined the presence of community features (e.g., senior centers, parks), research characterizing engagement in these resources or changes in resources availability over time is needed. To bridge this gap, researchers can (1) integrate qualitative research methods and survey measures to quantify how often participants engage with specific local amenities and (2) assess changes in the environment over time (e.g., desegregation, gentrification) using longitudinal public archival data to better estimate changes in community-level factors.

Translating Research into Community-Level Interventions

Researchers are now beginning to test community-level interventions that may be helpful for preventing or delaying the onset of AD/ADRD. One of these community-level interventions has taken place in Japan, and involved examining the effects of opening salons (i.e., community centers) on the onset of cognitive disability (Hikichi et al., 2017). Community salons created spaces where residents could socialize and participate in exercises (e.g., light stretching) and engage in cognitively stimulating activities (e.g., crafts, playing instruments, games). The study found that the proportion of residents participating in salons increased over time and that the frequency of salon participation was associated with a lower incidence of cognitive disability. This study suggests that community-level investments that include creating spaces for social interaction may be an effective approach to preventing cognitive decline.

> **Implementation Takeaway #2**
> Creating community contexts that support cognitive health will require clinical neuropsychologists to collaborate with community partners. The AARP Livable Communities program provides a strong model of translating research into practice by funding small grants to support livability projects and sharing free toolkits to help researchers implement age-friendly improvements in their communities (AARP.org).

Other researchers have partnered with local YMCA branches for a multi-site clinical trial of a physical exercise intervention in adults with mild cognitive impairment (Shadyab et al., 2025). Participants demonstrated over 80% adherence to the intervention and sustained engagement over 12 months was associated with reduced brain volume loss. Implementing the intervention in local community fitness centers improved the external validity of the study and helped build an intervention model that could be easily translated to other communities using existing fitness facilities. The success of this intervention model demonstrates that leveraging local expertise and infrastructure, such as the YMCA, can help researchers to optimize intervention delivery to sustain behavioral changes, potentially even beyond the study's conclusion, and improve the brain health of older adults.

Researchers have also endeavored to design interventions that are effective and applicable across broad geographic and cultural contexts. The World Wide FINGERS research network is one example of a global collaboration between countries in North and South America, Europe, and Asia that are working together to test the efficacy of a multi-domain lifestyle intervention for dementia prevention consisting of physical activity, nutritional counseling, cognitive training, and psychosocial support. Importantly, these interventions are tailored to each country's unique cultural, socioeconomic, and healthcare context. For example, while the original FINGERS trial in Finland provided nutrition recommendations based on a healthy Nordic diet, the Latin American trial utilizes a Mediterranean-like diet composed of locally available ingredients and consistent with regional dietary habits (Crivelli et al., 2023).

This research marks an important step towards implementing individual interventions across diverse contexts. However, further work is needed to directly examine how environmental factors (e.g., social infrastructure, built environment, healthcare access) shape the successful implementation and adoption of these interventions.

Researchers and clinicians must also work to bridge the gap between science, public policy, and clinical practice to reduce the risk for AD/ADRD across communities. We have created a table with examples of how to integrate community context considerations into clinical practice for neuropsychologists to leverage when seeing patients (Table 7.1). At the individual-level, clinical neuropsychologist can begin to incorporate measures of community context into their assessments and reports by directly highlighting and addressing for medical providers how environmental resources and barriers may be impacting their patient's cognitive health. Taken together, advancing cognitive health and reducing the burden of AD/ADRD will require coordinated care efforts. Individual-level clinical practices with community-driven intervention and policy initiatives will ensure both personal and community factors are addressed in prevention and care.

Key Points in Review

1. **Community Context as a Modifiable Target for Intervention**: Features of the community context represent important modifiable targets for reducing the risk of AD/ADRD at the population level. However, further research is needed to clarify the biosocial mechanisms (e.g., stress, health behaviors) through which community features influence cognitive and brain health.
2. **Addressing Structural Inequalities to Promote Cognitive Health Equity:** Contextual resources are not distributed evenly. Racially/ethnically minoritized older adults often face community-level and individual-level barriers to accessing resources. Researchers and policymakers must address the structural drivers of inequality (e.g., residential segregation, redlining) through economic and social policy reform.
3. Additional resources:

   a. National Neighborhood Data Archive (https://nanda.isr.umich.edu/data/)
   b. IPUMS National Historical Geographic Information System data (https://www.nhgis.org/)
   c. Longitudinal Tract Database (https://s4.ad.brown.edu/projects/diversity/researcher/bridging.htm)
   d. AARP Livable Communities (https://www.aarp.org/livable-communities/)

Table 7.1 Integrating community context into clinical neuropsychology practice

Environmental factor	Clinical application
Neighborhood economic resources	Collect patients' residential addresses to assess neighborhood-level economic resources using tools like the Area Deprivation Index (ADI). This information can inform decisions regarding the appropriateness of applying normative data, which are often based on high socioeconomic status populations
Educational access and quality	Assess the quality of the patient's education beyond years of school attended. Ask questions about class sizes, school resources, geographic context (e.g., rural vs urban), and whether the school was segregated or desegregated during their attendance. A deeper understanding of educational quality can provide greater context to performance on cognitive testing
Healthcare access and quality	Identify barriers to healthcare access such as transportation, insurance coverage, or provider availability. Offering telethealth may help improve the accessibility of neuropsychological services. Research studies such as the Washington Heights and Inwood Community Aging project (WHICAP) have implemented home visits and field-based cognitive assessments to improve the representativeness of their research samples by ensuring older adults with transportation or mobility limitations are included (Manly et al., 2005)
Built environment	Consider how characteristics of the built environment (e.g., safety, walkability, availability of recreation centers/grocery stores) may influence whether patients are able to implement lifestyle recommendations. For example, patients who live in a low-resource neighborhood may not be able to join a gym, participate in clubs at a recreation center, or shop for healthy foods. Recommending online exercise classes, virtual social groups, and meals on wheels may improve the feasibility of interventions for this population
Social and community context	Leverage multiple family members (with patient consent) to address care needs during feedback sessions. Connecting patients with a care ecosystem service where a care professional helps to manage their providers and medical appointments can also help reduce the burden on individual family members and overcome barriers for patients with limited social support

Acknowledgements We would like to acknowledge Asmi Dhotre for her assistance in preparing the table and supporting the development of this chapter.

References

Adkins-Jackson, P. B., George, K. M., Besser, L. M., Hyun, J., Lamar, M., Hill-Jarrett, T. G., Bubu, O. M., Flatt, J. D., Heyn, P. C., Cicero, E. C., Zarina Kraal, A., Pushpalata Zanwar, P., Peterson, R., Kim, B., Turner, R. W., II., Viswanathan, J., Kulick, E. R., …, Babulal, G. (2023). The structural and social determinants of Alzheimer's disease related dementias. *Alzheimer's & Dementia, 19*(7), 3171–3185. https://doi.org/10.1002/alz.13027

AARP. (n.d.). *AARP livable communities*. https://www.aarp.org/livable-communities/

Barnes, L. L., Lewis, T. T., Begeny, C. T., Yu, L., Bennett, D. A., & Wilson, R. S. (2012). Perceived discrimination and cognition in older African Americans. *Journal of the International Neuropsychological Society, 18*(5), 856–865. https://doi.org/10.1017/S1355617712000628

Barrington, W. E., Stafford, M., Hamer, M., Beresford, S. A. A., Koepsell, T., & Steptoe, A. (2014). Neighborhood socioeconomic deprivation, perceived neighborhood factors, and cortisol responses to induced stress among healthy adults. *Health & Place, 27*, 120–126. https://doi.org/10.1016/j.healthplace.2014.02.001

Berg, K. A., Dalton, J. E., Gunzler, D. D., Coulton, C. J., Freedman, D. A., Krieger, N. I., Dawson, N. V., & Perzynski, A. T. (2021). The ADI-3: A revised neighborhood risk index of the social determinants of health over time and place. *Health Services and Outcomes Research Methodology, 21*(4), 486–509. https://doi.org/10.1007/s10742-021-00248-6

Besser, L. M. (2021). Outdoor green space exposure and brain health measures related to Alzheimer's disease: A rapid review. *British Medical Journal Open, 11*(5), Article e043456. https://doi.org/10.1136/bmjopen-2020-043456

Besser, L. M., Jimenez, M. P., Reimer, C. J., Meyer, O. L., Mitsova, D., George, K. M., Adkins-Jackson, P. B., & Galvin, J. E. (2023). Diversity of studies on neighborhood greenspace and brain health by racialized/ethnic group and geographic region: A rapid review. *International Journal of Environmental Research and Public Health, 20*(9). https://doi.org/10.3390/ijerph20095666

Besser, L. M., McDonald, N. C., Song, Y., Kukull, W. A., & Rodriguez, D. A. (2017). Neighborhood environment and cognition in older adults: A systematic review. *American Journal of Preventive Medicine, 53*(2), 241–251. https://doi.org/10.1016/j.amepre.2017.02.013

Besser, L. M., Rodriguez, D. A., McDonald, N., Kukull, W. A., Fitzpatrick, A. L., Rapp, S. R., & Seeman, T. (2018). Neighborhood built environment and cognition in non-demented older adults: The Multi-Ethnic Study of Atherosclerosis. *Social Science & Medicine, 200*, 27–35. https://doi.org/10.1016/j.socscimed.2018.01.007

Bronfenbrenner, U. (1977). Toward an experimental ecology of human development. *American Psychologist, 32*(7), 513–531. https://doi.org/10.1037/0003-066X.32.7.513

Burstin, H., Leatherman, S., & Goldmann, D. (2016). The evolution of healthcare quality measurement in the United States. *Journal of Internal Medicine, 279*(2), 154–159. https://doi.org/10.1111/joim.12471

Chan, O. F., Liu, Y., Guo, Y., Lu, S., Chui, C. H. K., Ho, H. C., Song, Y., Cheng, W., Chiu, R. L. H., Webster, C., & Lum, T. Y. S. (2023). Neighborhood built environments and cognition in later life. *Aging & Mental Health, 27*(3), 466–474. https://doi.org/10.1080/13607863.2022.2046697

Clark, A. L., Thomas, K. R., Ortega, N., Haley, A. P., Duarte, A., O'Bryant, S., for the HABS-HD Study Team. (2024). Empirically derived psychosocial-behavioral phenotypes in Black/African American and Hispanic/Latino older adults enrolled in HABS-HD: Associations with AD biomarkers and cognitive outcomes. *Alzheimer's & Dementia, 20*(2), 1360–1373. https://doi.org/10.1002/alz.13544

Clark, A. L., Weigand, A. J., Clay, O. J., Owens, J., Fiala, J., Crowe, M., Marsiske, M., & Thomas, K. R. (2022). Associations between social determinants of health and 10-year change in everyday functioning within Black/African American and White older adults enrolled in ACTIVE. *Alzheimer's & Dementia, 14*(1), Article e12385. https://doi.org/10.1002/dad2.12385

Clarke, P. J., Ailshire, J. A., House, J. S., Morenoff, J. D., King, K., Melendez, R., & Langa, K. M. (2012). Cognitive function in the community setting: The neighbourhood as a source of 'cognitive reserve'? *Journal of Epidemiology and Community Health, 66*(8), 730–736. https://doi.org/10.1136/jech.2010.128116

Clarke, P. J., & Melendez, R. (2023). *The National Neighborhood Data Archive (NaNDA): 2016–2020 neighborhood sociodemographic measures technical documentation on index creation.* https://doi.org/10.7302/7033

Clarke, P. J., Morenoff, J., Debbink, M., Golberstein, E., Elliott, M. R., & Lantz, P. M. (2014). Cumulative exposure to neighborhood context: Consequences for health transitions over the adult life course. *Research on Aging, 36*(1), 115–142. https://doi.org/10.1177/0164027512470702

Clarke, P. J., & Nieuwenhuijsen, E. R. (2009). Environments for healthy ageing: A critical review. *Maturitas, 64*(1), 14–19. https://doi.org/10.1016/j.maturitas.2009.07.011

Clay, O. J., Ball, K. K., Wheeler, K. M., Crowe, M., Marsiske, M., Dean, L. T., Thorpe, R. J., Jones, R., Owens, J. H., Rebok, G. W., & Willis, S. L. (2022). Evaluating social determinants of health domains and their predictive validity within Black/African American and White older adults from the ACTIVE Trial. *Journal of Aging and Health, 35*(9_suppl), 11S–18S. https://doi.org/10.1177/08982643221111205

Crivelli, L., Calandri, I. L., Kimie Suemoto, C., Salinas, R. M., Velilla, L. M., Yassuda, M. S., Caramelli, P., Lopera, F., Nitrini, R., Sevlever, G. E., Sosa, A. L., Acosta, D., Baietti, A. M. C., Cusicanqui, M. I., Custodio, N., De Simone, S. D., Derio, C. D., Duque-Peñailillo, L., Duran, J. C., … & Allegri, R. F. (2023). Latin American initiative for lifestyle intervention to prevent cognitive decline (LatAm-FINGERS): Study design and harmonization. *Alzheimer's & Dementia: The Journal of the Alzheimer's Association, 19*(9), 4046–4060. https://doi.org/10.1002/alz.13101

Crowe, M., Clay, O. J., Martin, R. C., Howard, V. J., Wadley, V. G., Sawyer, P., & Allman, R. M. (2013). Indicators of childhood quality of education in relation to cognitive function in older adulthood. *The Journals of Gerontology: Series A, 68*(2), 198–204. https://doi.org/10.1093/gerona/gls122

Diez Roux, A. V., & Mair, C. (2010). Neighborhoods and health. *Annals of the New York Academy of Sciences, 1186*(1), 125–145. https://doi.org/10.1111/j.1749-6632.2009.05333.x

Estrella, M. L., Durazo-Arvizu, R. A., Gallo, L. C., Isasi, C. R., Perreira, K. M., Vu, T.-H.T., Vasquez, E., Sachdeva, S., Zeng, D., Llabre, M. M., Tarraf, W., González, H. M., Daviglus, M. L., & Lamar, M. (2020). Associations between perceived neighborhood environment and cognitive function among middle-aged and older women and men: Hispanic Community Health Study/Study of Latinos Sociocultural Ancillary Study. *Social Psychiatry and Psychiatric Epidemiology, 55*(6), 685–696. https://doi.org/10.1007/s00127-019-01829-0

Finlay, J., Esposito, M., Langa, K. M., Judd, S., & Clarke, P. J. (2022). Cognability: An ecological theory of neighborhoods and cognitive aging. *Social Science & Medicine, 309*, Article 115220. https://doi.org/10.1016/j.socscimed.2022.115220

Finlay, J., Esposito, M., Li, M., Kobayashi, L. C., Khan, A. M., Gomez-Lopez, I., Melendez, R., Colabianchi, N., Judd, S., & Clarke, P. J. (2021a). Can neighborhood social infrastructure modify cognitive function? A mixed-methods study of urban-dwelling aging Americans. *Journal of Aging and Health, 33*(9), 772–785. https://doi.org/10.1177/08982643211008673

Finlay, J., Yu, W., Clarke, P. J., Li, M., Judd, S., & Esposito, M. (2021b). Neighborhood cognitive amenities? A mixed-methods study of intellectually-stimulating places and cognitive function among older Americans. *Wellbeing, Space and Society, 2*, Article 100040. https://doi.org/10.1016/j.wss.2021.100040

Frank, L. D., Bigazzi, A., Hong, A., Minaker, L., Fisher, P., & Raine, K. D. (2022). Built environment influences on healthy eating and active living: The NEWPATH study. *Obesity, 30*(2), 424–434. https://doi.org/10.1002/oby.23352

George, K. M., Lutsey, P. L., Kucharska-Newton, A., Palta, P., Heiss, G., Osypuk, T., & Folsom, A. R. (2020). Life-course individual and neighborhood socioeconomic status and risk of dementia in the Atherosclerosis Risk in Communities Neurocognitive Study. *American Journal of Epidemiology, 189*(10), 1134–1142. https://doi.org/10.1093/aje/kwaa072

Glymour, M. M., Kawachi, I., Jencks, C. S., & Berkman, L. F. (2008). Does childhood schooling affect old age memory or mental status? Using state schooling laws as natural experiments. *Journal of Epidemiology & Community Health, 62*(6), 532–537. https://doi.org/10.1136/jech.2006.059469

Glymour, M. M., & Manly, J. J. (2008). Lifecourse social conditions and racial and ethnic patterns of cognitive aging. *Neuropsychology Review, 18*(3), 223–254. https://doi.org/10.1007/s11065-008-9064-z

Griffith, D. M., Towfighi, A., Manson, S. M., Littlejohn, E. L., & Skolarus, L. E. (2023). Determinants of inequities in neurologic disease, health, and well-being: The NINDS Social Determinants of Health Framework. *Neurology, 101*(7 Supplement 1), S75–S81. https://doi.org/10.1212/WNL.0000000000207566

Gustavsson, A., Norton, N., Fast, T., Frölich, L., Georges, J., Holzapfel, D., Kirabali, T., Krolak-Salmon, P., Rossini, P. M., Ferretti, M. T., Lanman, L., Chadha, A. S., & van der Flier, W. M. (2023). Global estimates on the number of persons across the Alzheimer's disease continuum. *Alzheimer's & Dementia, 19*(2), 658–670. https://doi.org/10.1002/alz.12694

Gutierrez, S., Whitmer, R. A., Soh, Y., Peterson, R., George, K. M., Lor, Y., Barnes, L. L., Mayeda, E. R., Allen, I. E., Torres, J. M., Glymour, M. M., & Gilsanz, P. (2024). School-based racial segregation, social support, and late-life cognitive function in the Study of Healthy Aging in African Americans (STAR). *Alzheimer's & Dementia, 20*(9), 6257–6267. https://doi.org/10.1002/alz.14112

Hamlin, A. M., Kraal, A. Z., Sol, K., Morris, E. P., Martino, A. G., Zaheed, A. B., & Zahodne, L. B. (2022). Social engagement and its links to cognition differ across non-Hispanic Black and White older adults. *Neuropsychology*. https://doi.org/10.1037/neu0000844

Hamlin, A. M., Weigand, A. J., Clay, O. J., Marsiske, M., Wallace, G., Dadson, D., Thomas, K. R., & Clark, A. L. (2025). The independent and interactive effects of economic stability and healthcare access on 10-Year cognitive trajectories of Black/African American and White older adults from the ACTIVE Study. *The Journals of Gerontology. Series B, Psychological Sciences and Social Sciences, 80*(2). https://doi.org/10.1093/geronb/gbae196

Hamlin, A. M., Weigand, A. J., Marsiske, M., Sisco, S., Tarraf, W., Thomas, K. R., & Clark, A. L. (in press). Locus of control moderates the effects of residential segregation on everyday functioning in Black older adults from the ACTIVE Study. *Neuropsychology*.

Hargraves, J. L., & Hadley, J. (2003). The contribution of insurance coverage and community resources to reducing racial/ethnic disparities in access to care. *Health Services Research, 38*(3), 809–829. https://doi.org/10.1111/1475-6773.00148

Hikichi, H., Kondo, K., Takeda, T., & Kawachi, I. (2017). Social interaction and cognitive decline: Results of a 7-year community intervention. *Alzheimer's & Dementia: Translational Research & Clinical Interventions, 3*(1), 23–32. https://doi.org/10.1016/j.trci.2016.11.003

Hill, C. V., Pérez-Stable, E. J., Anderson, N. A., & Bernard, M. A. (2015). The National Institute on aging health disparities research framework. *Ethnicity & Disease, 25*(3), 245–254. https://doi.org/10.18865/ed.25.3.245

Hunt, J. F. V., Buckingham, W., Kim, A. J., Oh, J., Vogt, N. M., Jonaitis, E. M., Hunt, T. K., Zuelsdorff, M., Powell, R., Norton, D., Rissman, R. A., Asthana, S., Okonkwo, O. C., Johnson, S. C., Kind, A. J. H., & Bendlin, B. B. (2020). Association of neighborhood-level disadvantage with cerebral and hippocampal volume. *JAMA Neurology, 77*(4), 451–460. https://doi.org/10.1001/jamaneurol.2019.4501

Hunt, J. F. V., Vogt, N. M., Jonaitis, E. M., Buckingham, W. R., Koscik, R. L., Zuelsdorff, M., Clark, L. R., Gleason, C. E., Yu, M., Okonkwo, O., Johnson, S. C., Asthana, S., Bendlin, B. B., & Kind, A. J. H. (2021). Association of neighborhood context, cognitive decline, and cortical change in an unimpaired cohort. *Neurology, 96*(20), e2500–e2512. https://doi.org/10.1212/WNL.0000000000011918

Juster, R.-P., McEwen, B. S., & Lupien, S. J. (2010). Allostatic load biomarkers of chronic stress and impact on health and cognition. *Neuroscience & Biobehavioral Reviews, 35*(1), 2–16. https://doi.org/10.1016/j.neubiorev.2009.10.002

Kind, A. J. H., & Buckingham, W. R. (2018). Making neighborhood-disadvantage metrics accessible—The Neighborhood Atlas. *The New England Journal of Medicine, 378*(26), 2456–2458. https://doi.org/10.1056/NEJMp1802313

Kirby, J. B., & Kaneda, T. (2005). Neighborhood socioeconomic disadvantage and access to health Care. *Journal of Health and Social Behavior, 46*(1), 15–31. https://doi.org/10.1177/002214650504600103

Kraal, A. Z., Sharifian, N., Zaheed, A. B., Sol, K., & Zahodne, L. B. (2019). Dimensions of religious involvement represent positive pathways in cognitive aging. *Research on Aging, 41*(9), 868–890. https://doi.org/10.1177/0164027519862745

Kuo, W., Bratzke, L. C., Oakley, L. D., Kuo, F., Wang, H., & Brown, R. L. (2019). The association between psychological stress and metabolic syndrome: A systematic review and meta-analysis. *Obesity Reviews, 20*(11). https://doi.org/10.1111/obr.12915

Lamar, M., Lerner, A. J., James, B. D., Yu, L., Glover, C. M., Wilson, R. S., & Barnes, L. L. (2020). Relationship of early-life residence and educational experience to level and change in cognitive functioning: Results of the Minority Aging Research Study. *The Journals of Gerontology: Series B, 75*(7), e81–e92. https://doi.org/10.1093/geronb/gbz031

Lee, H., & Waite, L. J. (2018). Cognition in context: The role of objective and subjective measures of neighborhood and household in cognitive functioning in later life. *The Gerontologist, 58*(1), 159–169. https://doi.org/10.1093/geront/gnx050

Livingston, G., Huntley, J., Sommerlad, A., Ames, D., Ballard, C., Banerjee, S., Brayne, C., Burns, A., Cohen-Mansfield, J., Cooper, C., Costafreda, S. G., Dias, A., Fox, N., Gitlin, L. N., Howard, R., Kales, H. C., Kivimäki, M., …, Mukadam, N. (2020). Dementia prevention, intervention, and care: 2020 report of the Lancet Commission. *The Lancet, 396*(10248), 413–446. https://doi.org/10.1016/S0140-6736(20)30367-6

Logan, J. R., Xu, Z., & Stults, B. J. (2014). Interpolating U.S. decennial densus tract data from as early as 1970 to 2010: A longitudinal tract database. *The Professional Geographer*, *66*(3), 412–420. https://doi.org/10.1080/00330124.2014.905156

Lupien, S. J., Juster, R.-P., Raymond, C., & Marin, M.-F. (2018). The effects of chronic stress on the human brain: From neurotoxicity, to vulnerability, to opportunity. *Frontiers in Neuroendocrinology, 49*, 91–105. https://doi.org/10.1016/j.yfrne.2018.02.001

Manly, J. J., Schupf, N., Tang, M.-X., & Stern, Y. (2005). Cognitive decline and literacy among ethnically diverse elders. *Journal of Geriatric Psychiatry and Neurology, 18*(4), 213–217. https://doi.org/10.1177/0891988705281868

Mantri, S., Nwadiogbu, C., Fitts, W., & Dahodwala, N. (2019). Quality of education impacts late-life cognition. *International Journal of Geriatric Psychiatry, 34*(6), 855–862. https://doi.org/10.1002/gps.5075

McCormack, G. R., & Shiell, A. (2011). In search of causality: A systematic review of the relationship between the built environment and physical activity among adults. *International Journal of Behavioral Nutrition and Physical Activity, 8*(1), 125. https://doi.org/10.1186/1479-5868-8-125

Meyer, O. L., Sisco, S. M., Harvey, D., Zahodne, L. B., Glymour, M. M., Manly, J. J., & Marsiske, M. (2017). Neighborhood predictors of cognitive training outcomes and trajectories in ACTIVE. *Research on Aging, 39*(3), 443–467. https://doi.org/10.1177/0164027515618242

Michael, Y. L., Senerat, A. M., Buxbaum, C., Ezeanyagu, U., Hughes, T. M., Hayden, K. M., Langmuir, J., Besser, L. M., Sánchez, B., & Hirsch, J. A. (2024). Systematic review of longitudinal evidence and methodologies for research on neighborhood characteristics and brain health. *Public Health Reviews, 45*, 1606677. https://doi.org/10.3389/phrs.2024.1606677

Mullins, M. A., Bynum, J. P. W., Judd, S. E., & Clarke, P. J. (2021). Access to primary care and cognitive impairment: Results from a national community study of aging Americans. *BMC Geriatrics, 21*(1), 580. https://doi.org/10.1186/s12877-021-02545-8

Nelson, A. (2002). Unequal treatment: Confronting racial and ethnic disparities in health care. *Journal of the National Medical Association, 94*(8), 666–668.

Office of Disease Prevention and Health Promotion. (n.d.). *Social Determinants of Health—Healthy People 2030|health.gov*. Retrieved October 16, 2023, from https://health.gov/healthypeople/priority-areas/social-determinants-health

Padeiro, M., de São José, J., Amado, C., Sousa, L., Roma Oliveira, C., Esteves, A., & McGarrigle, J. (2022). Neighborhood attributes and well-being among older adults in urban areas: A mixed-methods systematic review. *Research on Aging, 44*(5–6), 351–368. https://doi.org/10.1177/0164027521999980

Petersen, M. E., Zhou, Z., Hall, J. R., Phillips, N., Meeker, K. L., Borzage, M. T., Braskie, M. N., Clark, A. L., Shi, Y., Rissman, R. A., Zhang, F., Vintimilla, R., Casas, A., Rhodes, J., Barber, R. C., Johnson, L., Yaffe, K., Toga, A. W., O'Bryant, S. E., for the HABS-HD Study Team. (2025). Health and Aging Brain Study-Health Disparities (HABS-HD) methods and partner characteristics. *Alzheimer's & Dementia: Translational Research & Clinical Interventions, 11*(3), Article e70140. https://doi.org/10.1002/trc2.70140

Powell, W. R., Buckingham, W. R., Larson, J. L., Vilen, L., Yu, M., Salamat, M. S., Bendlin, B. B., Rissman, R. A., & Kind, A. J. H. (2020). Association of neighborhood-level disadvantage with Alzheimer disease neuropathology. *JAMA Network Open, 3*(6), Article e207559. https://doi.org/10.1001/jamanetworkopen.2020.7559

Rakesh, D., Seguin, C., Zalesky, A., Cropley, V., & Whittle, S. (2021). Associations between neighborhood disadvantage, resting-state functional connectivity, and behavior in the Adolescent Brain Cognitive Development Study: The moderating role of positive family and school environments. *Biological Psychiatry: Cognitive Neuroscience and Neuroimaging, 6*(9), 877–886. https://doi.org/10.1016/j.bpsc.2021.03.008

Rebok, G. W., Gellert, A., Coe, N. B., Clay, O. J., Wallace, G., Parisi, J. M., Aiken-Morgan, A. T., Crowe, M., Ball, K., Thorpe, R. J., Marsiske, M., Zahodne, L. B., Felix, C., & Willis, S. L. (2023). Effects of cognitive training on Alzheimer's disease and related dementias: The moderating role of social determinants of health. *Journal of Aging and Health, 35*(9_suppl), 40S–50S. https://doi.org/10.1177/08982643231203755

Seblova, D., Eng, C., Avila-Rieger, J. F., Dworkin, J. D., Peters, K., Lapham, S., Zahodne, L. B., Chapman, B., Prescott, C. A., Gruenewald, T. L., Arpawong, T. E., Gatz, M., Jones, R. J., Glymour, M. M., & Manly, J. J. (2023). High school quality is associated with cognition 58 years later. *Alzheimer's & Dementia: Diagnosis, Assessment & Disease Monitoring, 15*(2), Article e12424. https://doi.org/10.1002/dad2.12424

Shadyab, A. H., Aslanyan, V., Jacobs, D. M., Salmon, D. P., Morrison, R., Katula, J. A., Jin, S., Thomas, R. G., LaCroix, A. Z., Pa, J., Cotman, C. W., Feldman, H. H., Baker, L. D., for the ADCS EXERT Study Group. (2025). Effects of exercise versus usual care on older adults with amnestic mild cognitive impairment: EXERT versus ADNI. *Alzheimer's & Dementia, 21*(4), Article e70118. https://doi.org/10.1002/alz.70118

Sharifian, N., Spivey, B. N., Zaheed, A. B., & Zahodne, L. B. (2020). Psychological distress links perceived neighborhood characteristics to longitudinal trajectories of cognitive health in older adulthood. *Social Science & Medicine, 258*, Article 113125. https://doi.org/10.1016/j.socscimed.2020.113125

Sisco, S., Gross, A. L., Shih, R. A., Sachs, B. C., Glymour, M. M., Bangen, K. J., Benitez, A., Skinner, J., Schneider, B. C., & Manly, J. J. (2015). The role of early-life educational quality and literacy in explaining racial disparities in cognition in late life. *The Journals of Gerontology: Series B, 70*(4), 557–567. https://doi.org/10.1093/geronb/gbt133

Small, M. L., & McDermott, M. (2006). The presence of organizational resources in poor urban neighborhoods: An analysis of average and contextual effects. *Social Forces, 84*(3), 1697–1724. https://doi.org/10.1353/sof.2006.0067

Swope, C. B., & Hernández, D. (2019). Housing as a determinant of health equity: A conceptual model. *Social Science & Medicine, 243*, Article 112571. https://doi.org/10.1016/j.socscimed.2019.112571

Vassilaki, M., Aakre, J. A., Castillo, A., Chamberlain, A. M., Wilson, P. M., Kremers, W. K., Mielke, M. M., Geda, Y. E., Machulda, M. M., Alhurani, R. E., Graff-Radford, J., Vemuri, P., Lowe, V. J., Jack, C. R., Jr., Knopman, D. S., & Petersen, R. C. (2023). Association of neighborhood socioeconomic disadvantage and cognitive impairment. *Alzheimer's & Dementia, 19*(3), 761–770. https://doi.org/10.1002/alz.12702

Weathers, E. S., & Sosina, V. E. (2022). Separate remains unequal: Contemporary segregation and racial disparities in school district revenue. *American Educational Research Journal, 59*(5), 905–938. https://doi.org/10.3102/00028312221079297

Weden, M. M., Carpiano, R. M., & Robert, S. A. (2008). Subjective and objective neighborhood characteristics and adult health. *Social Science & Medicine, 66*(6), 1256–1270. https://doi.org/10.1016/j.socscimed.2007.11.041

Williams, D. R., & Collins, C. (2001). Racial residential segregation: A fundamental cause of racial disparities in health. *Public Health Reports, 116*(5), 404–416. https://doi.org/10.1093/phr/116.5.404

Wolinsky, F. D., Andresen, E. M., Malmstrom, T. K., Miller, J. P., Schootman, M., & Miller, D. K. (2012). Childhood school segregation and later life sense of control and physical performance in the African American Health cohort. *BMC Public Health, 12*(1), 827. https://doi.org/10.1186/1471-2458-12-827

Yannatos, I., Stites, S., Brown, R. T., & McMillan, C. T. (2023). Contributions of neighborhood social environment and air pollution exposure to Black-White disparities in epigenetic aging. *PLoS ONE, 18*(7), Article e0287112. https://doi.org/10.1371/journal.pone.0287112

Yen, I. H., Michael, Y. L., & Perdue, L. (2009). Neighborhood environment in studies of health of older adults: A systematic review. *American Journal of Preventive Medicine, 37*(5), 455–463. https://doi.org/10.1016/j.amepre.2009.06.022

Yu, W., Esposito, M., Li, M., Clarke, P., Judd, S., & Finlay, J. (2023). Neighborhood 'disamenities': Local barriers and cognitive function among Black and white aging adults. *BMC Public Health, 23*(1), 197. https://doi.org/10.1186/s12889-023-15026-x

Zaheed, A. B., Sharifian, N., Kraal, A. Z., Sol, K., Hence, A., & Zahodne, L. B. (2019). Unique effects of perceived neighborhood physical disorder and social cohesion on episodic memory and semantic fluency. *Archives of Clinical Neuropsychology, 34*(8), 1346–1355. https://doi.org/10.1093/arclin/acy098

Zeki Al Hazzouri, A., Haan, M. N., Osypuk, T., Abdou, C., Hinton, L., & Aiello, A. E. (2011). Neighborhood socioeconomic context and cognitive decline among older Mexican Americans: Results from the Sacramento Area Latino Study on Aging. *American Journal of Epidemiology, 174*(4), 423–431. https://doi.org/10.1093/aje/kwr095

Chapter 8
Cognitive Function as the Sixth Vital Sign: Integrating Cognitive Disorder Management into Primary Care

Heather Cuevas

Executive Summary
This chapter emphasizes the critical role of cognitive health in chronic care management, proposing cognition as a "6th vital sign" in patient care. To minimize disease complications, coordination and continuity of care require continuous progress monitoring, which can be achieved with the use of the Chronic Care Model to track disease-specific indicators over time. Cognitive monitoring, particularly in primary care settings, is essential to this approach. The Medicare Annual Wellness Visit offers an opportunity to implement regular cognitive assessments and ensure that cognitive health is integrated into routine management.

Cognitive Function in Non-Dementia-Related Chronic Disease

Chronic non-neurologic conditions show clear associations with lower cognitive performance among adults (Kim et al., 2019). For example, hypertension and diabetes are linked to diminished memory and executive function, while chronic kidney disease—both non-dialysis and hemodialysis populations—is repeatedly related to declines in global cognition, executive function, attention, and memory (Lee et al., 2025). Inadequately treated chronic conditions such as hypothyroidism or congestive heart failure are well known to cause cognitive dysfunction due to mechanisms such as reduced levels of T3 uptake or decreased blood flow to the brain (Goh et al., 2022; Shaji & Joel, 2022). Other treatments for chronic conditions can have detrimental

H. Cuevas (✉)
School of Nursing, The University of Texas at Austin, Austin, TX, USA
e-mail: hcuevas@mail.nur.utexas.edu

M. Lanca and R. Fallows (eds.), *Advancing Neuropsychology Through Population Health*, https://doi.org/10.1007/978-3-032-22457-6_8

effects on memory, including opioids for chronic pain, certain antidepressants, sleep aids, and anticholinergics (Wouters et al., 2020). Many of these chronic diseases, especially when they are not well managed, can foster cognitive impairment leading to poorer health outcomes, increased hospitalizations, or more severe symptoms of the chronic condition.

Studies report that the presence of several chronic diseases correlates with poorer self-management and increased functional dependency (Cuevas et al., 2022b; Hill et al., 2021). As such, it is necessary to assess individuals for these impairments because neurocognitive impairments can lead to poorer outcomes in all facets of healthcare. For example, patients hospitalized with dementia and other comorbidities such as diabetes or heart failure are more likely to be readmitted or die after discharge than those with dementia only (Martín et al., 2019). Multiple reviews have found that early recognition and management of cognitive problems can lead to better care, including implementation of pharmacological interventions (e.g., cholinesterase inhibitors for Alzheimer's disease) and nonpharmacological therapies (e.g., cognitive training, lifestyle modifications) (Hilsabeck et al, 2024).

Implementation Takeaway #1

Common cognitive symptoms associated with specific chronic illnesses:

	Common cognitive deficits	Clinical manifestation examples
Diabetes Biessels and Whitmer (2020), Yu et al. (2025)	Memory decline	Forgetting to check blood glucose at home
	Visuospatial ability impairment	Inability to administer insulin
	Impaired executive function	Unable to correlate food intake to glucose levels
Cardiovascular disease Goh et al. (2022), Wee et al. (2023)	Decreased attention	Inability to follow instructions
	Memory decline Executive dysfunction	Forgetting medications
	Motor speed decline	Taking a longer time to stand up from a sitting position
	Impaired executive function	Inability to plan and follow a prescribed diet

(continued)

(continued)

	Common cognitive deficits	Clinical manifestation examples
Hypothyroidism Shaji and Joel (2022)	Memory decline/Executive dysfunction	Forgets thyroid medication several times a week
	Impaired executive function	Inability to time thyroid medication properly (i.e., apart from food and other pills)
Rheumatoid Arthritis Chaurasia et al. (2020)	Decline in short-term memory	Asking the same questions repeatedly
	Problems with phonetic fluency	Inconsistent pronunciation or difficulty with complex words
	Visuospatial ability impairment	Difficulty physically navigating the environment independent of joint issues or pain
Chronic Obstructive Pulmonary Disease Morris et al. (2019)	Information processing deficits	Trouble, unrelated to dyspnea, in keeping up with conversations
	Verbal memory decline	Remembering names of medications
	Decreased attention	Inability to follow the conversation
Chronic Kidney Disease Pépin et al. (2024)	Impaired executive function	Difficulty linking diet with decreased kidney function
	Memory decline	Changes in memory that parallel decline in kidney function
	Decreased attention	Changes in attention that parallel decline in kidney function
Cancer Lange et al. (2019)	Memory decline	Brain fog or "chemo brain"
	Decreased attention	Taking longer than usual to do routine tasks
	Impaired executive function	Difficulty implementing specialist's instructions

Cognitive Monitoring in Primary Care

Screening for cognitive problems should become the 6th vital sign (the other five being temperature, heart rate, respiratory rate, blood pressure, and oxygen saturation) in people with chronic conditions, as these conditions are linked to higher rates of cognitive impairment. If present, cognitive impairment can lead to worse medical outcomes, decreased levels of daily functioning, decreased ability to self-manage chronic conditions, and decreased quality of life (Cuevas et al., 2024; Lovett et al., 2020). A recent systematic review and meta-analyses ($n = 91$, representing 800,297 participants) examining associations of cognitive dysfunction with any health condition showed that healthy controls outperformed participants with chronic conditions in all tested cognitive domains—including those with conditions that did not arise from the central nervous system (e.g., diabetes, asthma) (Schretlen et al., 2024). Of course, some chronic diseases can cause more severe cognitive impairment than others; but the presence of mild or moderate cognitive problems should also be considered, because such problems can reduce individuals' independence, disease self-management, or relationships. For example, in a meta-synthesis of qualitative studies investigating the impact of non-dementia-related chronic illness on cognitive function, participants described a process of adapting to new changes as they navigated new ways of working with symptoms, relationships, and the healthcare system (Cuevas et al., 2024). In other words, it was a process of adapting to new realities and making the best of situations despite some sense of loss. The unexpected nature of cognitive dysfunction was problematic for these participants, many of whom stated that they wished "they had been told sooner" about the possibility of cognitive problems related to chronic illness.

Early cognitive screening can detect the possibility of cognitive concerns which can allow for not just timely diagnosis, but also a way to document any changes before mild neurocognitive disease onset. Documentation of cognitive decline can then enable health care providers to develop cognitive strategies and medical interventions to maximize treatment adherence (Choukou et al., 2023). With the increasing recognition of the importance of screening for cognitive dysfunction, the frequency of cognitive assessments has grown, especially in primary care settings. While it is likely not practical for every primary care provider to be an expert in fully assessing cognitive function, training in recognition of risk factors, understanding conditions associated with cognitive impairment, and knowing when to consult with neuropsychology can be helpful.

Unfortunately, some patients with cognitive complaints may not seek treatment for potential chronic conditions because they fear a diagnosis of a dementia and thus skip tests that could reveal other chronic conditions early when treatments are sometimes most effective (Birt et al., 2020). However, people diagnosed with chronic conditions may be more likely to report cognitive problems to their health care providers (National Association of Chronic Disease Directors, 2018) since they have more frequent medical appointments with their providers and likely more established, comfortable relationships with them. In these situations, routine medical visits can be used to detect cognitive dysfunction early. One way to do this is to include an inventory of cognitive symptoms in the usual review of systems that includes memory changes and confusion. This inventory can trigger health care providers to assess and discuss symptoms related to cognitive function. For example, adding one question related to each cognitive domain in the neurologic or mental health sections of the review of systems may be helpful. Questions could include, "Do you forget recent events or conversations (memory)?"; "Do you struggle to find common words (language)?"; or "Can you use appliances or devices as well as you used to (executive function)?" (Collum & Karlawish, 2020). Community surveys have shown that the prevalence of cognitive complaints is double that reported in primary care provider medical records (National Association of Chronic Disease Directors, 2018).

Inquiring about cognitive health at medical visits is important. Studies have shown that about 75% of people diagnosed with dementia are diagnosed in the primary care setting (Ford et al., 2021). However, early symptoms are sometimes missed, which can delay correct diagnoses and treatment. The United States Preventive Services Task Force (USPSTF) recommends against blanket screening of the entire population for cognitive dysfunction due to lack of evidence of benefit. Instead two groups have been prioritized for screening: (1) people with subjective memory complaints, and (2) older adults with physical frailty and/or chronic conditions (USPSTF, 2020). But USPSTF's recommendation does not necessarily mean that screening adults over 65 years of age, as the Centers for Medicare and Medicaid (CMS) recommend, is not beneficial. USPSTF's approach is to focus and summarize the available evidence and the implications of those results are of concern especially in primary care. The absence of evidence may result in inaction in a primary care setting that is already challenged by lack of time. In fact, other national organizations such as the Alzheimer's Association and the Alzheimer's Foundation have stated that the USPSTF report does not adequately consider the possible improved health outcomes resulting from screening, the disparities in dementia care that may increase from a lack of early detection, and early detection and treatment of mild cognitive impairment (MCI) can slow progression to dementia (Tzeng et al., 2024).

Additionally, patients and clinicians alike might be concerned that an implication of USPSTF's report is that screening is not valuable. Ignoring the value of cognitive screening in primary care overlooks the potential value of having knowledge of a patient's cognitive function—either positive or negative—that leads to treatment or reassurance. Primary care practices are well positioned to screen because providers often have established relationships with patients and families and are familiar with their living conditions and other comorbidities. However, the administration of these screening tests is not limited to physicians; studies show that allied health professionals can utilize cognitive screeners in their practice settings (Bandini et al., 2022). Risk-scoring algorithms are available to determine who might be at the highest risk for cognitive dysfunction (Daunt et al., 2021). Ideally, the cognitive evaluation should be an easily administered, validated, performance-based tool that is reliable and sensitive to change over time, just as measures of blood pressure, weight, and temperature. Cognitive function would thus be measured when other important health metrics are gathered. The cognitive results could be included in the patient's medical record and potentially used to inform patients about risks for problems with disease self-management. Cognitive function would no longer be scored as pass/fail but would be measured as fluctuating over time.

Screening Tools for Cognitive Impairment

Various tools are available for screening cognitive impairments in primary care. These tools can be broadly categorized as brief cognitive screening measures, cognitive assessments, or comprehensive neuropsychological evaluations. For primary care settings, the emphasis is often placed on brief, easy-to-administer screening measures that identify individuals at risk who may need further assessment. Selecting the appropriate screening tool depends on several factors like time constraints, the patient's cognitive status, and language. Brief screens are most popular, though there are a host of other cognitive screens for consideration. Negative findings can occur in individuals experiencing subtle decline and/or individuals who have high cognitive reserve, and thus patient background must be taken into consideration. For the average medically/neurologically stable patient, a normal cognitive screening test implies continued monitoring by repeating the test every 4 years in people aged between 50 and 70 and then every 2 years in those over 70 (USPSTF, 2020). Decisions about more comprehensive cognitive testing and/or referring for neuropsychological testing are wide-ranging and beyond the scope of this chapter (see Roebuck-Spencer et al., 2017).

Brief Cognitive Screening Tools

These measures are designed to be quick and easy to administer, to provide an initial indication of cognitive impairment. Many do not require additional training and are widely available for clinicians to incorporate into their practices. Unfortunately, most of the research for these measures continues to be driven by utility in evaluating risk for mild cognitive impairment or dementia and research with other conditions impacting cognition is less robust. The ability of these measures to detect symptom exaggeration or the impact of psychological distress is limited. Further, while several of the measures have been translated into different languages, clinicians should be mindful that some measures offer only direct translation, which may result in use of a word that is not common to some regions/dialects within that language family. Finally, educational adjustments to total scores are often times limited to those with lower than 12 years of education, broadly. This creates complications with individuals who are illiterate or have low education (may overestimate their degree of cognitive difficulty) as well as those with high education (may underestimate, or not identify until someone is more progressed into cognitive decline).

Implementation Takeaway #2

There are several common brief cognitive screens which can be considered, such as:

- **Mini-Mental State Examination (MMSE)**: Assesses a range of cognitive domains, including orientation, attention, memory, language, and visuospatial skills. The MMSE is useful for detecting moderate to severe dementia, but its ability to detect early cognitive decline or MCI is limited (Arevalo-Rodriguez et al., 2021). The MMSE takes about 5–10 min to complete.
- **Montreal Cognitive Assessment (MoCA)**: The MoCA assesses a wider range of cognitive domains and is suitable for detecting MCI, Alzheimer's disease, and other forms of dementia (Dautzenberg et al., 2022). It takes 10–12 min to complete and requires the user to complete a certification program.
- **Clock Drawing Test (CDT)**: This simple test asks patients to draw a clock face, indicating a specific time and usually takes less than a minute to complete. It evaluates spatial and executive function and has been found effective for detecting early cognitive changes (Park et al., 2018). The **Mini-Cog** augments this CDT by having the patient learn three semantically unrelated words, complete the CDT, and then freely recall the three words.
- **Short Test of Mental Status (STMS)**: This brief 5-min test is designed to evaluate orientation, short-term memory, and simple problem-solving abilities. It is shorter than the MMSE, but it still offers valuable insights into cognitive function (Townley et al., 2019).
- **The Geriatric Depression Scale (GDS)**: Though not a cognitive test per se, the GDS is a 5–7-min test used to screen for depression, a common condition that often coexists with cognitive decline. Since depression can mimic or exacerbate cognitive issues, differentiating between the two is critical for accurate diagnosis (Abdullah et al., 2022). The GDS is also available in a short form, which comprises 15 items.

Cognitive Assessments

When screening tools suggest possible cognitive impairment, more comprehensive assessments may be warranted. These assessments typically involve longer tests and interviews, with additional diagnostic tests. Neuropsychological testing provides a thorough assessment of cognitive function across various domains, such as memory, executive function, language, and attention while considering the interaction of various individual demographic factors and psychological and social effects. It is typically used when there is uncertainty about the diagnosis, when the cognitive issues are complex, or when a definitive diagnosis of dementia is required (Kiselica et al., 2024). For the non-neuropsychologist, there are some cognitive assessment tools to use prior to referral to neuropsychology referral which may be of use. These include the Clinical Dementia Rating (CDR) scale, The Alzheimer's Disease Assessment Scale—Cognitive Subscale (ADAS-Cog), or the National Institute of Health (NIH) toolbox. To improve diagnostic results, screening tests should also be chosen with patients' educational levels in mind. Tests like the Money Test or Phototest, for example, were developed to decrease bias related to educational levels (Dreo et al., 2024). Digital cognitive screening tools in addition to the NIH toolbox are under development and can also be helpful, because they may increase access and capacity, as well as include a variety of languages in one application (Hilsabeck et al., 2024).

Challenges in Screening for Cognitive Problems

The benefits of early identification of cognitive problems are clear, but there are several challenges:

1. **Subtle Onset of Symptoms**: Cognitive impairments often present with subtle symptoms that can be easily overlooked by patients, families, or even clinicians. Symptoms such as forgetfulness, difficulty with concentration, or occasional confusion can be attributed to normal aging (Mattke et al., 2023). Patients with chronic diseases frequently experience subjective cognitive dysfunction, which affects their healthcare interactions, self-perception, and relationships (Cuevas et al., 2024). Cognitive impairment can also complicate the use of chronic illness self-management interventions if not detected (Vogeley et al., 2024).
2. **Stigma and Denial**: Research suggests that stigma associated with chronic illnesses can significantly impact older adults' self-concept and illness management (Earnshaw et al., 2022). Stigma can also lead to poor medication adherence and health risk behaviors. For example, someone with type 2 diabetes may not check their glucose prior to eating a meal at a restaurant. This highlights the need for interventions in primary care to address chronic illness, including dementia, stigma to improve patient outcomes. Patients may resist screening due to the implications of such a label.

   Denial also plays a role in chronic illness management. Initially older adults may feel overwhelmed by their diagnosis, but over time, they tend to deny being identified as sick (Patierno et al., 2023). Similarly, family members may be in denial about their loved one's cognitive difficulties, making it harder to initiate screening (Brownell et al., 2024; Cuevas et al., 2021). This may be compounded by research suggesting that those with more than one diagnosis experience more stigma and, therefore, more treatment barriers in comparison to those with a single diagnosis (Islam et al., 2022). Of note, anosognosia, or lack of insight, is present in 20-80% of people with Alzheimer's (Hanseewu et al., 2020). This is sometimes confounded with denial however they are distinct phenomena. Anosognosia is considered organic in nature, linked to brain injury and executive dysfunction, while denial is a psychological defense mechanism (Prigatano et al., 2024).
3. **Lack of Training**: Many primary care clinicians may not feel adequately trained to identify or assess cognitive impairment (Tierney et al., 2014). This can lead to under-recognition, delays in diagnosis, and inappropriate management. Further, although screening tools are available in a wide array of languages, providers

may not be well versed in working with interpreters for cognitive screening. In these cases, it is also essential to consider cultural factors such as quality of education and beliefs around aging and illness, beyond language alone.

4. **Complexity of Diagnosis**: Cognitive problems are multifactorial, and differentiating among normal aging, depression, treatment side-effects, early-stage dementia, or other conditions that can mimic cognitive impairment can be challenging. A single screening tool may not provide a definitive diagnosis. For example, some studies have shown that sometimes as many as 30% of people with a "normal" MMSE result have executive function impairment (Arevalo-Rodriguez et al., 2021).

Tracking Disease-Specific Indicators Over Time

Tracking cognitive changes in people with chronic diseases is a complex task requiring careful consideration of assessment methods and reliable, and clinically relevant approaches (i.e., how to cognitive test score translate to problems in daily life). Some screening tests have score changes that are considered clinically significant (e.g., a change in score of 1.4 to 3 points in the MMSE) (Muir et al., 2024). Longitudinal studies show cognitive function can remain stable or follow distinct trajectories in those primarily affected by age, education, and exercise tolerance (Park, 2018). Identifying these predictors over time may enable clinicians to target at risk patients. Reliable measurement of cognitive change over repeated administrations must account for factors such as practice effects, demographic influences, and consistency in administration (Gates et al., 2021). Self-reported cognitive function is often assessed using heterogeneous measures and may not closely correlate with neuropsychological test results, but it is frequently associated with other patient-reported outcomes (Cuevas et al., 2022a). Regular cognitive screening in primary care settings can identify patients who are at risk, but there is a need for more standardized approaches, such as those recommended by professional organizations, to facilitate cross-study comparisons when chronic conditions are non-neurological (Park, 2018).

In addition to the various general cognitive screening tools, there are emerging brief, disease-specific, technology-based measures. Researchers are exploring innovative approaches to tracking cognitive changes in older adults, particularly those at risk for Alzheimer's disease. The Cognitive Function Instrument (CFI) shows promise in detecting early cognitive decline in preclinical stages, with both self and partner reports providing valuable insights (Amariglio et al., 2015). Integrating such data into population health models can enhance our understanding of cognitive change at both individual and population levels, although challenges remain for accessing confidential health records. These approaches show promise for providing more comprehensive, sensitive measures of cognitive function that will enable early detection and intervention in chronic disease.

The Cognition in Primary Care program, adapting the GSA KAER Toolkit, offers a comprehensive approach with provider training, electronic health record (EHR) tools, and in-clinic workflow support (Raetz et al., 2023). The Toolkit was developed for primary care practices and involves four steps: Kickstart, Assess, Evaluate, and Refer. It includes practice integration resources as well as strategies to initiate cognitive health conversations with patients, choose cognitive screening tests, implement steps in the diagnostic process, and refer to specialty providers and community resources (Gerontological Society of America, 2025). Additionally, computerized cognitive assessments show potential for use in primary care settings, although further validation is needed.

Implementation Takeaway #3

Attitudes regarding screening for cognitive problems and management of those conditions may vary among groups based on intersectionality of their individual diversity factors. For example, participants in one study ($n = 29$; 100% Latino) screened for MCI and Alzheimer's and related dementias were interested in sharing results with family, and close to half of the participants in that study made lifestyle changes on the basis of those results (Cabrera et al., 2021). Similarly, qualitative work has found participants ($n = 30$; 100% Latino) were interested in "brain health"; however, there are concerns about equitable access to these resources as only one participant in that study had ever had a health care provider who discussed brain health with them. Among Latino participants, maintaining cognitive health was based on family responsibilities and perceived societal roles (Cuevas et al., 2021). Given these considerations, clinicians should consider these recommendations when working with Latino adults on their cognition and health: (1) Due to the diversity of languages and dialects, modify health information to match the community's characteristics (Quiroz et al., 2022); (2) Implement health literacy programs to increase dementia awareness, address misperceptions, and empower Latino adults to take action now to reduce their later risk (Light et al., 2024); and (3) Emphasize the benefits lifestyle modifications for other chronic illnesses will have on dementia risk. Linking this information can increase patient empowerment and activation (Vila-Castelar et al., 2022).

Integrating Cognitive Screening Using the Chronic Care Model

The Annual Wellness Visit (AWV) for Medicare beneficiaries includes a requirement to assess cognitive impairment (Centers for Medicare and Medicaid Services, 2024). To guide primary care providers, recommendations for cognitive assessment during AWVs have been developed, including the use of structured tools like those previously mentioned. Additionally, informant reporting tools such as the Short Informant Questionnaire on Cognitive Decline in the Elderly are also recommended when reliable informants are available (Jorm, 1994). Despite these recommendations, a survey of Medicare beneficiaries found that only about half reported having an AWV, and fewer than one-third received a structured cognitive assessment. Medicare Advantage enrollees were more likely to report both AWVs and cognitive assessments than were FFS Medicare beneficiaries (Jacobson et al., 2020).

AWVs that integrate screening for cognitive problems according to the Chronic Care Model (CCM) offer greater early detection and better management of cognitive problems. This model, originally developed to improve the quality of care for patients with chronic conditions (Wagner, 2019), provides a comprehensive framework that can be adapted to address the complexities of cognitive health. The CCM emphasizes a proactive, patient-centered approach that includes clinical and community resources, to improve health outcomes and reduce costs. Cognitive screening within the framework of the CCM has the potential to improve outcomes by addressing cognitive issues early in their development and providing better long-term care management. Below, we explore how cognitive screening can be seamlessly incorporated into each of the CCM's six key elements: (1) community resources and policies; (2) health systems; (3) self-management support; (4) delivery system design; (5) decision support; and (6) clinical information systems.

Community Resources and Policies

The integration of cognitive screening begins with ensuring that adequate resources are available to support individuals with cognitive impairments—educational programs, support groups, and resources to help them manage their conditions. This includes access to screening tools, educational programs for both patients and caregivers, and policies promoting awareness about cognitive health. For example, healthcare providers could collaborate with local organizations to offer training for caregivers and family members on how to recognize early signs of cognitive decline. Policy initiatives could encourage insurance coverage for regular cognitive screenings, particularly for high-risk populations such as the elderly or those with a family history of dementia. Community-based resources, such as memory clinics, support groups, and advocacy organizations, should be leveraged to provide patients with ongoing support after problems are identified.

Health System

The healthcare environment should support well-coordinated care, including access to specialized care and the appropriate use of technology. Incorporating cognitive screening into the health system requires ensuring all healthcare providers are trained to recognize and screen for cognitive issues. The integration of cognitive screening measures in EHRs can facilitate this process by prompting healthcare providers during routine visits (Hilsabeck et al., 2024). Screening tools like the Mini-Cog, the MoCA, or the MMSE can be embedded into the EHR system so providers can quickly assess cognitive function during regular visits. This integration would help ensure cognitive problems are detected early, and facilitate patients receiving appropriate referrals for further neuropsychological evaluation or specialized care as needed. The health system should also offer integrated care models that bring together primary care providers, neurologists, geriatric specialists, neuropsychologists and other healthcare professionals to create a comprehensive care plan for patients with cognitive impairments.

Self-Management Support

The self-management component of the CCM focuses on empowering patients to manage their own health and care. For patients with cognitive impairments, this is particularly challenging, because cognitive decline can affect memory, decision-making, and the ability to follow treatment plans. To support self-management, healthcare providers can offer strategies to help patients with early cognitive decline maintain independence as long as possible. For example, providers might recommend cognitive exercises, memory aids, and modifications to the home environment to reduce risk and enhance safety.

Patients and their caregivers can also be supported by education on how to adapt their daily routines to compensate for cognitive challenges. Resources such as memory training programs, online platforms, or mobile apps designed to improve cognitive function can be beneficial. Several interventions developed for a variety of chronic conditions (e.g., "chemo brain," type 2 diabetes, heart failure) have shown improvement not only in specific cognitive domains, but also in self-management of chronic conditions (Pressler et al., 2022; Stuifbergen et al., 2018; Von Ah & Crouch, 2020). These interventions were led by registered nurses, which allowed for increased accessibility.

Another crucial aspect of self-management support is the involvement of family members or caregivers in the care process. This might include training caregivers on how to communicate effectively with patients who are experiencing cognitive difficulties and providing them with strategies for managing behavioral symptoms that may arise (Riffin et al., 2025).

Delivery System Design

Organization of care delivery should be designed to be more efficient, with an emphasis on team-based care and proactive management (Passmore et al., 2024). Cognitive problems require a multidisciplinary approach to care, and the CCM encourages a team-based delivery system. For individuals with cognitive impairments, this might involve a primary care provider working with neurologists, neuropsychologists, occupational therapists, social workers, and other specialists. Coordinated care is key to addressing the various aspects of cognitive impairment from diagnosis to management and support.

The delivery system should also be designed to facilitate regular monitoring of cognitive function, especially for patients with a higher risk of cognitive decline, such as those with a history of stroke or diabetes (Kanne et al., 2023). Regular follow-up visits, annual cognitive screening, and ongoing evaluations of patients' needs can help healthcare providers adjust care plans as necessary.

Decision Support

Evidence-based guidelines and tools should be used to assist healthcare providers in making informed decisions. Integrating cognitive screening into the decision support component of the CCM means using evidence-based guidelines and decision-making tools to aid clinicians in managing patients with cognitive impairments. Tools like the CDR for diagnosing dementia and Alzheimer's disease can be incorporated into clinical workflows to assist providers in making accurate diagnoses and treatment decisions (Nosheny et al., 2023). Decision support tools can help healthcare providers identify when to refer patients to specialists or initiate more advanced diagnostic testing (Sutton et al., 2020). Decision support systems can also provide reminders for providers to monitor cognitive health in patients with chronic conditions that may affect cognition, such as diabetes, hypertension, or heart disease.

Clinical Information Systems

Clinical information systems play a crucial role in the integration of cognitive screening into the CCM. By utilizing EHRs and other health information technologies, providers can track cognitive screening results over time, identify patterns of decline, and monitor the efficacy of interventions. Cognitive screening data can be used to generate alerts for clinicians when a patient may require additional evaluation or intervention. These systems can also track medication adherence, monitor for changes in behavior or functioning, and ensure that the patient's care plan remains aligned with the patient's needs (Sutton et al., 2020). Clinical information systems can also help to integrate information from multiple sources, including specialists, caregivers, and community resources, to provide a holistic approach to care for patients with cognitive impairments.

Interventions Following Positive Screening

Ultimately, research evidence shows there are modifiable risk factors associated with both chronic medical conditions and dementia (e.g., body composition, physical inactivity, smoking, and sleep disturbance) such that early intervention may slow disease progression and improve quality of life in several ways (Jones et al., 2024). Some of the more impactful interventions following early detection include:

1. **Care Planning**: Early cognitive diagnosis allows for advanced care planning, including decisions about driving, living arrangements, financial matters, and end-of-life preferences. It also gives patients and families time to adjust and seek support resources. In a qualitative study ($n = 65$) of older adults and their caregivers, participants supported early identification of declining health and cognitive problems for the reasons listed above (Kendell et al, 2020). Additionally, they focused on establishing links to community resources as part of the planning process and a personalized approach involving primary care providers.
2. **Reducing Caregiver Burden**: Family caregivers often report high levels of stress and emotional strain when cognitive decline is not identified early. By diagnosing cognitive issues sooner, providers can guide families toward resources and support networks to reduce the burden not only of cognitive dysfunction, but also co-existing chronic illnesses (Lara-Ruiz et al, 2019; Lindeza et al, 2024).
3. **Preventing Secondary Complications**: Cognitive decline is often accompanied by other medical and psychological issues, such as depression, anxiety, and functional impairment. Early identification helps prevent these from worsening, impacting quality of life, and complicating the overall treatment plan (Mukherjee et al., 2024). For example, for pulmonary patients, cognitive screening and subsequent psychoeducation reduced 30-day hospital readmission rates by 50% (Ketterer et al., 2019). In diabetes care, early diagnosis of cognitive impairment can lead to tailored glucose-lowering treatments, reducing the risk of hypoglycemia and improving treatment adherence (Biessels & Whitmer, 2020).
4. **Public Health Implications**: Given the projected rise in the number of people with dementia worldwide, screening for cognitive problems also plays a role in public health initiatives aimed at improving care coordination and resource allocation (World Health Organization, 2021). Findings from a systematic review and meta-analysis (32 studies; 9069 participants with chronic conditions) showed that interdisciplinary teams in care coordination improved patient activation and appropriate use of the health care system (Cuevas et al., 2021).

Conclusion

Integrating screening for cognitive problems into the CCM offers a structured, systematic approach to early detection and ongoing management of cognitive impairments. By addressing the needs of individuals with cognitive decline within the

CCM framework, healthcare providers can improve outcomes, enhance quality of life, and reduce the burden of these conditions on both patients and the healthcare system. This integration requires collaboration across multiple levels of the healthcare system, from community resources to the use of clinical decision-making tools. By embracing the CCM's principles, healthcare systems can ensure that cognitive issues are not overlooked and that individuals receive the care and support they need to maintain their independence and well-being.

Key Points in Review

1. Cognitive function can be measured as other health metrics are gathered. Those results could be potentially used to inform risks for problems with disease chronic disease self-management.
2. The Annual Wellness Visit can be structured around the Chronic Care Model and offer a way to achieve early detection and better management of cognitive problems.
3. Additional Resources
    a. National Institute on Aging: Alzheimer's and Related Dementias Resources for Professionals
    b. Alzheimer's Association: Cognitive Screening and Assessment
    c. Centers for Medicare & Medicaid Services: Cognitive Assessment & Care Plan Services

References

Abdullah, S., Critchfield, M., Maltby, J., & Mukaetova-Ladinska, E. B. (2022). Improving diagnosis of functional cognitive impairment in younger adults in primary care: Validation of cognitive screening tools and the 4-item geriatric depression scale. *Journal of Alzheimer's Disease, 86*(4), 1797–1804.

Amariglio, R. E., Donohue, M. C., Marshall, G. A., Rentz, D. M., Salmon, D. P., Ferris, S. H., ... & Sperling, R. A. (2015). Tracking early decline in cognitive function in older individuals at risk for Alzheimer disease dementia: the Alzheimer's Disease Cooperative Study Cognitive Function Instrument. *JAMA neurology, 72*(4), 446–454.

Arevalo-Rodriguez, I., Smailagic, N., Roqué-Figuls, M., Ciapponi, A., Sanchez-Perez, E., Giannakou, A., Pedraza, O. L., Bonfill Cosp, X., & Cullum, S. (2021). Mini-Mental State Examination (MMSE) for the early detection of dementia in people with mild cognitive impairment (MCI). *Cochrane Database Systematic Reviews, 7*(7), CD010783. https://doi.org/10.1002/14651858.CD010783.pub3

Bandini, J. I., Schulson, L. B., Ahluwalia, S. C., et al. (2022). Primary care providers' barriers to early detection of cognitive impairment: A systematic review. *Journal of the American Geriatrics Society, 70*(10), 2932–2942. https://doi.org/10.1111/jgs.17840

Biessels, G. J., & Whitmer, R. A. (2020). Cognitive dysfunction in diabetes: How to implement emerging guidelines. *Diabetologia, 63*, 3–9. https://doi.org/10.1007/s00125-019-04977-9

Birt, L., Poland, F., Charlesworth, G., Leung, P., & Higgs, P. (2020). Relational experiences of people seeking help and assessment for subjective cognitive concern and memory loss. *Aging & Mental Health, 24*(8), 1356–1364. https://doi.org/10.1080/13607863.2019.1592111

Brownell, M., Sehar, U., Mukherjee, U., & Reddy, P. H. (2024). Creating cultural and lifestyle awareness about dementia and co-morbidities. *Journal of Alzheimer's Disease Reports, 8*(1), 747–764. https://doi.org/10.3233/ADR-240043

Cabrera, L. Y., Kelly, P., & Vega, I. E. (2021). Knowledge and attitudes of two Latino groups about Alzheimer disease: A qualitative study. *Journal of Cross-Cultural Gerontology, 36*(3), 265–284.

Centers for Medicare & Medicaid Services. (2024). Cognitive assessment & care plan services. Retrieved September 10, 2024, from https://www.cms.gov/medicare/payment/fee-schedules/physician/cognitive-assessment

Chaurasia, N., Singh, A., Singh, I. L., Singh, T., & Tiwari, T. (2020). Cognitive dysfunction in patients of rheumatoid arthritis. *Journal of Family Medicine and Primary Care, 9*(5), 2219–2225. https://doi.org/10.4103/jfmpc.jfmpc_307_20

Choukou, M.-A., Olatoye, F., Urbanowski, R., Caon, M., & Monnin, C. (2023). Digital health technology to support healthcare professionals and family caregivers caring for patients with cognitive impairment: Scoping review. *JMIR Mental Health, 10*, Article e40330. https://doi.org/10.2196/40330

Collum, L., & Karlawish, J. (2020). Cognitive impairment evaluation and management. *Medical Clinics of North America, 104*(5), 807–825. https://doi.org/10.1016/j.mcna.2020.06.007

Cuevas, H., Heitkemper, E., & Haque, B. (2022a). Relationships among perception of cognitive function, diabetes self-management, and glucose variability in older adults: A mixed methods study. *Research in Gerontologic Nursing, 15*(4), 203–212. https://doi.org/10.3928/19404921-20220609-02

Cuevas, H., Danesh, V., & Henneghan, A. (2022b, Mar 31). Self-reported cognitive function in persons with non-neurologic chronic diseases: A systematic review. *Journal of Aging Research*, 5803337.

Cuevas, H., Heitkemper, E., & Kim, J. (2024). Subjective cognitive dysfunction in chronic illness: A systematic review and meta-synthesis. *Western Journal of Nursing Research, 46*(9), 708–724. https://doi.org/10.1177/01939459241272039

Cuevas, H., Heitkemper, E., Huang, Y. C., Jang, D. E., Garcia, A. A., & Zuniga, J. A. (2021). A systematic review and meta-analysis of patient activation in people living with chronic conditions. *Patient Education and Counseling, 104*(9), 2200–2212.

Daunt, P., Ballard, C. G., Creese, B., Davidson, G., Hardy, J., Oshota, O., … & Alzheimer's Disease Neuroimaging Initiative. (2021). Polygenic risk scoring is an effective approach to predict those individuals most likely to decline cognitively due to Alzheimer's disease. *The Journal of Prevention of Alzheimer's Disease, 8*(1), 78–83.

Dautzenberg, G. M., Lijmer, J. G., & Beekman, A. T. (2022). The montreal cognitive assessment (MoCA) with a double threshold: Improving the MoCA for triaging patients in need of a neuropsychological assessment. *International Psychogeriatrics, 34*(6), 571–583.

Dreo, J., Jug, J., Pavlovčič, T., Ogrin, A., Demšar, A., Aljaž, B., Agatić, F., & Marusic, U. (2024). Comparative Performance of Five Cognitive Screening Tests in a Large Sample of Seniors. *Dementia and Geriatric Cognitive Disorders, 53*(6), 289-298.

Earnshaw, V. A., Watson, R. J., Eaton, L. A., Brousseau, N. M., Laurenceau, J. P., & Fox, A. B. (2022). Integrating time into stigma and health research. *Nature Reviews Psychology, 1*, 236–247. https://doi.org/10.1038/s44159-022-00034-2

Ford, E., Sheppard, J., Oliver, S., Rooney, P., Banerjee, S., & Cassell, J. A. (2021). Automated detection of patients with dementia whose symptoms have been identified in primary care but have no formal diagnosis: A retrospective case-control study using electronic primary care records. *British Medical Journal Open, 11*(1), Article e039248. https://doi.org/10.1136/bmjopen-2020-039248

Gates, T. M., Kamminga, J., Jayewardene, A., Vincent, T., Quan, D., Brew, B. J., Bloch, M., & Cysique, L. A. (2021). An examination of reliable change methods for measuring cognitive change with the Cogstate computerized battery: Research and clinical implications. *Archives of Clinical Neuropsychology, 36*(4), 597-612.

Gerontological Society of America. (2025). *KAER Toolkit*. Retrieved June 17, 2025, from https://www.kaerbrain.org/

Goh, F. Q., Kong, W. K. F., Wong, R. C. C., et al. (2022). Cognitive impairment in heart failure—a review. *Biology, 11*(2), 179. https://doi.org/10.3390/biology11020179

Hanseewu, B. J., Scott, M. R., Sikkes, S. A. M., Properzi, M., Gatchel, J. R., Salmon, E., Marshall, G. A., & Vannini, P. (2020). Evolution of anosognosia in Alzheimer's Disease and its relationship to amyloid. *Annals of Neurology, 87*(2), 267–280. https://doi.org/10.1002/ana.25649

Hill, N, L., Bhargava, S., Brown, M. J., Kim, H., Bhang, I., Mullin, K., Phillips, K. & Mogle, J. (2021). Cognitive complaints in age-related chronic conditions: A systematic review. *PLOS One*. https://doi.org/10.1371/journal.pone.0253795

Hilsabeck, R. C., Perry, W., Lacritz, L., et al. (2024). Improving early detection of cognitive impairment in older adults in primary care clinics: Recommendations from an interdisciplinary geriatrics summit. *Annals of Family Medicine, 22*(6), 543–549. https://doi.org/10.1370/afm.3174

Islam, S. S., Neargarder, S., Kinger, S. B., Fox-Fuller, J. T., Salazar, R. D., & Cronin-Golomb, A. (2022). Perceived stigma and quality of life in Parkinson's disease with additional health conditions. *General Psychiatry, 35*(3), Article e100653.

Jacobson, M., Thunell, J., & Zissimopoulos, J. (2020). Cognitive assessment at Medicare's annual wellness visit in fee-for-service and Medicare advantage plans. *Health Affairs, 39*(11), 1935–1942. https://doi.org/10.1377/hlthaff.2019.01795

Jones, A., Ali, M. U., Kenny, M., Mayhew, A., Mokashi V., He, H., Lin, S., Yavari, E., Paik, K., Subramanian, D., Dydynsky, R., Aryal, K., Correia, R. H., Dash, D., Manis, D. R., O'Connell, M., Liu-Ambrose, T., Taler, V., McMillan, J. M., … & Griffith, L. (2024) Potentially modifiable risk factors of dementia and mild cognitive impairment: An umbrella review and meta-analysis. *Dementia and Geriatric Cognitive Disorders, 53*(2), 91–106. https://doi.org/10.1159/000536643

Jorm, A. F. (1994). A short form of the Informant Questionnaire on Cognitive Decline in the Elderly (IQCODE): Development and cross-validation. *Psychological Medicine, 24*(1), 145–153.

Kanne, G. E., McConnell, E. S., Disco, M. E., Black, M. C., Upchurch, G., Matters, L. M., Halpern, D. J., White, H. K., & Helfin, M. T. (2023). The interagency care team: A new model to integrate social and medical care for older adults in primary care. *Geriatric Nursing, 50*, 72–79. https://doi.org/10.1016/j.gerinurse.2022.12.008

Kendell, C., Kotecha, J., Martin, M., Han, H., Jorgensen, M., & Urquhart, R. (2020). Patient and caregiver perspectives on early identification for advance care planning in primary healthcare settings. *BMC Family Practice, 21*(1), 136. https://doi.org/10.1186/s12875-020-01206-w

Ketterer, M. W., Ouellette, D., & Jennings, J. (2019). Psychoeducation for chronic cognitive impairment and reduced early readmissions amongst pulmonary inpatients. *Psychology, Health, & Medicine, 24*(10), 1207–1212. https://doi.org/10.1080/13548506.2019.1601749

Kim, J. S., Park, E., & Minjeong, A. N. (2019). The cognitive impact of chronic diseases on functional capacity in community-dwelling adults. *Journal of Nursing Research, 27*, Article e3. https://doi.org/10.1097/jnr.0000000000000272

Kiselica, A. M., Karr, J. E., & Mikula, C. M. (2024). Recent advances in neuropsychological test interpretation for clinical practice. *Neuropsychology Reviews, 34*(2), 637–667. https://doi.org/10.1007/s11065-023-09596-1

Lange, M., Joly, F., Vardy, J., Ahles, T., Dubois, M., & Castel, H. (2019). Cancer-related cognitive impairment: An update on state of the art, detection, and management strategies in cancer survivors. *Annals of Oncology, 30*, 1925–1940. https://doi.org/10.1093/annonc/mdz410

Lara-Ruiz, J., Kauzor, K., Nakhala, M., Banuelos, D., Woo, E., & Razani, J. (2019). The functional ability of MCI and Alzheimer's patients predicts caregiver burden. *Journal of Gerontopsychology and geriatric psychiatry, 32*(1), 31–39. https://doi.org/10.1024/1662-9647/a000200

Lee, K. G. R., Ghadge, A., Raut, B., Veighey, K., Amin, J., Capasso, G., Cockwell, P., Kalra, P. A., Pepin, M., Phillips, T., Taal, M., Unwin, R. & Fraser, S. D. S. (2025). Cognitive impairment and health outcomes in non-dialysis chronic kidney disease: A systematic review and meta-analysis. *Clinical Kidney Journal, 18*(6), sfaf150. https://doi.org/10.1093/ckj/sfaf150

Lindeza, P., Rodrigues, M., Costa, J., Guerreiro, M., & Rosa, M. M. (2024). Impact of dementia on informal care: A systematic review of family caregivers' perceptions. *BMJ Supportive & Palliative Care, 14*(e1), e38–e49. https://doi.org/10.1136/bmjspcare-2020-002242

Light, S. W., Sideman, A. B., Vela, A., & Wolf, M. S. (2024). Introducing a brain health literacy framework to promote health equity for Latinos: A discussion paper. *Patient Education and Counseling, 124*, Article 108254.

Lovett, R. M., Curtis, L. M., Persell, S. D., et al. (2020). Cognitive impairment no dementia and associations with health literacy, self-management skills, and functional health status. *Patient Education & Counseling, 103*(9), 1805–1811. https://doi.org/10.1016/j.pec.2020.03.013

Martín, J., Padierna, A., Anton-Ladislao, A., Moro, I., & Quintana, J. M. (2019). Predictors of mortality during hospitalization and 3 months after discharge in elderly people with and without dementia. *Aging & Mental Health, 23*(8), 1057–1065. https://doi.org/10.1080/13607863.2018.1459471

Mattke, S., Jun, H., Chen, E., Liu, Y., Becker, A., & Wallick, C. (2023). Expected and diagnosed rates of mild cognitive impairment and dementia in the US Medicare population: Observational analysis. *Alzheimer's Research & Therapy, 15*(1), 128.

Morris, C., Mitchell, J. W., Moorey, H., Younan, H. C., Tadros, G., & Turner, A. M. (2019). Memory, attention, and fluency deficits in COPD may be a specific form of cognitive impairment. *ERJ Open Research, 5*(2), 00229–02018. https://doi.org/10.1183/23120541.00229-2018

Mukherjee, U., Sehar, U., Brownell, M., & Reddy, P. H. (2024). Sleep deprivation in dementia comorbidities: Focus on cardiovascular disease, diabetes, anxiety/depression, and thyroid disorders. *Aging, 16*(21), 13409–13429. https://doi.org/10.18632/aging.206157

Muir, R. T., Hill, M. D., Black, S. E., & Smith, E. E. (2024). Minimal clinically important difference in Alzheimer's disease: Rapid review. *Alzheimer's & Dementia, 20*(5), 3352–3363.

National Association of Chronic Disease Directors. (2018). *Subjective cognitive decline—a public health issue*. Centers for Disease Control and Prevention. https://www.cdc.gov/healthy-aging-data/media/pdfs/subjective-cognitive-decline-508.pdf

Nosheny, R. L., Yen, D., Howell, T., et al. (2023). Evaluation of the electronic clinical dementia rating for dementia screening. *JAMA Network Open, 6*(9), Article e2333786. https://doi.org/10.1001/jamanetworkopen.2023.33786

Passmore, R. C., Iqbal, A., Rader, T. L., et al. (2024). Team-based approach to successful annual wellness visits. *Journal of Primary Care and Community Health, 15*, 21501319241249400. https://doi.org/10.1177/21501319241249400

Park, S. K. (2018). Trajectories of change in cognitive function in people with chronic obstructive pulmonary disease. *Journal of Clinical Nursing, 27*(7–8), 1529–1542.

Park, J., Jeong, E., & Seomun, G. (2018). The clock drawing test: A systematic review and meta-analysis of diagnostic accuracy. *Journal of Advanced Nursing, 74*(12), 2742–2754.

Patierno, C., Fava, G. A., & Carrozzino, D. (2023). Illness denial in medical disorders: A systematic review. *Psychotherapy and Psychosomatics, 92*(4), 211–226. https://doi.org/10.1159/000531260

Pépin, M., Levassort, H., & Massy, Z. A. (2024). The impact of chronic kidney disease on cognitive function. *Current Opinion in Nephrology and Hypertension, 33*(6), 566–572. https://doi.org/10.1097/MNH.0000000000001017

Pressler, S. J., Jung, M., Gradus-Pizlo, I., Titler, M. G., Smith, D. G., Gao, S., Lake, K. R., Burney, H., Clark, D. G., Wierenga, K. L., Dorsey, S. G., & Giordani, B. (2022). Randomized controlled trial of a cognitive intervention to improve memory in heart failure. *Journal of cardiac failure, 28*(4), 519-530.

Prigatano, G. P., Russell, S., & Meites, T. M. (2024). Studying lack of awareness of cognitive decline in neurodegenerative diseases requires measures of both anosognosia and denial. *Frontiers in Aging Neuroscience, 15*, 1325231. https://doi.org/10.3389/fnagi.2023.1325231

Quiroz, Y. T., Solis, M., Aranda, M. P., Arbaje, A. I., Arroyo-Miranda, M., Cabrera, L. Y., ... & Sexton, C. (2022). Addressing the disparities in dementia risk, early detection and care in Latino populations: Highlights from the second Latinos & Alzheimer's Symposium. *Alzheimer's & Dementia, 18*(9), 1677-1686.

Raetz, J., Fitzpatrick, A., Belza, B., McKiddy, S., Hsu, A., Liao, J., Park, C., & Gaster, B. (2023). The cognition in primary care program: A step-by-step clinic workflow putting the GSA KAER toolkit into action. *Innovation in Aging, 7*(Supplement_1), 920–920.

Riffin, C., Brody, L., Wolff, J. L., & Pillemer, K. A. (2025). A pilot trial evaluating collaborative healthcare encounters with caregivers: A checklist-based intervention for primary care. *Journal of Applied Gerontology,, 44*(12), 07334648251323688.

Roebuck-Spencer, T. M., Glen, T., Puente, A. E., Denney, R. L., Ruff, R. M., Hostetter, G., & Bianchini, K. J. (2017). Cognitive screening tests versus comprehensive neuropsychological test batteries: A national academy of neuropsychology education paper†. *Archives of Clinical Neuropsychology : The Official Journal of the National Academy of Neuropsychologists, 32*(4), 491–498. https://doi.org/10.1093/arclin/acx021

Schretlen, D. J., Finley, J.-C. A., Del Bene, V. A., & Varvaris, M. (2024). The ubiquity of cognitive impairment in human illness: A systematic review of meta-analyses. *Archives of Clinical Neuropsychology, acae113*. https://doi.org/10.1093/arclin/acae113

Shaji, B., & Joel, J. J. (2022). Impact of hypothyroidism on metabolic and cognitive dysfunction: A comprehensive review. *Journal of Young Pharmacists, 14*(4), 349–354. https://doi.org/10.5530/jyp.2022.14.71

Stuifbergen, A. K., Becker, H., Perez, F., Morrison, J., Brown, A., Kullberg, V., & Zhang, W. (2018). Computer-assisted cognitive rehabilitation in persons with multiple sclerosis: Results of a multi-site randomized controlled trial with six-month follow-up. *Disability and Health Journal, 11*(3), 427–434.

Sutton, R. T., Pincock, D., Baumgart, D. C., Sadowski, D. C., Fedorak, R. N., & Kroeker, K. I. (2020). An overview of clinical decision support systems: Benefits, risks, and strategies for success. *NPJ Digital Medicine, 3*, 17. https://doi.org/10.1038/s41746-020-0221-y

Tierney, M. C., Naglie, G., Upshur, R., Jaakkimainen, L., Moineddin, R., Charles, J., & Ganguli, M. (2014). Factors associated with primary care physicians' recognition of cognitive impairment in their older patients. *Alzheimer Disease & Associated Disorders, 28*(4), 320–325.

Townley, R. A., Syrjanen, J. A., Botha, H., Kremers, W. K., Aakre, J. A., Fields, J. A., ... & Boeve, B. F. (2019, August). Comparison of the short test of mental status and the montreal cognitive assessment across the cognitive spectrum. In *Mayo clinic proceedings* (Vol. 94, No. 8, pp. 1516–1523). Elsevier.

Tzeng, H. M., Raji, M. A., Shan, Y., Cram, P., & Kuo, Y. F. (2024). Annual wellness visits and early dementia diagnosis among Medicare beneficiaries. *JAMA Network Open, 7*, Article e2437247. https://doi.org/10.1001/jamanetworkopen.2024.37247

U.S. Preventive Services Task Force. (2020). Screening for cognitive impairment in older adults: U.S. Preventive Services Task Force recommendation statement. *JAMA, 323*(8), 757–763. https://doi.org/10.1001/jama.2020.0435

Vila-Castelar, C., Fox-Fuller, J. T., Guzmán-Vélez, E., Schoemaker, D., & Quiroz, Y. T. (2022). A cultural approach to dementia—insights from US Latino and other minoritized groups. *Nature Reviews Neurology, 18*(5), 307–314.

Vogeley, A., Cecil, P., Opsasnick, L., Curtis, L. M., Yoshino-Benavente, J., Bonham, M., Russell, A., O'Conor, R., Wolf, M. S., & Lovett, R. (2024). Associations between 10-year depressive symptom trajectories, cognitive function, and self-management capacity skills among older primary care patients. *Alzheimer's & Dementia,* 20(s3), e088300.

Von Ah, D., & Crouch, A. (2020). Cognitive rehabilitation for cognitive dysfunction after cancer and cancer treatment: implications for nursing practice. In *Seminars in oncology nursing* (Vol. 36, No. 1, p. 150977). WB Saunders.

Wagner, E. H. (2019). Organizing care for patients with chronic illness revisited. *The Milbank Quarterly, 97*(3), 659–664. https://doi.org/10.1111/1468-0009.12416

Wee, J., Sukudom, S., Bhat, S., Marklund, M., Peiris, N. J., Hoyos, C. M., Patel, S., Naismith, S. L., Dwivedi, G., & Misra, A. (2023). The relationship between midlife dyslipidemia and lifetime incidence of dementia: A systematic review and meta-analysis of cohort studies. *Alzheimer's & Dementia, 15*(1), e12395. https://doi.org/10.1002/dad2.12395

World Health Organization. (2021). *Global status report on the public health response to dementia.* https://www.who.int/publications/i/item/9789240033245

Wouters, H., Hilmer, S. N., Gnjidic, D., et al. (2020). Long-term exposure to anticholinergic and sedative medications and cognitive and physical function in later life. *The Journals of Gerontology: Series A, 75*(2), 357–365. https://doi.org/10.1093/gerona/glz019

Yu, X., He, H., Wen, J., Xu, X, Ruan, Z., Hu R, Wang F., & Ju, H. (2025). Diabetes-related cognitive impairment: Mechanisms, symptoms, and treatments. *Open Medicine, 20*(1), 20241091. https://doi.org/10.1515/med-2024-1091

Part III
Change in Action: Creating Neuropsychology Models to Meet Population Health Demands

Chapter 9
Leading Systems-Level Change in a Model of Population Health

Robert Fallows and Margaret Lanca

Executive Summary
This chapter explores the tools and strategies necessary for promoting and leading system-level change within a model of population health. It begins by examining how healthcare systems evolve, to emphasize the importance of understanding and applying change management processes. Within that process, specific quality improvement tools are integrated leaning on implementation science as a powerful tool for effecting reliable change. Finally, the chapter addresses the development of leadership skills in health management by discussing the essential skills required for effective leadership. Specifically, the contrast of a manager versus a leader is emphasized with a call to action for those stepping into leadership.

R. Fallows (✉)
Samaritan Medical Group, Corvallis, OR, USA
e-mail: rfallows@samhealth.org

M. Lanca
Cambridge Health Alliance; Harvard Medical School, Cambridge, MA, USA
e-mail: margaret_lanca@hms.harvard.edu

M. Lanca and R. Fallows (eds.), *Advancing Neuropsychology Through Population Health*, https://doi.org/10.1007/978-3-032-22457-6_9

Systems and Change

The Evolution of Healthcare Systems: How Does It Happen?

Population health management is a relatively novel approach for healthcare and can be conceptualized as a framework for realizing the promises of population health, which continues to evolve within dynamic, changing systems. As neuro/psychologists know, change can be challenging for individuals and organizations alike, as we all seek homeostasis, including healthcare systems. Effective implementation of a population health mission requires that healthcare leaders refine their skills to understand change management processes specifically for a population health context. Leaders must learn how to sustain a healthy workforce in a time of high burnout rates and know how to lead within and outside of healthcare organizations through models such as collective impact.

Much has been written on the topic of change in healthcare, and both external and internal forces are recognized to be integral. Externally, healthcare is a highly regulated sector. In one study, the American Hospital Association (2017) reported that there were 629 discrete federal regulatory requirements and that an average hospital needs to dedicate 59 full time employees to manage compliance of these regulations, costing $39 billion a year, industry wide. When new rules are enacted, systems are expected to pivot how they report out their work by a certain date and sometimes with incomplete information as regulatory requirements are not always clear. Depending on whether it is a healthcare system or a hospital, innovations in healthcare can also serve as external drivers. The introduction of GLP-1 pharmaceuticals, for example, had ripple effects throughout healthcare starting with upstream prevention benefits for obesity to chronic disease management. This single drug class undoubtedly was felt with greater significance for the primary care provider, but spread throughout healthcare, especially for bariatric surgeons (Lin et al., 2024). But ripple effects are also felt by neuropsychology, as the neuropsychologist must also consider how they adapt their feedback and understanding of this treatment for patients with questions about how weight loss may or may not be protective against neurodegenerative conditions.

External drivers do not imply that health systems merely wait around for something to happen to them and then respond accordingly. Rather, there are tools that healthcare systems employ to manage or even mitigate external drivers of change. Mitigation efforts can range from hiring lobbyists or political advisors to influence the upcoming regulatory process, to hiring the right team to monitor the external environment and then implement the change within the system. It also generally includes a guiding philosophy, either spoken or unspoken, about how and when new treatments and innovations are taken on in the adoption cycle. Interestingly, the process of responding to external drivers and understanding the organization adoption cycle is key to sparking internal change as well. As demonstrated below, leaders who promote meaningful systems of change often follow key change management principles, being thoughtful of team design and employing evidence-based techniques to drive an outcome.

Change Management: Principles, Teams, and Methods for Internal Systems Change

John Kotter was a pioneer of change management, and his change management principles originally published in 1995 and memorialized in his 1996 book persist even in the face of rapidly evolving healthcare and technology (Kotter, 1996). Central to his change management principles was appreciating how change management interacts with leadership style. A leader that fails to consider change management principles and who adopts an authoritarian leadership style is likely to get work done on paper only, see few results, and wonder why the team reports burnout or is 'not on the same page.' Often these authoritarian leaders (if they have some awareness of the lack of change) may feel like a "health system in motion stays in motion," and that they are the only individual trying to effect change or who cares and may ultimately develop resentment toward their team. At the other extreme, an overly democratic leader who needs to ensure that all of their team members are 'on board' before proceeding is likely to wallow in the stagnant waters of "analysis paralysis." Further, as will be shown below, these overly democratic leaders are unlikely to truly get all members of their entire team 'on board' before being able to make change. Ultimately, the goal of change management should be to understand how change happens, drive this from an authoritative and empowering leadership style (that can flex to authoritarian or democratic, only when judicious to do so) and use empirically supported methods that drive this change. Leadership style is incredibly important to attend to and will be covered in the second half of this chapter; however, leadership style without effective change management makes for an incomplete, and sometimes incompetent leader.

The first step in Kotter's eight-step model for change management is to create a sense of urgency. This may be a learning edge for neuro/psychologists who do not typically have formal training in leadership, including knowing how to advocate for their projects/innovations in business settings. Rather, neuro/psychologists typically work with relatively small teams embedded within other teams (e.g., epilepsy) and/or departments (e.g., neurology, psychiatry) in larger healthcare organizations. To truly advocate and create that sense of urgency, the neuro/psychologist leader needs to act as an interpreter. That is, in advocating their project/innovation to administration, they can't speak in straightforward clinical terms and need to be able to discuss concepts related to financial outcomes and the regulatory environment. If the public needs to be engaged, they must be able to translate complex concepts in way that is engaging to the public. Ultimately, the message creating the sense of urgency should have consistency so that it feels genuine and clear; however, it must be adapted to the diverse stakeholders engaged in the project.

To illustrate these concepts, the change management and quality improvement process of a fictitious healthcare system whose goal was to improve evidence-based suicide prevention in their communities is elaborated. In this fictitious health system, a Medical Director who is a psychologist, Dr. Shield, not only identified a critical need in the healthcare organization for suicide prevention but recognized fertile timing for implementation, as the institution was in the second year of adopting a High Reliability Organization (HRO) operating system that prioritized safety. An HRO approach is an evidence-based strategy derived from high risk environments such as nuclear power plants and airline pilots, since adopted to healthcare, that includes five key pillars: preoccupation with failure, reluctance to simplify interpretations, sensitivity to operations, commitment to resilience, and deference to expertise. Within this environment, Dr. Shield created a sense of urgency by crafting the following major talking points to the two main stakeholders:

(1) **Healthcare administration**: "As part of our HRO journey, we need to recognize the impact of suicide on our healthcare system and communities. Our state has one of the highest suicide rates in the country and providers are often not well equipped to mitigate risk and direct individuals to effective treatment. Consequently, patients are often sent to overloaded emergency departments where their symptoms are not fully addressed, leaving them feeling unheard and dissatisfied. Although suicide prevention is complex, we have committed to a reluctance to simplify interpretations and defer to expertise. With that in mind, there are established evidence-based approaches, which exist for driving that change, including grant funding to help us implement this work."

(2) **Primary care and integrated behavioral health colleagues**: "Most patients who die by suicide saw a healthcare provider in the month preceding their death. For many of those patients, that was not a behavioral health provider. Patients trust their primary care teams and by building skill in mitigating risk and starting meaningful treatment, we can empower each other and our patients, save lives and reduce burnout."

Once the sense of urgency was established by providing a succinct, but emotionally powerful and data driven message (and getting ahead of the funding question), it was time for the second stage of Kotter's work: build the guiding coalition. Here, Dr. Shield leaned on another time-tested principle. In his 1962 text, *Diffusion of Innovations*, Everett Rogers described the *adoption curve,* which remains an integral part of understanding strategy in effecting internal change (Rogers, 1962). This curve can also be used to understand the different types of employees within an organization, division, or department and their likelihood of adopting change (see Fig. 9.1). While employees don't generally remain in one category for all new processes, team member's persona is critical. For example, the "innovator" on a specific project is often key to getting that project off the ground. These individuals will be the first to adopt a new process, are more tolerant of risk, and may be enthusiastic with personal stakes in the new process. Ultimately though, they make up a small part of

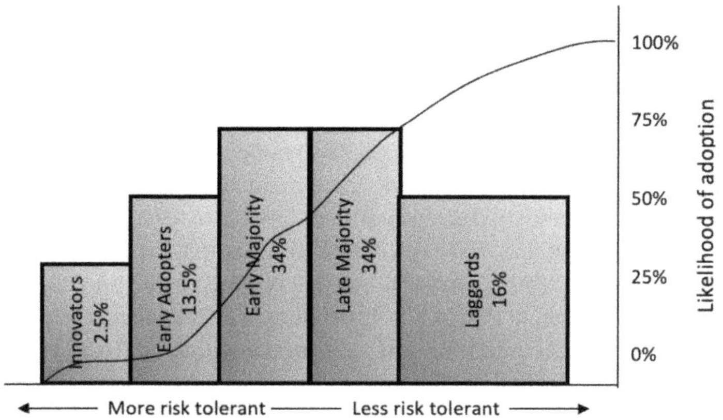

Fig. 9.1 The adoption curve

the team and designing a project with just them in mind is likely to fail. Instead, smart leaders are thoughtful to include early adopters and early majority individuals, in the initial change management cycle. Early adopters are influential individuals, sometimes opinion leaders in the group, who are willing to take some measured risks. The "early majority" is comprised of individuals who are more cautious and pragmatic, wanting to see some early proof of success. Understanding who in the group fits these categories and ensuring diversity of opinion in the design of a new process is more likely to ensure success; however, being neglectful of the right side of the curve is also a recipe for disaster. As a leader speaks to members of the late majority, that is, those individuals who are skeptical and typically only move forward with more substantial evidence of benefit/effect, a leader must take into consideration some of these team members' reservations and figure out how you address them in order to move forward.

With these principles in mind, it became very clear to Dr. Shield early on that there was no consistency across primary care clinics in this healthcare organization. Some had a 'red phone' procedure while others diverted calls to the integrated behavioral health provider. Some clinics were aware of the challenge and had formed their own internal committees (innovator/early adopter) while others were deferring to healthcare administrative leaders with frustration, to fix the problem (late majority/laggards). In developing the team, Dr. Shield identified a need to have a team representative of both stages of development as well as diversity in terms of role in the clinic. The team needed to also be small enough to be agile in getting the work done. As a result, an eight-person team with a primary care physician, a nurse practitioner, an integrated neuro/psychologist, a medical assistant, a manager, a front office/call center employee, and a policy writer was established, pulling heavily from clinics that were innovators to early majority but consulting with late majority clinic staff in the process.

The third and fourth phase of the change management process included developing a vision and strategy and effectively communicating that vision. This puts the leader in the position of needing to clearly define what the outcome of the work should be and creating a path toward achieving it while driving a compelling message for the importance of the work. In this case, Dr. Shield identified the critical points of intervention to improve the system, while recognizing the intervention must proceed systematically. They established an early framework for assessing and managing risk where the majority of patients were reaching out for help—primary care. Dr. Shield gathered his team who crafted a communique that outlined that within three, one-hour meetings, a risk management Policy and Procedure (P&P) in primary care was going to be developed which included training and implementation. To increase meeting efficiency, Dr. Shield asked team members to complete a training on evidence-based suicide risk management strategies in advance of their first meeting—ensuring that they were all working from a similar framework. In the first meeting, the takeaways from the training and challenges were reviewed within their roles, as well as discussing some templates of P&Ps from other organizations. Integrating that feedback, Dr. Shield and a policy writer constructed a draft framework and shared it in advance of a second meeting, where process was critiqued, and definitions clarified to facilitate training. Between the second and third meeting the leads worked to finalize language and flow and disseminate it to the group for a final review. In their third meeting, they edited final critiques, emphasizing the goal of not letting "perfect be the enemy of good," and started discussing how to train and implement this policy and procedure.

Just as the team developed a clear understanding of what their work was and the urgency behind it, the leader also needed to ensure that administrative leaders were onboard for the fifth element of change management (removing obstacles) to have the highest likelihood of success. In order to secure administrative support, it was again important to have a clear and compelling vision of what the team was trying to accomplish. While the priority in an HRO system is ultimately "no harm," the team decided to focus on subgoals that align with the process work. Recognizing that screening and mitigating risk was a primary reason for the P&P work, updates that reflect the success of that work was pivotal. An example of a key measure adopted by the team was the conversion percentage of "positive" depression screening (i.e., Patient Health Questionnaire—9 [PHQ-9] greater than 10 or with a question 9 greater than 0) to a more formal risk assessment tool (i.e., Columbia Suicide Severity Rating Scale [C-SSRS]). Sharing this change to administration while working with the team to define and understand barriers in early pilot testing was deemed the best strategy for Dr. Shield to have the greatest likelihood of success by meaningfully breaking down barriers. For example, if a barrier was identified by the team that primary care staff needed training, but didn't have time, it was decided that an engaged administrative staff would be more likely to help out if they better understood the potential benefits of such an investment. While the next step was Kotter's sixth strategy in change management of creating and celebrating short term wins (e.g., the creation of the P&P), two realities needed to be underscored:

1. Dr. Shield could not roll this program out system wide on Day One and expect spontaneous adoption, and
2. Adoption of new ideas and the nature of human behavior lead to variability in adoption, even in innovator/early adopter clinics. Patience is a virtue.

To address these realities, the skilled Dr. Shield implemented quality improvement techniques and ensured adherence to them. Here, Dr. Shield identified their early adopter and innovator clinics and took the information from the team to begin training and rolling out the policy and procedure as a pilot. They defined their metric of PHQ-9 to C-SSRS conversion rate and repeated the first six steps in Kotter's change management strategy with the target clinic to determine impact on that outcome. Outcome metrics are an essential part of the change management process. If Dr. Shields went to the team and presented the information in table format, the September 2024 meeting would have been quite uncomfortable as they would have seen a downward trend in August (see Table 9.1).

Consequently, Dr. Shields presented the data in a control chart, demonstrating normal variation, or noise in the month of August (see Fig. 9.2). Ultimately, by combining these change management and quality improvement strategies, they were able to track the effect of different interventions with the team over time as they repeated change management cycles. For example, say in August 2024 Dr. Shield and the primary care clinic team conduct stakeholder interviews and decide that challenges related to stigma in the medical assistants may be contributing to a challenge in screening. Further, they find that physicians may be reluctant to instruct their team to screen, since resources for follow up are limited (e.g., "why ask questions for something I can't provide effective treatment for?").

Table 9.1 Hypothetical presentation of PHQ-9 to C-SSRS conversion rates

Month/Year	Conversion Rate (%)	Month/Year	Conversion Rate (%)	Month/Year	Conversion Rate (%)
Jan 2024	10.6	**April 2024**	14.0	**Jul 2024**	17.2
Feb 2024	18.0	**May 2024**	14.9	**Aug 2024**	14.9
Mar 2024	15.1	**Jun 2024**	17.1		

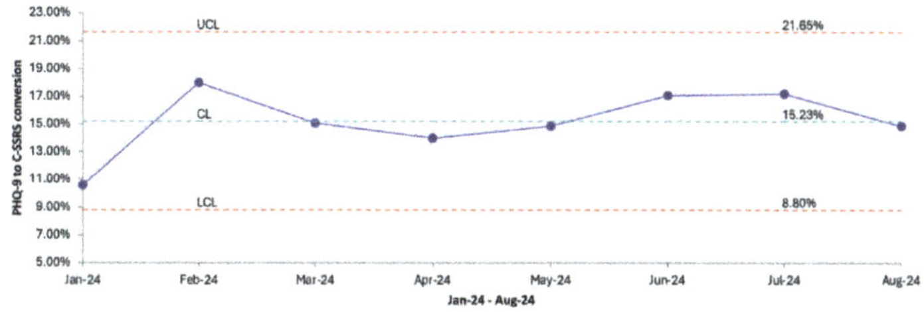

Fig. 9.2 Control chart presentation of PHQ-9 to C-SSRS conversion rates

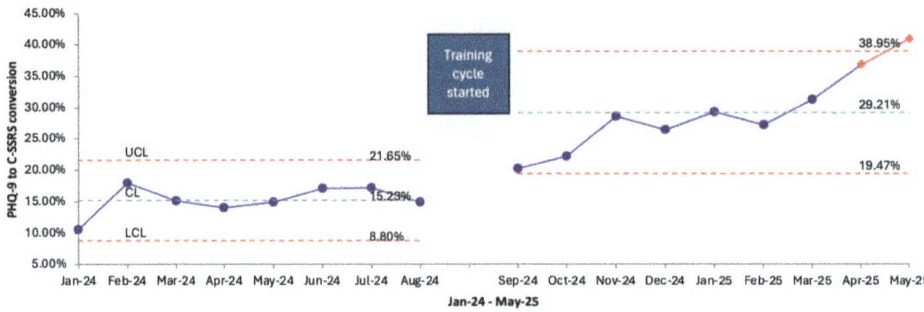

Fig. 9.3 Control chart presentation of PHQ-9 to C-SSRS conversion rates following clinic intervention

Based on this feedback, the team came back together to develop and implement two resources: a gatekeeper training proven to reduce stigma for the support staff (Question, Persuade, Refer [QPR]) and a physician training on why suicide risk reduction techniques work and clarifying what their role in the treatment process is (20 min lunch and learn). These change management cycles again lead the team to re-analyze the control chart to determine if the intervention was successful (see Fig. 9.3). In doing so, they create a break where the intervention occurred and find that not only was there some consistent evidence of upward improvement, but that the change may have extended further over time. Ultimately, these kinds of thoughtful implementations and working through the change management cycle helps the group succeed in Kotter's final steps in change management: sustaining momentum and anchoring the change in the culture.

For our psychologist, Dr. Shield, who was leading the charge, the change management process in Fig. 9.4 shows how the nature of this work was built on itself over time to sustain that change. In this graphic, Dr. Shields is using the Plan-Do-Study-Act (PDSA) cycle which included the following components: Plan (team agrees to two trainings to address a perceived barrier with a plan to measure the impact), Do (provide the trainings), Study (re-run the analysis in the control charts and examine the impact), and Act (based on the results, determine effectiveness of intervention and decide to persist or change course).

Change Management & Implementation Science Summary

Change can happen by either internal or external forces, but rarely if ever does positive internally driven change happen by accident. Rather, leaders need to be intentional about understanding the dynamics of the larger system, have a framework for understanding how change occurs and is sustained, and be able to articulate that change and the value of change to the different stakeholders. Their focus is on building that sense of urgency, creating high functioning teams that carry out the work

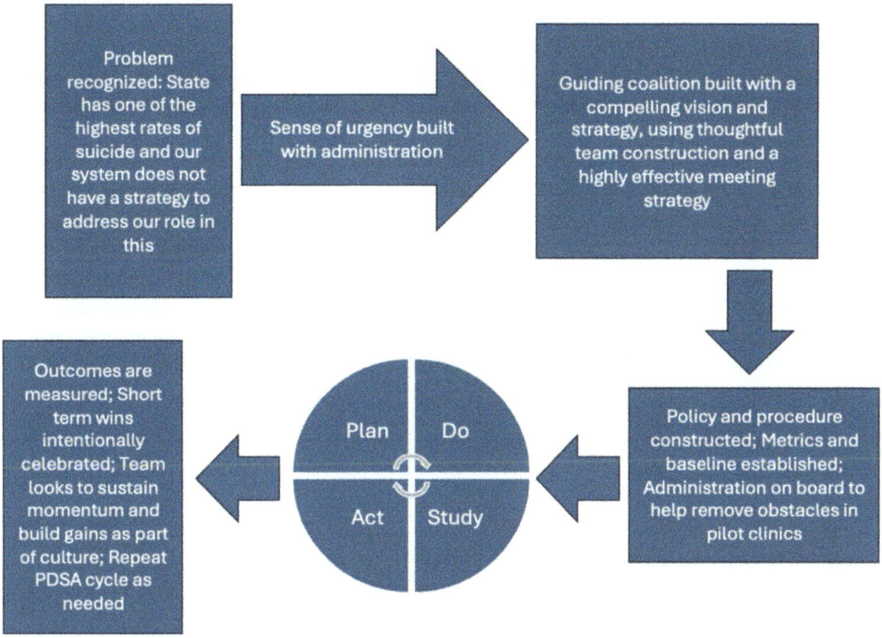

Fig. 9.4 Overview of the change management process for Dr. Shield

effectively while reducing waste, and sustaining change once it is gained. Leaders in these situations often find themselves playing the role of interpreter, educator, facilitator, and vision holder while pulling in multiple evidence-based tools to drive the outcome.

While neuro/psychologists have many foundational tools inherent to help them be successful in quality improvement (QI) work, there are other skills they will need to develop and graduate programs would be wise to adopt teaching of these techniques into curriculum (Arredondo et al., 2025). Examples of these methods include QI methodologies such as the Plan-Do-Study-Act (PDSA) cycle or the Define, Measure, Analyze, Improve, and Control (DMAIC) method. Given the psychometrics training neuro/psychologists receive in graduate school, they are well equipped to interpret when a PDSA/DMAIC cycle is effective and can relay to their administrative counterparts that change management involves some degree of normal variation. To do this, control charts (also called Shewhart charts and process improvement charts) can help the administrative team to understand that the fluctuation that is observed is simply 'noise' by examining when observations exceed the upper or lower control limit or follow above or below the mean in a consecutive series (e.g., rule of 7 consecutively falling above or below the mean). These charts are easy to understand once simple education is provided and provide more meaningful discussion with whichever team the neuro/psychologist is working with.

Implementation Takeaway #1

Change management cycles are typically implemented for large projects that healthcare systems are trying to undertake, such as the fictitious hospital's suicide prevention initiative. However, they do not have to occur on such a large scale and these principles work well when scaled down. For example, neuropsychology clinic wait lists are often quite significant as demonstrated in Chaps. 5 and 6. When services are inaccessible, they are less likely to be utilized and work arounds that may be less effective are likely to be sought. The neuro/psychologist seeking to streamline access in their clinic while creating space for neuro/psychologists and their colleagues to focus on primary and secondary prevention components can follow a similar process as outlined above. Additional reading on these techniques is encouraged, and many healthcare systems have dedicated quality or process improvement teams that can aid in rolling out these strategies.

Neuro/Psychologists Leading Healthcare Change

Building a Case for Leadership as a Complimentary, but Distinct Skill Set

Change management strategies are essential in healthcare leadership, and an integral skill set of an effective leader. Managers are typically key to driving initiatives and implementations. Specifically, a manager can direct projects, lead constructive conversations to create a product, and measure outcomes following a PDSA cycle. When a leader does this work, they are engaging their team in a different way that helps to evolve the culture of the group. The leader does this by understanding where the work aligns within their larger vision, has a guiding philosophy for how they go about executing that vision by engaging others, and uses personal reflection and continuous learning to improve/develop their skill set.

In the complex world of modern healthcare transitioning toward population health, emerging evidence has shown that healthcare organizations led by clinicians may have better patient outcomes (Goodall, 2011; Tasi et al., 2019) and staff retention (Bäker & Goodall, 2021). And while clinicians spend years attaining and refining their clinical expertise through independent self-study, coursework, continuing education, supervised work experience and other methods, very few clinical programs emphasize leadership development as part the training curriculum. Experts note that changes need to occur to clinical training curriculum to foster important leadership development skills (Berwick et al., 2008); however, for some the absence of training is likely driven by a belief that all the expertise gained in medical or graduate school simply translates to leadership skills; this is often referred to as "Expert Leadership" (Goodall et al., 2015). There are four driving factors as to why these experts perform better than non-clinician management. These include acknowledgement that the clinician is immediately viewed as part of the group of other clinicians, not an outsider, and has an inherent appreciation of the values and motivations of their colleagues they lead. Further, Goodall suggests that these expert leaders are better able to drive translational medicine by tying together academics and clinical delivery and that well established clinician experts may also be able to attract better candidates into the organization. While these attributes may certainly be true, researchers examining clinician leadership uniformly acknowledge that clinicians need to develop other skills in order to thrive as leaders (Looi et al., 2023; Stoller, 2014).

Whether leading a small team or a large organization, it is important for neuro/psychologists to recognize that not all of the skills gained in their clinical training are immediately transferable to leadership. In comparing and contrasting some of the core competencies of neuro/psychologists (American Board of Professional Psychology, 2025; American Psychological Association, 2011) versus skills required for clinician leaders (Angood & Falcone, 2023) (see Table 9.2), one can appreciate the need for additional training to foster development of these essential attributes. Specifically, in their clinical practices, neuro/psychologists may be working in collaborative environments with multi-disciplinary teams. They focus their work on evidence-based assessment and intervention methods to meet the needs of the diverse communities they serve while also addressing the questions of the clinical care team. They are self-reflective and monitor their ethical decision making, and how their practice and ethics interact with different values and ethics of colleagues. As the neuro/psychologist steps into leadership, additional skills are needed. Leaders build business acumen including finance and strategic knowledge while embracing and guiding organizations through complex legal and regulatory landscapes. They recognize that they are not often the sole decision maker but collaborate with teams to drive outcomes. They become excellent communicators that are forward thinking, developing a vision and communicating in a way that attracts and empowers others. In both situations, they recognize that their clinical and leadership skills need continued improvement, being aware of their boundaries of competence and committed to lifelong learning.

Ultimately, leadership training should be incorporated earlier in careers, as opposed to learning through trial and error. The latter may risk development of a dominance style of leadership (i.e., authoritarianism) which may naturally rise out of a clinician's directive/expert role in their practice. Specifically, within an individual practice, some degree of "command and control" may be employed as the expert; however, as a clinician leader, expertise must often be balanced with collaboration and influence and there are some leadership styles that emphasize substantial humility to the extent of countering "command and control" (Angood & Falcone, 2023; Looi et al., 2023).

Table 9.2 Commonalities and differences In neuro/psychologist vs leadership training

	Psychologist based training skills	Leadership based training skills
Professionalism	Reflecting the values and ethics of psychology, taking personal responsibility and working proactively to monitor and resolve professional challenges	Develop, communicate, and execute a vision that helps all employees connect their individual work with the larger picture of the organization. Lead through collaboration and influence
Ethics/Legal	Uses advanced knowledge of professional ethics codes and models ability to apply ethical decision making into work	Steer organizations through complex and frequently changing regulatory and legal requirements; balance many ethical codes simultaneously
Reflective Practice	Engages in reflection around professional activity and is aware of limitations in knowledge/ability, develops plans to address gaps. Monitors need for self-care and supervision/consultation	Understanding that leadership is a skill that will require ongoing development and maintenance. Commitment to strong emotional intelligence and self-evaluation of outcomes
Relationships	Manages difficult communication and has developed skill with verbal and non-verbal methods of communication. Engaged in a variety of relationships and evaluates effectiveness to engage in those relationships	Ability to operate within a dyad or triad model of leadership, being paired with an administrative or nurse leader. Be able to understand the priorities and language of other leaders (e.g., legal, finance, human resources)
Supervision	Has knowledge of different supervision models and delivers effective supervision, while self-monitoring any limits in competency to meet supervisee's needs	Driving a culture of wellness and safety, intentionally addressing burnout and violence in healthcare. Able to engage in feedback, coaching, and mentoring of others
Management-Administration	Provides constructive feedback and operates within the management hierarchy. Shows ability to administer programs and participates in change efforts	Ability to engage in strategic planning and budgeting, prioritizing the often limited resources of healthcare organizations to drive outcomes

Building a Pathway for Clinician Leaders

Acquiring leadership training in a neuro/psychologist's career, either during training or subsequently, will equip them to take on leadership roles which may create significant benefit for the systems in which they operate. The impetus is not solely on the provider to develop these skills, though. It also benefits healthcare organizations to build a strong pipeline of clinician leaders to remain competitive/viable in a tumultuous US healthcare landscape (Angood & Falcone, 2023). Not dissimilar from the skills required to develop clinical expertise, clinicians benefit from outcomes based training programs that are multi-modal, including coursework, simulation, and feedback through coaching and mentoring (Geerts et al., 2020). Out of this necessity, several training programs for clinician leaders have improved over the past decade, ranging from professional organizations (e.g., the American Association for Physician Leadership), to workshop-based programs adopted by healthcare organizations, to executive master's degree programs for clinicians. Continuing education and numerous books on the topic of leadership also serve to augment the clinician leader's ability to grow their skill.

Implementation Takeaway #2

1. All clinicians are leaders. Even the solo practitioner in a growing outpatient clinic of a hospital system carries expertise that others will defer to; it is therefore important to understand how to grow and manage expert leadership.
2. Neuro/psychologists have clinical training which prepares them well for formal leadership roles; however, to thrive as a leader, they should seek both formal and informal training to hone their skills in business acumen, change management, management of others, communication, and vision/strategy development and execution.

Additional Considerations Regarding Healthcare Clinician Leadership Styles

There are various prominent leadership philosophies and often skilled leaders will blend theories for specific purposes, values, and expectations within the context of the group/organization they are leading. The most prominent styles are transactional, servant, and transformational. Each of these can be successful, but its success is often shaped by the workplace context and what it demands, as well as the leader's own personality style. Regardless of the style of leadership, having a solid set of principles to guide a leader is critical. Further, leaders must maintain flexibility to adapt to the situation and environment, especially when considering the longevity of one's leadership journey. Ensuring that one is engaged in reflection and intentional about methods is crucial to the integrity and effectiveness as a leader.

Transactional leadership remains a prevalent leadership orientation in the structure of healthcare (Burns, 1978). It is based on the concept of clear structure with accountability toward goals. Meeting goals, such as productivity requirements, is rewarded by the system and leader; however, failure to meet a goal can result in punishment. The goal of this style of leadership is to drive performance and there is a strong sense of order; however, the consequence of this leadership style is that employees can feel negatively engaged when punishments occur, and that the leadership structure can feel stifling to creativity. Further, the leader skilled only in a transactional style really does not have very many tools from which to lead, with the exception of coming up with new incentives or punishments. *Servant* leaders tend to be relationally focused leaders who emphasize psychological trust and safety while downplaying their own contributions and promoting the needs of the people they lead (Greanleaf, 1977). These leaders tend to be empathetic and focus on a positive workplace environment with mentoring, active listening, and focusing on collaboration and continual learning. While this leadership style can be an asset in many environments, in some systems this type of leader may be regarded as overly passive and not the one to go to in case of an emergency. Servant leaders also tend to adhere to a more democratic style of leadership which can create delays in making decisions. The *transformational* leader is generally a charismatic leader who may be described by their team as a visionary or inspirational (Bass, 1985). These types of leaders are typically quick thinking, adaptable, and create a sense of enthusiasm in those they lead. Still, this leader type has some weaknesses associated with them as well, including perception that the leader may be "all talk" that they are creating too much competition among their direct reports, or that the organization is overly dependent on their vision alone.

Given the strengths and weakness associated with all types of leaders, dogmatic adherence to one leadership style can be limiting, and akin to rigid adherence to a psychological theory. Even the strictest of cognitive behavioral therapists typically recognizes the suitability of other theoretical perspectives as needed (e.g., the presence of transference and countertransference in their work with patients). This is not unlike a neuro/psychologist who typically adopts a fixed-flexible approach a neuropsychological evaluation. The same flexibility is needed in leadership; learning and applying various leadership approaches is important—ones that fit a personal style and work setting, but also applying other styles as needed. Further, critical to leadership development is the opportunity to seek mentorship, coaching, and/or 360 evaluative feedback that provides a truer barometer of performance.

Rarely Leading Alone: Healthcare Organizational Structure and Leadership

Healthcare is a relatively non-descript term for a huge, multifaceted industry. To some, it can be a small private or group practice, and to others, it is associated with being a part of a very large conglomerate system. It can also refer businesses associated with pharmaceuticals/medical devices, technology start-ups, electronic medical record systems, and patient advocacy groups, etc. Given that healthcare is such a diverse industry, leaders are going to encounter different organizational structures for leadership.

Some of the most prominent organizational structures have leadership structures that are either: (1) flat; (2) hierarchical; and/or (3) matrixed, but there are other structures too. Flat leadership does not necessarily refer to the absence of a hierarchical structure or organizational chart. Rather, it is focused on the intentional distribution of the decision making process, as opposed to a more directive approach. Further, while there often is still an organizational chart, efforts tend to be made to reduce the distance between the individual workers and the higher leaders in the organization. Collaboration is highly valued and there is a strong need for psychological safety and trust as employees are placed into smaller teams which often align with their areas of passion. Within these teams, democratic styles or a deference to expertise depending on the make-up of the team is preferred. While empowering to team members, these structures can be harder to sustain in larger organizations and can create confusion for some about who to report to for which projects/needs. Still, even within larger organizations, it is not uncommon to see projects adopt a flat leadership structure. In our fictitious hospital developing a suicide prevention platform, it would likely behoove Dr. Shield to employ a flat leadership structure in this situation, even if they work in a hierarchical organization. By doing so, deference to various types of expertise within the small, but diverse team is valued to drive the outcome. For example, the medical assistant will be able to speak more directly to the screening process and barriers compared to the front office staff member and the psychologist will be more adept at discussing the psychometrics/validity of tools than the medical assistant. Thus, a flat team that acknowledges these areas of expertise and values them by intentionally seeking them out, brings out the best chance of a policy reflective of the work that needs to be done while catching and addressing potential blind spots early on.

Other organizational structures can include hierarchical and division types, which are common among medium to large healthcare organizations. Here, specialists are grouped according to their areas of expertise (e.g., hospitalists vs. primary care) to better support specific goals that reflect their work (e.g., lowering re-admission rate for hospitalists vs. access metrics for primary care). Within these divisions or service lines, smaller teams (e.g., a specific clinic) tend to report to medical or regional directors, flowing then to the chief or senior medical director and onward to the chief medical officer. While some organizations task their medical directors with administrative tasks, others employ a dyad leadership model where a healthcare administrator is paired with the clinician leader. While these structures tend to promote reporting line clarity, decision making can sometimes become over centralized and carry a top-down philosophy instead of ensuring that bottom-up communication is flowing effectively.

Matrixed organizations are characterized by two or more entities within one organization working together to drive an outcome. Often used to foster collaboration on important projects, this structure combines the efforts and knowledge of the separate entities to drive an outcome. For example, a graduate medical education (GME) program reports up through the hospital leadership structure; however, they operate within a medical group service area to complete their outpatient required hours which is not under hospital leadership. In this situation, the GME director and the medical group vice president collaborate on strategies to grow the success of both programs. Other potential benefits to matrixed organizations is that projects tend not to be siloed, potentially allowing for recognition of challenges (and hopefully earlier fixes) sooner in the project lifecycle. Like flat leadership structures, individuals can sometimes become confused about who they report to and collaborators can struggle with decision making processes. Tools such as RACI matrices (responsible, accountable, consulted, and informed) used early on in collaboration can be beneficial.

Two Key Issues for Leaders in the Current Healthcare Climate

There are many areas worthy of a leader's attention and time. The cost of healthcare in the United States is increasing, inflation has risen in an industry whose costs are primarily driven by labor and supply, and the overall quality of care has not kept pace with similar resourced countries as was noted in Chap. 1. These population health challenges demand that clinician leaders be well versed in business principles including financial concepts that were not a part of their training. However, it is equally important to understand that resolutions to these challenges will take time. Leaders in healthcare directing a population health agenda must address burnout in healthcare, a long enduring and worsening problem, alongside adoption of strategies for leading population health such as the collective impact model.

Burnout in Healthcare

It is not uncommon to hear administrative messaging of "no margin, no mission"; however, with no workforce, there is also clearly no mission. The rates of burnout across healthcare have increased post-COVID and this remains a notable challenge for managers and leaders. Drivers such as "work outside of work" (i.e., time spent in the electronic medical record outside of normal work hours), higher patient acuity, and greater demand with less resources remain pertinent and enduring themes for leaders to address. The impact of burnout on patient safety is worthy of consideration, the cost of replacing burnt out clinicians is high, and the impact to access is crucial to address. Consequently, leaders should be encouraged to ensure that their vision and subsequent strategies embrace the spirit of the Quadruple Aim (Bodenheimer & Sinsky, 2014). That is, in addition to focusing on patient experience, population health, and cost of care, leaders much ensure they are bringing clinician wellness into the picture for improving the global healthcare system. As with most change management strategies, approaching burnout from a top-down perspective is problematic. Doing so assumes that the leader knows what is best and does not honor the lived experience of their team members. Instead, leaders should consider that "effective change occurs when both [systems and individuals] develop in an integrated fashion" (Maslach et al., 2001, pg. 419). Other important factors include ensuring that addressing burnout with one group does not unexpectedly burden another group (e.g., shifting work from neuro/psychologists to their overloaded technicians), or that employees are being individually blamed. Rather, systems need to address burnout with by understanding systemic pressures, and initiating programs to address (e.g., wellness initiatives not solely focused on personal resilience). Understanding burnout as a function of societal and professional factors, the role of the organization in addressing those factors, and ensuring fidelity to efforts (e.g., avoiding well intentioned strategies turning into lip service at the individual unit level due to other priorities) is key to driving a successful outcome.

Collective Impact: Leading Beyond Healthcare's Four Walls

Healthcare organizations are being tasked with driving more outcome metrics in the pursuit of creating equitable opportunity for individuals to attain and sustain health. No longer can hospitals solely focus on bed capacity or average length of stay alone. Rather their value based contracts (see Chap. 3), and Medicare reporting standards require that they attend to a broad range of metrics in order to optimize their reimbursement (e.g., preventative care screening such as cancer and depression screening or chronic condition management such as diabetes or hypertension control). However, from a population health perspective, much of what defines health occurs outside the four walls of a healthcare system. In response to this demand, organizations and their leaders are revising their organizational values, mission, and vision, and reassessing their strengths and weaknesses. This process, often called a SWOT analysis (strengths, weaknesses, opportunities, and threats), is part of an organizational strategic planning process. Notably, it is not possible for an organization to singularly meet the full needs of what makes a community healthy and ensures that the opportunity for health is equitable. The Collective Impact model offers a potential framework for addressing these organizational gaps or weaknesses through partnering with other organizations for whom that area represents a strength (Kania & Kramer, 2011). This model posits five specific conditions that should exist for success, including having a common agenda among organizations, common measurement system and definition of success, ensuring that the activities are mutually reinforcing (not redundant or overly separated), continuous communication with each other using a shared vocabulary, and a supporting infrastructure (i.e., backbone organization).

Small opportunities frequently arise for implementation of collaborative frameworks, such as the Collective Impact model. In Oregon, for example a Medicaid waiver allowing for clinicians to 'prescribe food' in recognition that food insecurity is a driver of poor health outcomes was enacted. While many hospitals have cafeterias with nutritionists/dieticians that provide oversight of nutritional needs, they likely lack the framework for allocating, building, and making available food boxes for their community. Partnering with organizations for whom this is a strength (e.g., community food pantries) allows the healthcare system to help drive that outcome; however, this is still secondary prevention and not addressing the root cause. Thinking outside the box at the root cause of those issues (e.g., food insecurity being driven by living in a food desert in low income, marginalized communities), healthcare leaders can bring about even more innovative platforms for primary prevention. One example from the Boston Medical Center was identified in Chap. 1; however, many other similar examples exist. One such example is the partnership between Highland Hospital and Mandela MarketPlace in Oakland in 2018 which created opportunity to not only purchase healthier food within the community, but classes to learn how to use the fresh produce to effect lifestyle change (Novotny, 2018). The enduring impact of this work is worthy of consideration for other healthcare leaders, ensuring that it's not just checks for community impact that flow out the door, but true partnership addressing the drivers for health.

Conclusion

Much like the practice of neuro/psychology or any other health discipline, there is no one single path to becoming an effective leader. Positions can be posted, but true leaders are not appointed. Leadership is part skill and part art form, one that requires intentionally seeking out education, mentorship, coaching, and feedback within a framework of embracing continual improvement and commitment to life-long learning. Leaders are intentional about embracing and driving forth their organizational mission and vision, more often than not driving population health as part of their healthcare strategy. True leaders understand their core values and personal vision, facilitating outcomes through integrity. They maintain flexibility and integrate the facets of leadership theory that best match both their own style and the environment they operate in. Finally, they make sure they are thoughtful about how you go about the change process in recognition that the status quo in healthcare is 'no longer' sustainable, there is a dire sense of urgency for change. Change in healthcare is necessary and population health using established leadership tools that reduce waste provides a viable framework for leaders to point toward in order to help effect that change.

Key Points in Review

1. Change management principles are key to the success of the leader. These include understanding Kotter's principles of change management, the dynamics of team construction, and infusing those strategies with other essential tools that reduce waste and improve outcomes.
2. Lean Six Sigma offers several tools that should be considered by the neuro/psychologist trying to drive a population health outcome. Specifically, PDSA or DMAIC cycles provide the ability to pilot and measure outcomes of interventions. Control charts allow for better understanding of normal variability and differentiating noise and signal. Neuro/psychologists, given their expertise in research and psychometrics, are in a strong position to use these tools to improve healthcare.
3. While these tools are important in helping to drive an outcome in healthcare, they need to be accompanied by strong leadership skills which have not historically been a part of healthcare clinician training. Attending to leadership style while knowing thyself is essential to a leader's success. Further, there are several enduring trends that are important to monitor in healthcare beyond cost and access, including burnout, population health and collective impact, and the role of technology and the patient in healthcare delivery.

References

American Board of Professional Psychology. (2025). *Competency requirements—Foundational and functional.* https://abpp.org/application-information/competency-requirements/

American Hospital Association. (2017). *Regulatory overload: Assessing the regulatory burden on health systems, hospitals, and post-acute care providers.* https://www.aha.org/sites/default/files/regulatory-overload-report.pdf

American Psychological Association. (2011). *Benchmarks evaluation system.* https://www.apa.org/ed/graduate/benchmarks-evaluation-system?tab=3

Angood, P.B., & Falcone, C.M. (2023). *Preparing physician leaders for the future* (White paper). American Association for Physician Leadership and Korn Ferry. https://www.physicianleaders.org/articles/doi/10.55834/wp.3106435376

Arredondo, K., Caloudas, A. B., Wittkower, L. D., Caloudas, S. G., Godwin, K. M., Cully, J. A., & Ecker, A. H. (2025). *Psychology in health care: How psychologists' training translates to quality improvement.* Advance online publication. https://doi.org/10.1037/ser0000961

Bäker, A., & Goodall, A. H. (2021). Do expert clinicians make the best managers? Evidence from hospitals in Denmark, Australia and Switzerland. *BMJ Leader, 5*, 161–166.

Bass, B. M. (1985). *Leadership and performance beyond expectations.* Free Press.

Berwick, D. M., Nolan, T. W., & Whittington, J. (2008). The triple aim: Care, health, and cost. *Health Affairs (Project Hope), 27*(3), 759–769. https://doi.org/10.1377/hlthaff.27.3.759

Bodenheimer, T., & Sinsky, C. (2014). From triple to quadruple aim: Care of the patient requires care of the provider. *Annals of Family Medicine, 12*(6), 573–576. https://doi.org/10.1370/afm.1713

Burns, J. M. (1978). *Leadership.* Harper & Row.

Geerts, J. M., Goodall, A. H., & Agius, S. (2020). Evidence-based leadership development for physicians: A systematic literature review. *Social Science & Medicine (1982), 246*, 112709. https://doi.org/10.1016/j.socscimed.2019.112709

Goodall A. H. (2011). Physician-leaders and hospital performance: Is there an association? *Social Science & Medicine (1982), 73*(4), 535–539. https://doi.org/10.1016/j.socscimed.2011.06.025

Goodall, A. H., Bastiampillai, T., Nance, M., Roeger, L., & Allison, S. (2015). Expert leadership: Doctors versus managers for the executive leadership of Australian mental health. *Australian & New Zealand Journal of Psychiatry, 49*(5), 409–411. https://doi.org/10.1177/0004867415576977

Greenleaf, R.K. *(1977). Servant leadership: A journey into the nature of legitimate power and greatness.* Paulist Press.

Kania, J., & Kramer, M. (2011). *Collective impact.* https://ssir.org/articles/entry/collective_impact

Kotter, J. P. (1996). *Leading change.* Harvard Business School Press.

Lin, K., Mehrotra, A., & Tsai, T. C. (2024). Metabolic bariatric surgery in the era of GLP-1 receptor agonists for obesity management. *JAMA Network Open, 7*(10), Article e2441380. https://doi.org/10.1001/jamanetworkopen.2024.41380

Looi, J. C. L., Allison, S., Kisely, S. R., & Bastiampillai, T. (2023). Physician leadership during the current crisis in healthcare: A perspective drawn from anthropological and clinical leadership research. *Australasian Psychiatry: Bulletin of Royal Australian and New Zealand College of Psychiatrists, 31*(4), 463–465. https://doi.org/10.1177/10398562231169128

Maslach, C., Schaufeli, W. B., & Leiter, M. P. (2001). Job burnout. *Annual Review of Psychology, 52*(1), 397–422. https://doi.org/10.1146/annurev.psych.52.1.397

Novotny, L. (2018, May). *Hospital aims to fix Oakland food desert, boost population health.* https://www.alamedahealthsystem.org/hospital-aims-fix-oakland-food-desert-boost-population-health/

Rogers, E. (1962). *Diffusion of innovations.* The Free Press.

Stoller, J. K. (2014). Help wanted: Developing clinician leaders. *Perspectives on Medical Education: Journal of the Netherlands Association of Medical Education, 3*(3), 233–237.

Tasi, M. C., Keswani, A., & Bozic, K. J. (2019). Does physician leadership affect hospital quality, operational efficiency, and financial performance? *Health Care Management Review, 44*(3), 256–262. https://doi.org/10.1097/HMR.0000000000000173

Chapter 10
Using Digital Tools for Cognitive Assessment Across Levels of Care

Shifali Singh and Sara Weisenbach

Executive Summary
Digital tools for measuring cognition have incredible potential toward enabling more widespread screening for cognitive health and more precise and efficient measurement of cognitive skills. While there is growing interest in integrating such tools into clinical practice, there is still much work that needs to be done to ensure that they are equal to or better than current gold-standard measures of cognitive functioning. This chapter describes the expanding role of technology in cognitive assessment and considers important parameters for implementation, including balancing test results with good clinical reasoning. It also considers how digital tools can enhance health equity, and therefore overall population health, if utilized responsibly.

S. Singh
Department of Neuropsychology, McLean Hospital, Belmont, MA, USA

Institute for Technology in Psychiatry, McLean Hospital, Belmont, MA, USA

Digital Neuropsychology and Brain Health Laboratory, Belmont, MA, USA

Department of Psychiatry, Harvard Medical School, Boston, MA, USA

Department of Psychiatry, Mass General Brigham, Boston, United States
e-mail: ssingh@mclean.harvard.edu

S. Weisenbach (✉)
Department of Neuropsychology, McLean Hospital, Belmont, MA, USA

Department of Psychiatry, Harvard Medical School, Boston, MA, USA

Mood and Cognition in Aging Laboratory, Belmont, MA, USA

Department of Psychiatry, Mass General Brigham, Boston, United States
e-mail: sweisenbach@mclean.harvard.edu

M. Lanca and R. Fallows (eds.), *Advancing Neuropsychology Through Population Health*, https://doi.org/10.1007/978-3-032-22457-6_10

The Expanding Role of Technology Devices in Cognitive Assessment: A New Era for Neuropsychology

Clinical neuropsychology and neuropsychological evaluations rely on psychometrically robust assessments that target a wide range of domains, including memory, executive functioning, processing speed, working memory, attention, and reasoning skills (Harvey, 2019). While foundational and clinically invaluable, these tools have only seen modest innovation over the decades, often presenting as slight iterations or modifications of existing, older measures (Singh & Germine, 2021). Limitations in normative data, particularly in race/ethnicity (Elbulok-Charcape et al., 2014), are associated with largely homogenous samples upon which diagnostic conclusions are made. Despite this, neuropsychological assessments remain an unparalleled "gold standard" for quantifying, monitoring, and characterizing cognitive impairment (Casaletto & Heaton, 2017). Unlike other areas of medicine, neuropsychology provides a unique synthesis of behavioral, cognitive, and biological information, offering insights that are difficult to replace. This distinct expertise places neuropsychologists as leaders in the evaluation of brain health—in essence, imposing a strict *necessity* to critically reconsider how best to enhance methods such that they meet the vastly evolving needs of the growing population.

Digital tools for measuring cognitive health, or computerized neuropsychological assessment devices (CNADs) were defined in a joint position paper of the American Academy of Clinical Neuropsychology and the National Academy of Neuropsychology as "any instrument that utilizes a computer, digital tablet, handheld device, or other digital interface instead of a human examiner to administer, score, or interpret tests of brain function and related factors relevant to questions of neurologic health and illness" (Bauer et al., 2012, p. 178). CNADs present an opportunity not just for slight modifications to existing tests, or mere digitization of paper-and-pencil assessments. Rather they can enable a transformative shift in how we conceptualize, conduct, and administer cognitive assessments. With the potential to increase precision diagnostics, broaden accessibility, and personalize brain health monitoring, these tools offer promise perhaps even beyond what we can currently conceptualize given the nascence of digital tool utilization in the field (Bilder & Reise, 2019; Manly, 2008). More critically, neuropsychologists can promote equity and accessibility by leveraging CNADs (Manly, 2008), which in turn can ensure the sustainability of the field within the larger health care system. As healthcare moves toward value-based models and precision medicine that are central to population health, it is crucial that neuropsychology embraces technological innovations to remain relevant and clinically impactful.

The integration of CNADs into neuropsychological practice allows for enhancements that can enable richer data on patients than ever before. Mobile cognitive assessments and cloud-based data collection can facilitate real-time, scalable, and adaptive evaluations (Manly, 2008). Ecological momentary assessment (EMA), for example, can be utilized to provide assessments longitudinally over multiple time-points in individuals' everyday environments. Performances on digital cognitive tests can be readily monitored alongside other data sources, such as speech capture. Together, this type of multimodal data collection goes beyond our highly controlled clinic settings, offering unique within- and between-person insights on individuals' everyday cognitive status. A notable challenge with this methodology is providing the data in a way that is readily digestible for clinicians; however, AI is being used in our clinics to determine which variables are most sensitive and specific to brain health. More advances in passive data collection methods, including keyboard interactions and wearable sensor data can add nuance to these associations, enabling greater precision in quantifying and characterizing current brain health. By understanding which CNADs are most highly associated with cognitive impairment or fluctuations in cognitive status, we can determine which tools might serve as the best "co-pilots" for clinicians, as well as those that may surpass our current measures. Perhaps more importantly, these tools can aid in the development of a more proactive—rather than reactive—approach to brain health monitoring, enabling patients to see a neuropsychologist for routine brain health "check-ups" for example, even before they may notice any changes in their cognitive functioning (Chaytor et al., 2021; Germine et al., 2021; Hawks et al., 2023, 2024; Mascarenhas et al., 2023; Singh et al., 2023). These check-ups could include ultra-brief screening measures that flag more serious cases of cognitive impairment for follow-up with neuropsychological workup.

Large language models (LLMs), natural language processing (NLP), machine learning (ML), and artificial intelligence (AI) offer great potential in neuropsychology. These analytic tools enable larger-scale data collection using unobtrusive yet powerful measurements of cognitive functioning. AI and ML can help customize digital neuropsychological batteries based on the referral question, patient background/history, or even patient demographic features like race/ethnicity or socioeconomic status—enabling subtle patterns in cognitive status (such as within-test variability) that are not currently readily accessible to clinicians using our current metrics. Speech analysis, bolstered by ML and NLP techniques in particular offer a quick, low-cost method of assessing cognitive status.

Similarly, immersive technologies like virtual reality (VR) and augmented reality (AR) are beginning to create more lifelike testing environments, enabling cognitive assessments to more closely mimic everyday functional challenges (Parsons et al., 2013; Parsons & Barnett, 2017; Weitzner et al., 2021). This can be particularly useful for assessing functional outcome data in older adult populations, who may have increased physical difficulty completing everyday tasks (Vahia, 2024). Moreover, these tools have been demonstrated to detect cognitive changes earlier and more sensitively than many traditional tools (Agurto et al., 2023; Cakmak et al., 2021; Norel et al., 2020; Straus et al., 2023; Waisbren et al., 2025).

The inevitable expansion of CNADs brings along critical challenges and considerations, many of which clinicians have already anticipated. First, the field must continue rigorous psychometric validation of these new methods to ensure they meet the same or better standards of reliability, validity, sensitivity, and specificity as traditional tests. Ethical concerns, including data concerns, maintaining patient privacy, and preventing disparities in access, are key considerations as we begin to expand our technological toolkit. Indeed, the globalization of neuropsychological services has called out significant disparities that require immediate addressing. That being said, barriers in adoption considerations cannot be understated, as not only do new tools need to be psychometrically robust, but they also must be readily accessible and interpretable by clinicians. Patients may be similarly hesitant to adopt technologies due to accessibility issues; however, the time and resources required to complete digitally-based assessments versus visiting a clinic for a full neuropsychological workup may be appealing to some individuals, particularly those who otherwise may not have the ability to undergo an evaluation at a physical clinic. Many training programs lack the sufficient resources to implement new technologies, which can expand inequities between well-funded institutions and those serving underserved communities. Initiatives offering low-cost, accessible training, coupled with organizationally driven investment in digital infrastructure, are therefore essential for democratizing access to these innovations.

Finally, there is a subtle urgency that most neuropsychologists are not confronted with routinely but are nonetheless somewhat existential threats to our field; there are continual developments of novel cognitive/brain health direct-to-consumer applications, which are often free or low-cost tools that can be used in conjunction with routine medical care from physicians and other medical professionals. Neuropsychology must be a leader in the digital brain health innovation space or otherwise be replaced by apps that promise quick and convenient insights, without sufficient empirical validation. If the field fails to actively shape the future of cognitive health, neuropsychology risks being sidelined by technologies that prioritize convenience and scalability over clinical rigor. Certainly there will be a significant learning curve and comfort-level when adopting these tools. As a field, neuropsychologists will need to go through validating CNADs against traditional tools and provide accessible education about the types of tools available—as well as their unique use cases. As a potential starting point, clinicians might begin to: (1) adopt digital versions of traditional measures; (2) digitize data summary sheets so they can be uploaded to databases, which can then be used to develop novel tests; (3) if in a university-based setting, partner with local technology experts to explain what we do and ask how they might help using their technology-based tools; and (4) if in private practice or other non-university-based setting, reach out to local technology experts (e.g., Principal Investigators of technology laboratories) and ask how they could see their technologies improving our field in any capacity (Singh & Germine, 2021).

Thus, the field of neuropsychology stands at a threshold of a transformative paradigm shift. By thoughtfully integrating digital tools in neuropsychological research and practice, we can expand the reach, relevance, and impact of our work—ultimately delivering more personalized, accessible, and equitable care for the diverse populations we serve.

Technology as a Tool for Improving Health Equity

Clinical neuropsychologists are specialized healthcare providers with limited availability and resources, and ideally, referrals should be reserved for individuals who are most likely to benefit from a comprehensive cognitive assessment. At the same time, widespread and frequent cognitive health screening is essential. The Healthy Brain Initiative (HBI), launched in 2005 through a partnership between the Centers for Disease Control and Prevention (CDC) and the Alzheimer's Association (AA), aimed to develop a National Public Health Road Map to Maintaining Cognitive Health (CDC & AA, 2007). The initiative's overarching long-term goal is "to maintain or improve the cognitive performance of all adults." It outlines 44 evidence-based actions that emphasize prevention, adopt a population or community health perspective, and seek to reduce healthcare disparities among racial and ethnic groups. Now in its fourth edition, released in 2023, the HBI Road Map highlights opportunities for public health efforts across a continuum that includes risk reduction, early detection and diagnosis, and improving safety and quality of care.

Mobile digital technologies can enable more widespread cognitive assessment, particularly when they can be used remotely, in the patient's own home under the supervision of a health professional. For example, numerous CNADs have been developed that can be self-administered remotely. Examples of such batteries (though not an exhaustive list) include the CANTAB Mobile (Cormack et al., 2018), CNS Vital Signs (Gualitieri et al., 2005), and ImPACT (https://impacttest.com/). One drawback of such assessments is that the environment in which they are administered is less controlled than if a patient were taking the test in a clinical setting; for example, performance could be impacted by interruptions and the clinician has no way of knowing if the patient performed the test without the use of external aids. For that reason (and others discussed above) such tests should not be used as stand-alone measures to make a diagnosis. However, they can serve as important screening tools to suggest who might benefit most from a more comprehensive evaluation. Moreover, the use of wearables and other digital tools described in the first section of this chapter could be used to track cognitive health following a cognitive screen or comprehensive neuropsychological evaluation and serve as prognostic indicator as to when cognition should be re-assessed more formally. Ideally, tools used in real-world settings, such as EMA and at-home mobile cognitive tests, would be combined with evaluations performed in a more controlled setting to derive a comprehensive picture of a person's true abilities in various cognitive domains, along with how contextual variables influence their cognitive performance.

The Covid pandemic forced the field of neuropsychology to transition to a fully virtual model, and there have now been a number of studies demonstrating low or no effect of test modality on performance (Butterbrod et al., 2024; Haebich et al., 2025; Ng & Peterson, 2025). Moreover, high acceptability ratings have been achieved for virtual assessments by patients and clinicians alike (Sumpter et al., 2022). At the same time, following the lifting of Covid restrictions, most neuropsychologists returned to either in-person or hybrid models of care. The reasons for this return are complex, but some reasons include increased comfort with in-person administration, a greater availability of traditional measures that can be administered in-person versus those that can be administered digitally (i.e., some stimuli are not amenable to digital administration), greater control during in-person administration, and payor models that provide greater reimbursement for in-person models of care. Nevertheless, the availability of virtual evaluations is now possible for those who would otherwise have great difficulty or be entirely unable to access care, such as homebound seniors, people with disabilities, and those who live in rural areas.

Implementation Takeaway #1

Digital health tools can enable a transformative shift in how we conceptualize, conduct, and administer cognitive assessments. With the potential to increase precision, broaden accessibility, and personalize brain health monitoring, these tools offer promise perhaps even beyond what we can currently conceptualize given the nascence of digital tool utilization in our field while maintaining scientific rigor. However, the field must continue rigorous psychometric validation of these new methods to ensure they meet the same or better standards of reliability, validity, sensitivity, and specificity as traditional tests and be readily accessible and interpretable by clinicians. Moving toward a technology-based practice and collaborating with innovators from other fields will be an excellent starting point for digitizing neuropsychology.

Implementation of Digital Tools in Cognitive Screening and Assessment

CNADs can be conceptualized as belonging to three categories (Chen et al., 2023). The first class is reflective of a digital version of a paper-and-pencil test, which is directly comparable to one another, such as the electronic Montreal Cognitive Assessment (eMoCA; Berg et al, 2018) or the digital Clock Drawing Test (dCDT; Chan et al., 2022; Yuan et al., 2022). The second category encompasses tests that were developed to be administered in a digitized format, such as the CogState (https://www.cogstate.com/), the TabCAT (Sideman et al., 2024), and the NIH Toolbox (https://nihtoolbox.org/). The third category includes tests that measure outcomes not possible from paper-and-pencil tests, such as those administered in a virtual reality environment, like the Virtual Supermarket Program (Zygouris et al., 2015, 2022). While a review of all available CNADs is beyond the scope of this chapter, please refer to Marton et al. (in press) for a detailed and comprehensive review of available CNADs belonging to all three categories.

Advantages of CNADs Over Traditional Tests

Digital cognitive tools offer a number of advantages over traditional paper-and-pencil measures. First, when the measure can be administered directly on a digital device, instructions are consistent for every patient, eliminating any performance variations that can occur as a result of examiner variables, such as administration errors. Second, responses that are automatically coded and scored eradicate human scoring errors and eliminates scoring time entirely. Third, digitization enables more precise and consistent measurements of behavior and generation of new data points that may be relevant to functioning and prognosis, not possible by a human examiner. For example, the dCDT (Schejter-Margalit et al., 2021) enables the ability to quantify response time variability, which may be relevant for prognosis in dementia (Lu et al., 2020) and other conditions. CNADs also enable the incorporation of modern psychometric theory into clinical practice, such as computerized adaptive testing (CAT). CAT selects the most informative item for each trial based on the individual's estimated ability. For the initial trial, it assumes an average ability level and presents an item of median difficulty. Subsequent items are chosen dynamically, becoming easier or harder depending on whether the previous response was correct or incorrect. CAT is already implemented in many educational tests and results in more efficient test administration since items are customized to the individuals' ability level (Thissen & Mislevy, 2000). Finally, CNADs have the potential to enable more widespread and comprehensive screening for common conditions, potentially improving health equity in identifying cognitive health conditions at the population level. This is discussed in more detail below.

Considerations for Utilizing CNADs in Clinical Practice

As with every test that is utilized in clinical practice, it is the responsibility of the clinician to ensure that it has strong reliability and validity and was normed on a sample reflective of the examinee. Some additional and complimentary considerations are necessary when evaluating the introduction of a CNAD into clinical practice. First, even tests belonging to the digital versions of paper-and-pencil tests become a different test when translated to a digital format. Paper-and-pencil tests entail the interaction of an examinee with an examiner who is providing the examinee feedback in the form of voice intonations, varying facial expressions, and other non-verbal forms of communication even when administering the test in a standardized way. This experience is fundamentally different from a computerized assessment, in which verbal and non-verbal forms of communication are the same for every item across every examinee. An illustrative example of this comparison is that of the Wisconsin Card Sorting Test (WCST) in traditional (Grant & Berg, 1948) versus computerized (Heaton & Staff, 2003) formats. In the traditional format, the examinee is hearing the live examiner give them feedback of "correct" or "incorrect" as they try to understand how to sort the cards in a way that will result in a "correct" response from the examiner. When taking the WCST on a computer, the feedback may be received differently because it is from a machine, and not by the examiner who will be involved in the interpretation of performance. Also, computerized measures require that the examinee interact with one or more devices, such as a tablet or cell phone, or a computer with a mouse and keyboard. Ideally, CNADs of this nature have normative data that was obtained from a sample taking the test in the digitized format. For example, Pearson conducted equivalency studies on the WAIS-V Q-Interactive and WAIS-V paper-and-pencil versions ensured that the same norms can be used for both administration formats for every subtest except for Spatial Addition, in which case digital norms were adjusted using equating techniques (Raiford & Courville, 2024). This is not the case for the WCST, whereby the normative sample for the computerized and paper-and-pencil versions are based on the paper-and-pencil format version only (Heaton & PAR Staff, 1993).

Another important consideration for clinicians to keep in mind is that hardware and software limitations can result in errors, such as delays or non-intentional variability in stimulus presentation. Operating systems can result in timing errors when other functions usurp processing from the test being administered, and automatic updates can influence the performance of a CNAD. Moreover, screen resolution and size can vary from one device to another, resulting in confounds to performance relative to the normative sample. For a complete discussion of these issues, the reader is referred to Parsons and colleagues (2018), which comprehensively describes practice parameters for consideration when utilizing CNADs in clinical neuropsychological settings.

Balancing CNAD Output with Clinical Reasoning

With the ease of use inherent in CNADs also comes the risk of over-reliance on automated processes for clinical decision making. For instance, it would be irresponsible to make a diagnosis of attention deficit hyperactivity disorder (ADHD) by relying on a single objective digital tool for ADHD symptoms, such as QBTest (Ulberstad, 2012). The responsible/ethical clinician incorporates those results with information gathered about the patient's history, including onset, duration, and the context in which symptoms occur, ideally with corroborative sources of information. Similarly, dementia should not be diagnosed by relying solely on the results of a test such as TabCAT (Sideman et al., 2024). While objective cognitive data gathered by such a tool can certainly inform a diagnosis and subsequent treatment plan, additional information, including symptom trajectory, context, and consideration of alternative sources of cognitive decline, must be incorporated into the assessment.

Many CNADs that are commercially available integrate an automated interpretive algorithm that determines impairment on the test, although how that algorithm was created is often not apparent to the end-user, potentially resulting in biased decision-making. A striking example of the consequences of over-reliance on digital tools comes from an algorithmic risk assessment tool that was used in the US criminal justice system, whereby a computer program was used to predict the likelihood of criminals re-offending and recommended harsher sentences based on skin color. In one actual case, offender A, an 18-year-old Black woman briefly stole a child's bike and rode it down the street until the child's mother ran after her. Offender A had a history of misdemeanors as a juvenile, and a computer program predicting risk of future offenses deemed her to be at "high-risk." Offender B, a 41-year-old White male, stole $86.35 worth of tools from hardware store. He had been convicted of armed robbery and attempted armed robbery previously, but the computer program categorized him as "low risk." Two years after those arrests, Offender A had been charged with no new crimes, while Offender B was serving eight years in prison after illegally entering a warehouse and stealing electronics valued at thousands of dollars (Angwin et al., 2016). While this is an extreme example, one could imagine how algorithms applied to tools used in clinical practice to make decisions about prognosis and clinical decision making must be carefully assessed for potential sources of bias. Machine learning models that are used to develop such tools are only as good as the training set on which they were developed. If the training set is biased in some way (dependent upon implicit or explicit human bias), the resultant algorithm will be as well.

CNADs and Stepped Care Models in Neuropsychology

As a basic premise, stepped care in medicine involves offering a level of care (restrictivity, intensity, cost, time) that is best matched to the complexity and severity of the problem. In neuropsychology, this can be conceptualized as cognitive screening at the lowest level, progressing to brief evaluations, then comprehensive evaluations, and at the highest level, comprehensive evaluations with treatment (see Lanca, 2018). As described in Weisenbach (2025) CNADs enable the opportunity to implement stepped care models on a much broader scale, given that the availability of a trained administrator is not necessarily required for the most basic care levels. CNADs can also be integrated with more traditional tools to offer a more comprehensive understanding of a person's function and can help to indicate when a higher level of care might be needed. For example, computerized tools for cognitive screening can enable comprehensive screens outside of the traditional visit with a medical professional. Some, but not all, are designed to be self-administered and can even be completed in a person's own home. EMA platforms could complement traditional brief and comprehensive neuropsychological assessments by enabling the contextual assessment of cognition, allowing a better understanding of how environmental factors impact a person's cognition, potentially leading to more effective treatment plans for optimizing cognitive functioning. Speech metrics could one day be used adjunctively with traditional assessments, and could be used prognostically to inform when someone is in need of initial or re-evaluation. Passive sensors such as actigraphy offer the ability to understand how factors such a sleep, movement, etc. correlate with cognition and could also be used prognostically.

Implementation Takeaway #2
CNADs offer advantages over traditional measures, such as consistent instructions, automatically coded responses and scoring, more precise measurement of behavior and generation of new data points, the potential for incorporating modern psychometric theory, and the enablement of more widespread and comprehensive screening for common conditions. Enthusiasm must be tempered, however, by considerations around the validity and reliability of available tests, how they were designed to be used, how normative data was derived (and on whom), in addition to hardware and software limitations. Moreover, no tool can replace good clinical reasoning when it comes to diagnostic accuracy and treatment decision-making. Appendix 1 includes a checklist for clinicians to utilize in determining whether or not a CNAD is ready for clinical adoption.

Conclusion

The advent and implementation of CNADs across clinical settings has the potential to enable more widespread screening of cognitive health, such as we have witnessed with public health efforts toward addressing hypertension and diabetes (e.g., free screenings at pharmacies and in other public spaces and the capability for screening to occur at home). In the practice of clinical neuropsychology, digital tools that can enable a transformative shift in how we conceptualize, conduct, and administer cognitive assessments, and virtual assessments are now available to those who have may have difficulty or live too far away from a practice setting, increasing access and improving health equity. CNADs can enhance our ability to deploy stepped levels of care in neuropsychology and can compliment our existing approaches by offering complimentary data that enable the contextualization of cognitive functioning in everyday settings. At the same time, there are many issues that clinicians must continuously monitor to ensure that CNADs intended to replace traditional measures stand-up to or surpass existing paper-and-pencil measures that serve as the gold standard. Issues related to reliability, validation, normative data, hardware and software issues, and the potential of bias in diagnostic algorithms must be carefully considered when the choice is made to implement a CNAD in a clinical setting. Critically, the ease that comes with administration, scoring, and interpretation of CNADs cannot replace good clinical reasoning, and CNADs should not be used as standalone assessment measures. While technology has the potential to enable cognitive health metrics at the population level and to change the practice of cognitive assessment as we know it today, it must be used responsibly to inform good patient care and treatment decision-making.

Key Points in Review

1. CNADs can enable more precise measurement of behavior and increased health equity, but measures used in clinical settings need to align with or exceed traditional gold-standard measures of cognitive ability in reliability, validity, and availability of good normative data.
2. CNADs can be a strong tools in clinical practice but should never been used in isolation and can never replace good clinical reasoning.
3. Additional resources:
   a. American Academy of Clinical Neuropsychology Disruptive Technology Initiative: https://theaacn.org/disruptive-technology-initiative/
   b. Society for Clinical Neuropsychology Association of Neuropsychology Students in Training Neurotechnology Focus Group: https://theaacn.org/disruptive-technology-initiative/

References

Agurto, C., Cecchi, G. A., Wen, B., Fraenkel, E., Berry, J., Navar, I., & Norel, R. (2023). Remote inference of cognitive scores in ALS patients using a picture description. *IEEE International Conference on Digital Health (ICDH), 2023*, 50–56. https://doi.org/10.1109/ICDH60066.2023.00017

Angwin, J., Larson, J., Mattu, S., & Kirchner, L. (2016, May 23). *Machine Bias*. https://www.propublica.org/article/machine-bias-risk-assessments-in-criminal-sentencing

Bauer, R. M., Iverson, G. L., Cernich, A. N., Binder, L. M., Ruff, R. M., & Naugle, R. I. (2012). Computerized neuropsychological assessment devices: Joint position paper of the American Academy of Clinical Neuropsychology and the National Academy of Neuropsychology. *The Clinical Neuropsychologist, 26*(2), 177–196. https://doi.org/10.1080/13854046.2012.663001

Berg, J. L., Durant, J., Léger, G. C., Cummings, J. L., Nasreddine, Z., & Miller, J. B. (2018). Comparing the electronic and standard versions of the Montreal cognitive assessment in an outpatient memory disorders clinic: a validation study. *Journal of Alzheimer's Disease, 62*(1), 93–97. https://doi.org/10.3233/JAD-170896

Bilder, R. M., & Reise, S. P. (2019). Neuropsychological tests of the future: How do we get there from here? *The Clinical Neuropsychologist, 33*(2), 220–245. https://doi.org/10.1080/13854046.2018.1521993

Butterbrod, E., van den Heuvel, D. M. J., Zevenhoven, P., Waterink, L., van Leeuwenstijn, M., Jutten, R. J., van der Flier, W. M., & Sikkes, S. A. M. (2024). Tele-neuropsychology in memory clinic settings: Reliability and usability of videoconference-based neuropsychological testing. *Journal of the International Neuropsychological Association, 30*, 954–965. https://doi.org/10.1017/S1355617724000432

Cakmak, A. S., Alday, E. A. P., Da Poian, G., Rad, A. B., Metzler, T. J., Neylan, T. C., & Clifford, G. D. (2021). Classification and prediction of post-trauma outcomes related to PTSD using circadian rhythm changes measured via wrist-worn research watch in a large longitudinal cohort. *IEEE Journal of Biomedical and Health Informatics, 25*(8), 2866–2876. https://doi.org/10.1109/JBHI.2021.3053909

Casaletto, K. B., & Heaton, R. K. (2017). Neuropsychological assessment: Past and future. *Journal of the International Neuropsychological Society, 23*(9–10), 778–790. https://doi.org/10.1017/S1355617717001060

Centers for Disease Control and Prevention and the Alzheimer's Association. (2007). *The Healthy brain initiative: A National Public Health roadmap to maintaining cognitive health.* https://www.cdc.gov/aging-programs/media/pdfs/2024/06/TheHealthyBrainInitiative_MaintainingCognitiveHealth.pdf

Chan, J. Y. C., Bat, B. K. K., Wong, A., Chan, T. K., Huo, Z., Yip, B. H. K., et al. (2022). Evaluation of digital drawing tests and paper-and-pencil drawing tests for the screening of mild cognitive impairment and dementia: A systematic review and meta-analysis of diagnostic studies. *Neuropsychology Review, 32*(3), 566–576. https://doi.org/10.1007/s11065-21-09523-2

Chen, L., Zhen, W., & Peng, D. (2023). Research on digital tool in cognitive assessment: A bibliometric analysis. *Frontiers in Psychiatry, 14*, 1227261. https://doi.org/10.3389/fpsyt.2023.1227261

Cormack, F. K., Morris, H., Barnett, J. H., & Housden, C. (2018). Cantab Mobile: Experience of a digital memory assessment tool in UK primary care. *Alzheimer's & Dementia, 14*(7P1-504), 522–P523. https://doi.org/10.1016/j.jalz.2018.06.515

Chaytor, N. S., Barbosa-Leiker, C., Germine, L. T., Fonseca, L. M., McPherson, S. M., & Tuttle, K. R. (2021). Construct validity, ecological validity and acceptance of self-administered online neuropsychological assessment in adults. *The Clinical Neuropsychologist, 35*(1), 148–164. https://doi.org/10.1080/13854046.2020.1811893

CNS Vital Signs. (2025). *CNS Vital Signs: Computerized neurocognitive assessment software* [Test administration guide]. CNS Vital Signs, LLC. Retrieved from https://www.cnsvs.com/

Cogstate. (2025). *Cogstate: Simplifying the measurement of cognition* [Computer software]. Cogstate Ltd. Retrieved from https://www.cogstate.com/

Gualtieri, C., & Johnson, L. (2006). Reliability and validity of a computerized neurocognitive test battery, CNS Vital Signs. *Archives of Clinical Neuropsychology, 21*(7), 623–643. https://doi.org/10.1016/j.acn.2006.05.007

Elbulok-Charcape, M. M., Rabin, L. A., Spadaccini, A. T., & Barr, W. B. (2014). Trends in the neuropsychological assessment of ethnic/racial minorities: A survey of clinical neuropsychologists in the United States and Canada. *Cultural Diversity and Ethnic Minority Psychology, 20*(3), 353–361. https://doi.org/10.1037/a0035023

Engi Raiford, S., & Courville, T. (2024). Equivalence of Q-interactive and paper administration of cognitive tasks: WAIS-5. *Pearson Inc.* https://www.pearsonassessments.com/content/dam/school/global/clinical/us/assets/wais-5/q-interactive-wais-5.pdf?srsltid=AfmBOoqA8Wi88fMDRDM3q8BUXMdYastH01KTVE5zs2IYXvOD5jhQFx_n

Germine, L., Strong, R. W., Singh, S., & Sliwinski, M. J. (2021). Toward dynamic phenotypes and the scalable measurement of human behavior. *Neuropsychopharmacology, 46*(1), 209–216. https://doi.org/10.1038/s41386-020-0757-1

Grant, D. A., & Berg, E. A. (1948). A behavioral analysis of degree of reinforcement and ease of shifting to new responses in a Weigl-type card-sorting problem. *Journal of Experimental Psychology, 38*, 404–411. https://doi.org/10.1037/h005983

Haebich, K. M., Darke, H., Lami, F., Maier, A., Chisholm, A. K., Ure, A., Hogan, N. L., Eng, Y. F., Wrennall, J., Hearps, S. J. C., Efron, D., Joshua, N., Dabscheck, G., North, K. N., Anderson, V. A., & Payne, J. M. (2025). Agreement, reliability, feasibility, and acceptability of home-based telehealth versus face-to-face pediatric neuropsychological testing: A within-person crossover study. *Neuropsychology, 39*(2), 172–186. https://doi.org/10.1037/neu0000989

Harvey, P. D. (2019). Domains of cognition and their assessment. *Dialogues in Clinical Neuroscience, 21*(3), 227–237. https://doi.org/10.31887/DCNS.2019.21.3/pharvey

Hawks, Z. W., Beck, E. D., Jung, L., Fonseca, L. M., Sliwinski, M. J., Weinstock, R. S., Grinspoon, E., Xu, I., Strong, R. W., Singh, S., Van Dongen, H. P. A., Frumkin, M. R., Bulger, J., Cleveland, M. J., Janess, K., Kudva, Y. C., Pratley, R., Rickels, M. R., Rizvi, S. R., … Germine, L. T.

(2024). Dynamic associations between glucose and ecological momentary cognition in Type 1 Diabetes. *NPJ Digital Medicine, 7*, 59. https://doi.org/10.1038/s41746-024-01036-5

Hawks, Z. W., Strong, R., Jung, L., Beck, E. D., Passell, E. J., Grinspoon, E., Singh, S., Frumkin, M. R., Sliwinski, M., & Germine, L. T. (2023). Accurate prediction of momentary cognition from intensive longitudinal data. *Biological Psychiatry: Cognitive Neuroscience and Neuroimaging, 8*(8), 841–851. https://doi.org/10.1016/j.bpsc.2022.12.002

Heaton R.K., PAR Staff. (2003). Wisconsin card sorting test computer version 4: Odessa, FL: Psychological Assessment Resources.

ImPACT Applications, I. (n.d.). *ImPACT: Immediate Post-Concussion Assessment and Cognitive Testing*. https://impacttest.com/

Lanca, M. (2018). Integration of neuropsychology in primary care. *Archives of Clinical Neuropsychology, 33*(3), 269–279. https://doi.org/10.1093/arclin/acx135

Lu, K., Nicholas, J. M., James, S-N, Lane, C. A., Parker, T. D., Keshavan, A., Keuss, S. E., Buchanan, S. M., Murray-Smith, H., Cash, D. M., Sudre, C. H., Malone, I. B., Coath, W., Wong, A., Henley, S. M. D., Fox, N. C., Richards, M., Schott, J. M., & Crutch, S. J. (2020). Increased variability in reaction time is associated with amyloid beta pathology at age 70. *Alzheimer's & Dementia, 12*(1), e12076. https://doi.org/10.1002/dad2.12076

Manly, J. J. (2008). Critical issues in cultural neuropsychology: Profit from diversity. *Neuropsychology Review, 18*(3), 179–183. https://doi.org/10.1007/s11065-008-9068-8

Marton, K., Njoku, A., Clark, B., & Chen, M. (In Press). In S. Singh & S.L. Weisenbach (Eds.), *Neuropsychology in the age of digital health: exploration, application, and practical implementation.* Advancing cognitive health: Digital screening tools. Wiley Publishing.

Mascarenhas Fonseca, L., Strong, R. W., Singh, S., Bulger, J. D., Cleveland, M., Grinspoon, E., & Chaytor, N. S. (2023). Glycemic variability and fluctuations in cognitive status in adults with type 1 diabetes (GLUCOG): Observational study using ecological momentary assessment of cognition. *JMIR Diabetes, 8*, Article e39750. https://doi.org/10.2196/39750

Ng, R., & Peterson, R. K. (2025). A comparison of traditional face-to-face and remote administration of auditory attention and executive functioning measures in a cohort of clinically-referred pediatric patients. *The Clinical Neuropsychologist, 21*, 1–16. https://doi.org/10.1080/13854046.2025.2469338

NIH Toolbox. (2025). E. M. LaForte, J. N. Hook & A. K. Giella (Eds.), *National Institutes of Health (NIH) toolbox® V3 technical manual.* Toolbox Assessments, Inc. (Referenced in 2025 NIH Toolbox V3 documentation). https://nihtoolbox.org/

Norel, R., Agurto, C., Heisig, S., Rice, J. J., Zhang, H., Ostrand, R., & Cecchi, G. A. (2020). Speech-based characterization of dopamine replacement therapy in people with Parkinson's disease. *NPJ Parkinson's Disease, 6*, 12. https://doi.org/10.1038/s41531-020-0113-5

Parsons, T. D., Courtney, C. G., & Dawson, M. E. (2013). Virtual reality Stroop task for assessment of supervisory attentional processing. *Journal of Clinical and Experimental Neuropsychology, 35*(8), 812–826. https://doi.org/10.1080/13803395.2013.824556

Parsons, T. D., & Barnett, M. (2017). Validity of a newly developed measure of memory: Feasibility study of the Virtual Environment Grocery Store. *Journal of Alzheimer's Disease, 59*(4), 1227–1235. https://doi.org/10.3233/JAD-170295

Parsons, T. D., McMahan, T., & Kane, R. (2018). *The Clinical Neuropsychologist, 32*(1), 16–41. https://doi.org/10.1080/13854046.2017.1337932

Schejter-Margalit, T., Kizony, R., Shirvan, J., Cedarbaum, J. M., Bregman, N., Thaler, A., Giladi, N., & Mirelman, A. (2021). Quantitative digital clock drawing test as a sensitive tool to detect subtle cognitive impairments in early stage Parkinson's disease. *Parkinsonism & Related Disorders, 90*, 84–89. https://doi.org/10.1016/j.parkreldis.2021.08.002

Singh, S., & Germine, L. (2021). Technology meets tradition: A hybrid model for implementing digital tools in neuropsychology. *International Review of Psychiatry, 33*(4), 382–393. https://doi.org/10.1080/09540261.2020.1835839

Singh, S., Strong, R., Xu, I., Fonseca, L. M., Hawks, Z., Grinspoon, E., Jung, L., Li, F., Weinstock, R. S., Sliwinski, M. J., Chaytor, N. S., & Germine, L. T. (2023). Ecological momentary assessment of cognition in clinical and community samples: Reliability and validity study. *Journal of Medical Internet Research, 25*,. https://doi.org/10.2196/45028

Sideman, A. B., Nguyen, H. Q., Langer-Gould, A., Lee, E. A., Borson, S., Shen, E., Tsoy, E., Macias, M., Goode, C., & Rankin, K. (2024). Stakeholder-informed pragmatic trial protocol of the TabCAT-BHA for the detection of cognitive impairment in primary care. *BMC Primary Care, 25*(1), 286. https://doi.org/10.1186/s12875-024-02544-9

Straus, L. D., An, X., Ji, Y., McLean, S. A., Neylan, T. C., AURORA Study Group, & Koenen, K. C. (2023). Utility of wrist-wearable data for assessing pain, sleep, and anxiety outcomes after traumatic stress exposure. *JAMA Psychiatry, 80*(3), 220–229. https://doi.org/10.1001/jamapsychiatry.2022.4533

Sumpter, R., Camsey, E., Meldrum, S., Alford, M., Campbell, I., Bois, C., et al. (2022). Remote neuropsychological assessment: Acceptability and feasibility of direct-to-home teleneuropsychology methodology during the COVID-19 pandemic. *The Clinical Neuropsychologist, 37*(2), 432–447. https://doi.org/10.1080/13854046.2022.2056922

Thissen, D., & Mislevy, R. J. (2000). Testing algorithms. In H. Wainer (Ed.). *Computerized adaptive testing: A primer*. Lawrence Erlbaum Associate.

Ulberstad, F. (2012). *QbTest technical manual*. Stolckholm, Sweden Qbtech AB.

Vahia, I. V. (2024). Navigating new realities in aging care as artificial intelligence enters clinical practice. *The American Journal of Geriatric Psychiatry, 32*(3), 267–269. https://doi.org/10.1016/j.jagp.2024.01.011

Waisbren, S. E., Norel, R., Agurto, C., Singh, S., Connor, Z. A., Ebrahim, M. G., & Cecchi, G. A. (2025). Beyond neuropsychological tests: AI speech analysis in PKU. *Journal of Inherited Metabolic Disease, 48*(1), Article e12831. https://doi.org/10.1002/jimd.12831

Weisenbach, S. L. (2025). Empowering minds: Revolutionizing cognitive and emotional health assessment with stepped care and digital tools. *Journal of Clinical and Experimental Neuropsychology, 46*(6), 523–530. https://doi.org/10.1080/13803395.2025.2535584

Weitzner, D. S., Calamia, M., & Parsons, T. D. (2021). Test–retest reliability and practice effects of the Virtual Environment Grocery Store (VEGS). *Journal of Clinical and Experimental Neuropsychology, 43*(6), 547–557. https://doi.org/10.1080/13803395.2021.1960277

Yuan, J., Au, R., Karjadi, C., Ang, T. F., Devine, S., Auerbach, S., et al. (2022). Associations between the digital clock drawing test and brain volume: Large community-based prospective cohort (Framingham heart study). *Journal of Medical Internet Research, 24*, Article e34513. https://doi.org/10.2196/34513

Zygouris, S., Giakoumis, D., Votis, K., Doumpoulakis, S., Ntovas, K., Segkouli, S., Karagiannidis, C., Tzovaras, D., & Tsolaki, M. (2015). Can a virtual reality cognitive training application fulfill a dual role? Using the virtual supermarket cognitive training application as a screening tool for mild cognitive impairment. *Journal of Alzheimer's Disease, 44*(4), 1333–1347.

Zygouris, S., Segkouli, S., Triantafyllidis, A., Giakoumis, D., Tsolaki, M., Votis, K., & Tzovaras, D. (2022). Usability of the virtual supermarket test for older adults with and without cognitive impairment. *Journal of Alzheimer's Disease Reports, 6*(1), 229–234.

Chapter 11
Envisioning Contemporary Neuropsychology Practice in Population Health

Margaret Lanca and Robert Fallows

Executive Summary
This chapter argues that clinical neuropsychology must evolve from a model centered on individual, episodic assessment to one embedded within a population health framework that encompasses prevention and systems-level care. Traditional clinical practices with long waitlists, limited access, and cultural bias in tests and norms risk marginalizing the field and widening health inequities. Newer approaches that employ risk stratification, tiered service models, telehealth options, and measurement-based care (MBC) enable neuropsychologists to deliver more scalable, equitable, and context-responsive services. Advances in normative methods, such as regression-based norms and performance-based premorbid estimates, support fairer and more precise assessments across diverse populations. Improving the clinical neuropsychology workforce with multilingual and culturally responsive clinicians, and training/funding for interpreter-assisted evaluations are critical. Population health also compels neuropsychologists to consider broader social determinants, including built environment, and to move "upstream" by addressing modifiable risk factors. Over the lifespan of care, this means thinking about secondary prevention through reducing risk of a known neurological conditions; however, it also means applying frameworks that intervene early and beyond the clinic through partnerships with public health, community organizations, and policymakers. Finally, the Minnesota Guidelines position future neuropsychologists to lead within integrated systems, advocate for equity, and harness technology and implementation science to transform neuropsychology into a vital contributor to learning health systems and population-level cognitive health.

M. Lanca (✉)
Department of Psychiatry, Cambridge Health Alliance, Cambridge, MA, USA
e-mail: margaret_lanca@hms.harvard.edu

Department of Psychiatry, Harvard Medical School, Boston, MA, USA

R. Fallows
Samaritan Medical Group, Albany, OR, USA
e-mail: rfallows@samhealth.org

M. Lanca and R. Fallows (eds.), *Advancing Neuropsychology Through Population Health*, https://doi.org/10.1007/978-3-032-22457-6_11

Pulling It All Together: Neuropsychology and Population Health

Throughout this book, different concepts related to population health have been reviewed and the reader has hopefully appreciated that the field of clinical neuropsychology must evolve beyond the sole focus of the provision of neuropsychological assessment at the individual level. Failure to expand beyond this framework will relegate the profession to the medical classification equivalent of a laboratory/radiological test, soon to be put on a cost–benefit analysis by insurers against blood tests, neuroimaging and other emerging biomarkers and/or have need met through full or partial artificial intelligence automation. Similarly, failure to adopt a model of care to create increased access and significantly improve assessment that considers the diverse intersectionality of each patient will entrench perceptions that neuropsychology remains a niche service that is generally inaccessible, except for the privileged few. As we envision the 'neuropsychology of the future,' we must take into consideration some of the lessons from these chapters and a few other topics, to consider how the scope of neuropsychological clinical practice and research training for the next generation of neuropsychologists must evolve.

Evolving a Population Health-Informed Clinical Neuropsychology Practice

A justification for neuropsychological assessment no longer needs to be made. As demonstrated throughout this book, numerous studies have shown impact of many medical conditions and environmental factors on cognitive health. Further, there has been consistent demonstration of the cyclical cognitive ramifications these conditions have on overall health, if left unattended and untreated. Numerous provider specialties recognize the utility of neuropsychological testing and referrals for neuropsychological testing have surged to the point that there are long wait lists. Some of the primary challenges facing neuropsychology today are how to increase the access pipeline to assessment and improve the inequities in the process. This challenge requires a deeper understanding of the barriers and facilitators to equitable neuropsychology assessment. Ultimately, equity in care must involve re-envisioning how we fit the right neuropsychological service to the right person at the right time.

Risk stratification (a.k.a., triaging) is a systematic process by which healthcare providers integrate multiple pieces of information (e.g., medical history, acute symptoms, functional status, etc.) to make decision about a patient's likelihood of experiencing an adverse health outcome to guide decisions about the intensity and timing of a patient's care. This process is often paired with a panoply of available care options (also known as levels of care) to direct patients to the type of care that best meets their needs. These processes have secondary benefits of being able to provide more targeted care to a wider number of people. Although this practice is not widespread in neuropsychology, there have been more recent published papers of neuropsychology triage models and levels of care models (Hardy et al., 2017; Lanca, 2018). Some of these outcome studies have begun to show the benefits of targeting evaluations of differing lengths for different conditions. Hardy et al (2017), for example, outlined how brief, targeted evaluations tied to specific medical conditions (e.g., cancer, congenital disorders) can improve access and triage while maintaining clinical utility in a pediatric population.

Targeted evaluations that meet the specific needs of the patient, while also addressing the questions of the referring provider, supply an important reframe for the field of neuropsychology. When this is conducted within a system of care that can be designed/influenced by the neuropsychologist, there is a stronger potential for longitudinal tracking that can better ensure diagnostic accuracy and/or response to intervention. For example, Chapter 8 specifically discussed the value of routine cognitive screening for elders in primary care, and that cognition should be considered the 6th vital sign. For the neuropsychologist working at a healthcare system with routine cognitive screening for patients in primary care, they can use this information to help triage who may need a higher level of neuropsychological evaluation, such as a brief or more comprehensive neuropsychological evaluation. At a leadership level, neuropsychologists can also be involved in helping to implement a system-wide cognitive workflow in which patients who meet certain criteria get routine cognitive screening or another level of cognitive evaluation. This could be especially useful if dovetailed with the Medicare annual wellness visit for patients over 60. Neuropsychologists could also contribute to a workflow design that includes brief questions about functional status, incorporating feedback from collaterals if available. Patients without functional concerns may then get a brief cognitive screen (e.g., Mini-cog) while those with a positive response to the functional screen or the brief screen could get a more advanced screen (e.g., MoCA or SLUMS). Ultimately, even these tried-and-true paper and pencil screeners are likely to be replaced by ecological momentary assessment the patient can use within their day-to-day environment. Whether through paper and pencil screening or advanced at home assessments, serial screening over time allows the neuropsychologist to examine trends in cognitive and functional status and decide if they need to provide education on promoting cognitive health without further need for testing, provide a brief neuropsychological evaluation for confirmation of dementia (if screens show progressive decline in combination with functional decline), or provide a more robust neuropsychological evaluation if there are factors that may obscure a dementia diagnosis on screening (e.g., high premorbid ability, presence of psychiatric distress, etc.).

While dementia is commonly used as a key example for risk stratification/triage, other models such as the epilepsy triage model in Chapter 6 creates an opportunity for another subset of patients to benefit from some level of screening and/or education given the high prevalence of cognitive risk for that group. Similar models could be applied to other specialty neurology clinics, including those addressing movement disorders, multiple sclerosis, and other neurological conditions. Chapter 5 also demonstrated that this type of triaging can extend to youth populations, and that data sources can include information beyond the healthcare system. A child with a traumatic brain injury or neurodevelopmental disorder may have multiple episodes of school-based testing and numerous points of behavioral observations made by educational staff that can inform a more targeted evaluation.

Development of neuropsychological practice models that evaluate and extend service reach is essential. Borrowing from other specialties who have successfully completed this work, networking with community leaders where hard-to-reach patients live and work is critical in helping to understand and address barriers to care. Quality improvement (QI) or implementation studies (IS) are well poised to illuminate some of the barriers for these patients who remain largely unknown to neuropsychology practices. Hospital and large clinic practice leaders need to help fund and provide protected time to neuropsychology leaders to create better patient access pipelines by combining these efforts with larger accessibility efforts. These access barriers are often rooted in social determinants of health (SDOH) such as the distance one must travel to reach a neuropsychologist. In these cases, continued adoption of telehealth strategies to create more equitable access for those in rural and underserved areas is key. Acknowledging the historical harm caused by psychological/neuropsychological assessment to various communities is also essential. Fostering connections with trusted community centers and health centers leaders embedded in the patient's community may help improve working relationships, create opportunities for psychoeducation about the benefits of neuropsychology and serve to remove the burden of having the technology means and technological literacy from the patient to do their own health research. Continuing to invest in research to improve and advance technology tools for cognitive screening in primary care among other more sophisticated neuropsychological digital tools are important to extend brief cognitive evaluations to a wider group of patients. Rapid, reliable, and valid cognitive screening in primary care is particularly important since it is often the entry and access point for all of healthcare; consequently, it is essential for addressing healthcare gaps.

Culturally based barriers to care. Many neuropsychologists and other healthcare providers have recognized that healthcare has historically harmed diverse communities and that ongoing efforts are needed to improve culturally informed care. Understandably, many individuals from marginalized and underrepresented communities remain reticent to seek healthcare, may be refused, or receive substandard healthcare rooted in bias, or may arrive at a medical appointment with appropriate culturally based guardedness (Sue & Sue, 2022). Within one of our author's communities (RF), an individual who had a history of substance use and was unhoused was labeled as a "homeless" and reported to be treated poorly by a healthcare system, despite peer support from a respected organization accompanying this individual to the hospital for "shaking" that was not getting better on the previously prescribed Benadryl. Only through persistence of that peer support organization to push the healthcare system to recognize that this patient had been clean and sober for over a year and that the episodes of shaking were not a symptom of being unhoused did the person receive the care of a physician who truly heard them. Ultimately, the individual was diagnosed with Huntington's disease, a condition well known to have psychiatric distress as an early presenting symptom. Unfortunately, stigma around mental health, substance use, and being unhoused continues to be a significant challenge for many healthcare systems. Across ethnic, racial, gender, and linguistic groups, similar stories of delay in diagnosis and/or care at a rate that is higher than their English speaking, white, male counterparts are unfortunately plentiful. For the neuropsychologist driving a clinical practice that focuses on population health, they will intentionally seek to improve engagement with all of the communities in their area.

With the historical biases in neuropsychological assessment and research convincingly demonstrated, contemporary assessment practices are moving toward more valid and reliable neuropsychological practice and research within diverse populations. In a seminal paper, Manly (2020) reviewed evidence demonstrating that neuropsychological assessments contain systematic racial and cultural biases that stem not from inherent group differences but from structural inequities in education, language exposure, and life experiences. She reviewed that widely used neuropsychological tests—and the normative data underlying them—were developed primarily with White, English-speaking, highly educated samples, leading to misclassification and overdiagnosis of cognitive impairment in culturally and linguistically diverse populations. She advocated for abandoning simplistic race-based adjustments and instead developing norms and assessments grounded in education quality, acculturation, bilingualism, and sociocultural context, emphasizing that culturally valid testing is essential for accurate diagnosis, clinical equity, and ethical neuropsychological practice. This conclusion is underscored by other research studies revealing flawed data norming practices. Del Cacho-Tena et al (2024), conducted a systematic review of 412 studies published between 2000 and 2022 to evaluate trends, methods, and gaps in normative data development for neuropsychological tests. They found that most normative data studies focused on adults, relied heavily on regression-based methods, and most commonly examined predictors such as age, education, and sex, with verbal fluency being the most frequently normed test. They concluded that future work should expand normative data for children and incorporate more advanced or alternative statistical approaches to address current methodological limitations. Sex and gender-based norms are also under valid scrutiny. Grissom and Reyes (2019) reviewed sex and gender differences in core executive functions (EF) in the literature, including attention, working memory, impulsivity, decision-making, across both human and animal studies. Overall, there was little consistent evidence for robust, systematic sex or gender differences in EF; any apparent differences were small, subtle, and highly task-dependent rather than uniform across EF domains. They argued many reported differences likely reflect different strategies, developmental trajectories, or testing parameters, rather than innate differences in ability, meaning choice of tests, context, age, and environmental factors matter more than sex per se. Importantly, the review highlighted that EF performance was shaped by complex interactions of developmental programming, genotype, environmental exposures, and brain mechanisms, suggesting that future research should examine sex as a biological variable within this broader biopsychosocial context.

Emerging neuropsychological norms procedures are adopting new approaches to statistically calculating performance across variables of interest and abandoning static demographic corrections in favor of individual characteristics, contextual variables, and continuous modeling. For example, Gasquoine (2022) argued that instead of using race-based normative adjustments, neuropsychologists can reduce false positives by estimating an individual's premorbid ("preexisting") cognitive ability using performance-based "hold" measures (e.g., vocabulary or irregular-word pronunciation). This approach is applicable across all racial/ethnic groups and helps ensure that individuals with similar demographic backgrounds and true baseline abilities are assessed equivalently, focusing impairment classification on deviations from their own estimated baseline rather than group-average norms. Several normative systems incorporate such a process, such as the Montefiore Einstein Robust Geriatric Normative Project (Freilich et al., 2025), which uses a word reading test and occupational attainment, and the Calibrated Neuropsychological Normative System (Schretlen et al., 2010), which uses a word reading test that can be mixed with different demographic factors.

Regression-based normative approaches (RBNAs) estimate expected performance on cognitive tests by modeling scores as a function of multiple continuous predictors such as age, education, sex, and socioeconomic status, and then evaluating impairment based on residuals (i.e., the difference between observed and predicted scores) rather than relying on mean group comparisons. In a comprehensive methodological review, Christ et al. (2023) articulated best-practice standards for constructing RBNAs, emphasizing their superiority in flexibility, fairness, and interpretive transparency compared to traditional stratified norms. Building on this foundation, Oltra-Cucarella et al. (2025) advanced the methodology by advocating for raw-score modeling and cautioned against data transformations that reduce clinical interpretability or distort score distributions. More recent test-specific datasets further demonstrate how RBNAs can be applied in real-world neuropsychological assessment. Waggestad et al. (2025), for instance, derived regression-based norms for the Trail Making Test across the adult lifespan, while Stricker et al. (2025) produced comparable norms for remotely administered, self-guided cognitive measures suitable for telehealth contexts. Collectively, these contributions reflect a growing paradigm shift toward individualized, mechanism-based prediction models that move beyond demographic stratification and support more precise, equitable cognitive assessment.

Beyond normative systems, another known barrier for access to treatment is the need for treatment in another language of care. There is a growing need for neuropsychological services to be provided in a language other than English, given the rise of US and global immigration in the past several decades. This makes working with medical interpreters increasingly necessary, though sometimes there is minimal funding for hiring interpreters, and other times neuropsychologists have little experience in knowing how to work effectively with interpreters and/or having little access to tests normed and validated in other languages/cultures. Fortunately, there is growing literature on how neuropsychologists can work effectively with patients who need interpretive services (e.g., Lanca & Wilner, 2019). The European Consortium on Cross-Cultural Neuropsychology (ECCroN) task force conducted a conceptual literature review and provided practice guidelines for interpreter-mediated neuropsychological assessments (Nielsen et al., 2024). Secondarily, there needs to be greater training pipeline efforts for recruiting polyglot neuropsychologists; Rivera Mindt et al. (2010) issued a broad *"call to action"* for the field to expand multicultural training, recruit more diverse trainees, and build capacity to serve linguistically diverse populations, arguing that current services lag far behind demographic realities. Unfortunately, this process has been slow due to multifactorial complexities. Nguyen-Martinez et al. (2025) described the experiences of Asian neuropsychologists (many with varying levels of bilingualism), emphasizing persistent gaps in training opportunities, systemic barriers, and the need for targeted efforts to support a more culturally and linguistically responsive workforce. Additionally, more frequent cultural consultations are also needed, and when colleagues are sought out due to their expertise in providing care for specific linguistic and culturally diverse populations, healthcare systems should ensure that the consultant's time is respected and compensated by the healthcare system.

Contemporary neuropsychology has begun to recognize and address the biases embedded in traditional assessment practices, particularly for multicultural and multilingual populations. These providers develop and embrace newer models of clinical practice and assessment in order to reduce cultural barriers. This includes adopting better norming practices, which are foundational for the integrity of neuropsychology assessment, including emerging methods, which emphasize individualized modeling strategies, such as performance-based premorbid estimates and regression-based normative approaches. Collectively, this body of work illustrates a field-wide shift toward more equitable, accurate, and culturally valid neuropsychological assessment.

Implementation Takeaway #1

Neuropsychologists practicing within a population health framework are proactive to meet the needs of their communities. Understanding the composition of the provider's community is essential and several resources exist for doing so. Many electronic medical records have tools to analyze patient demographics, which can be explored by regions/zip codes. However, this may not capture all of the needed information (e.g., they don't capture those individuals in the community who are not seeking healthcare). This increases the imperative to consider regional demographics and how this might differ from clinic patient demographics. Resources for understanding these differences includes community health assessment and community health improvement plans (e.g., CHIP), which are required for many healthcare entities, and available to providers. Also, well-resourced foundations such as the Kaiser Family Foundation and the Ford Family Foundation can fund studies that result in community-focused reports, which often go beyond basic demographic data reported in census-style data and include rates of other health behaviors of interest, such as poverty indices and tobacco/alcohol use.

Documenting neuropsychological evaluations. One area of neuropsychology practice that will continue to develop is its documentation of evaluations. With expansion of reason for referral for neuropsychological assessments growing (e.g., pre- and post-neurosurgery evaluations, epilepsy, learning disabilities, dementia, forensic, etc.) and simultaneous expansion of neuropsychology beyond traditional general neurology/psychiatry departments, the variability and type of information needed to be conveyed has become greater and the number of different partners in care (patients/family members, neurologists, lawyers, school officials) has increased. As well, newer models of care with varying lengths of assessment (e.g., brief neuropsychological assessments) ultimately shape the length and structure of the report. Comprehensive neuropsychological reports were historically a central aspect of the neuropsychological assessment, in part because neuropsychologists very often were not conveyers of test results to patients, so there was a tendency to explain in greater length the rationale and justification for diagnoses. Appelbaum (1970) argued the psychological reports served as a "tool of persuasion" to the referral source. Before the era of managed care, neuropsychologists also had more time to write, and referral sources had more time to read lengthy reports (Donders, 1999). With increased pressures to shift more time in neuropsychological practice to evaluating patients and less time to documenting, the neuropsychological report has been getting shorter, particularly in non-forensic domain (Sweet et al., 2021), though child and adolescent reports continue to be longer than adult/geriatric reports. In one of the authors' research lab (ML), we showed that in a study with 426 medical providers, that the majority of surveyed providers asserted that they do not read the entire neuropsychological report because it is too long and that report turnaround is too long (Postal et al., 2017). We found that referring providers valued diagnostic impression and recommendations sections the most, and that they were least interested in lengthy descriptions of test results sorted by cognitive domains.

Over time, how neuropsychologists report their clinical evaluations will continue to evolve. Already available are artificial intelligence (AI) report writing tools that allow the provider to have a conversation with ambient technology listening, thus writing the report and freeing up the neuropsychologist's time to expand the number of individuals cared for. As evolution in technology continues and the use digital tools for neuropsychological testing become more pervasive, faster integration of test results using advanced data analytics to summarize and offer possible differential diagnoses will become possible. Advanced digital assessment tools will inevitably reduce the neuropsychologist's reliance on psychometrists/technicians. Rather, neuropsychologists can put their skills as an expert in brain behavior relationships to work by allowing them to make clinical decisions and guide treatment in a more efficient manner. It goes without saying that these technological advances will need to progress with thoughtfulness and with ethical guardrails. The APA's *Ethical Guidance for AI in the Professional Practice of Health Service Psychology* (Updated July 2025) outlines both the opportunities and the ethical risks associated with integrating AI into behavioral health, emphasizing improved decision-making, access, and workflow alongside the need for strong human oversight. The document highlights major ethical concerns—such as bias, transparency, data security, and limitations of current AI systems—and stresses that AI should augment, not replace, clinician judgment. For neuropsychology, this guidance underscores the importance of ensuring that AI-supported assessment, scoring, and diagnostic tools are used responsibly, with careful attention to validity, cultural fairness, and the preservation of clinician expertise in complex brain–behavior interpretation.

Expanding Research: Neuropsychologists Role in Population Health Studies and Implementation Science

Continued if not expanded neuropsychological research is critical to keep up with technological advances and population health efforts, particularly in improving health equity and access to neuropsychological evaluations as well as improving neuropsychological tests and norming procedures. As discussed in Chapters 4 and 7, SDOH substantially influence individuals' capacity to manage modifiable risk factors for cognitive decline and shapes overall neurocognitive functioning. For example, the SDOH effects on cognition persist even after accounting for vascular burden in adults (Amofa-Ho et al., 2025). In older adults, cumulative exposure to adverse SDOH, such as limited education, prolonged unemployment, food insecurity, and restricted access to healthcare is associated with accelerated cognitive decline (Yang et al., 2025). Related, children growing up in areas marked by socioeconomic deprivation, elevated crime rates, and lower educational opportunities experience worse health outcomes, including lower cognitive performance, higher BMI, and more sleep difficulties (Xiao et al., 2023). These findings underscore the importance of comprehensive SDOH data collection in both research and clinical practice to improve detection of cognitive abnormalities and to enhance diagnostic accuracy, treatment planning, and recommendations.

As discussed in Chapter 2 and illustrated in Chapter 9, measurement-based care (MBC) can strengthen both individual outcomes and health-system performance, but its success requires infrastructure, workflow integration, and IS research rather than simple deployment. To function at scale, cognitive MBC must be embedded into clinical workflows with appropriate data systems, clinician feedback loops, and organizational support. IS and QI research frameworks provide the methods to ensure sustainability—identifying barriers, tailoring strategies, evaluating adoption and fidelity, and iteratively refining processes through Plan-Do-Study-Act (PDSA) cycles. MBC also contributes to learning health systems by generating aggregated outcome data that reveal trends, disparities, and opportunities for system-level improvement. A remaining challenge, however, is integrating data from multiple cognitive MBC tools in ways that support meaningful triage across a provider's entire patient panel. This may be an area where AI will eventually offer powerful solutions. Continued QI and IS research can guide the implementation of cognitive screening by assessing readiness, selecting strategies (e.g., EMR integration, team training, clinical champions), and monitoring both implementation and clinical outcomes. Ultimately, cognitive MBC can shift neuropsychology from episodic, consultative evaluation toward continuous, data-informed care that enhances equity, early detection, and population-level cognitive health.

Next Generation Clinical Neuropsychologists: Cementing Cognitive Health as a Cornerstone to Population Health

The long-awaited revision to the competencies of neuropsychological practice, referred to as the Minnesota Conference Guidelines, aligns well with many aspects of population health in neuropsychological training (Stringer et al., 2025). The five foundational areas of the Minnesota Guidelines are neuroscience and brain-behavior relationships, integration of science and practice, ethics, standards, laws, and policies, diversity, and professional relationships. Within these guidelines, there is a focus on many areas discussed in this book, including equitable assessment and intervention, working within systems and consultation, health advocacy, administration/management, and technology/innovation. The inclusion of diversity as a core foundational neuropsychology competency (and captured in other foundational and functional competencies) was a significant development in the training guidelines for neuropsychologists from its last published iteration (i.e., Houston Guidelines, Hannay et al., 1998), reflecting the collaborative work of all the major neuropsychological organizations' efforts (e.g., AACN, SCN, NAN, ABN). The Minnesota guidelines explicitly broaden neuropsychology's traditional focus on individual assessment to include system-level competencies—such as cultural responsiveness, equity, and access—core principles of population health. By emphasizing training in culturally and linguistically informed practice, the guidelines acknowledge structural determinants of neuropsychological outcomes and the need for assessment models that work across diverse populations. The paper also promotes competency-based education that prepares clinicians to function effectively in integrated, interdisciplinary systems of care—an essential feature of population-health delivery models. Its attention to technology, telehealth, and scalable assessment practices supports broader reach and improved access to neuropsychological services at the community level. Collectively, the recommendations position future neuropsychologists to contribute not only to individual patient care but also to system redesign, workforce development, and upstream prevention efforts that improve cognitive health outcomes across populations. Further, the core competency of interdisciplinary systems awareness is clearly demonstrated throughout the practical applications in this book, examining how neuropsychologists use data from schools and primary care physicians, to how we collaborate within specialty interdisciplinary teams. A potential gap in this area of the Minnesota Guidelines is emphasis on how healthcare interacts with public health and the community to drive outcomes in order to address SDOH and better ensure distribution of health equity. Using models such as Collective Impact and working not only across departments in a healthcare organization, but across larger systems holds more promise in delivering on the promise of population health.

Health advocacy within systems, as was highlighted in Chapter 9, focusing on healthcare leadership, is essential in implementing the goals of population health within a healthcare system. Specifically, mere reliance on education to discuss with endocrinologists how diabetes impacts cognition and how those cognitive changes can impact adherence to treatment, especially compounded in different populations, is no longer sufficient. Identifying strategies on how to not just inform but implement change based on this foundational knowledge is required and neuropsychologists must move to adopt implementation science strategies. Within other domains of the Minnesota Guidelines are the focus on research and technology, thinking about how neuropsychologists create greater community access to services even when the neuropsychologist does not practice in the region. Evaluation of those digital strategies to not only examine how they align to current paradigms for cognitive testing but even serve to evolve those will be needed in order to more accurately and efficiently diagnose and treat cognitive disorders, while reducing the downstream impact of those disorders on other aspects of health. Ultimately, the Minnesota Guidelines serve as a guideline for preparation on entry into the field of neuropsychology and adherence to them will likely position early career neuropsychologists to advance population health. However, awareness of some of the continued training gaps and more frequent periodic updates of training guidelines and how they reflect the complex nature of care neuropsychologists provide will be important (Reyes et al., 2025).

Conclusion

Clinical neuropsychology must evolve beyond its traditional focus on individual evaluations to remain relevant within modern healthcare and population-health systems. The field faces growing pressure to increase access, address inequities, and design care models that match patients to the right level of neuropsychological service. Emerging triage and risk-stratification models, supported by targeted evaluations, serial cognitive screening, and system-wide workflows, demonstrate how neuropsychologists can guide early detection, streamline referrals, and embed cognitive health monitoring into primary care and specialty settings. Expanding digital tools and telehealth further enhances reach, particularly for underserved communities, while collaborations with community organizations can help reduce historically rooted, structural barriers to care. At the same time, the profession must adapt documentation practices and thoughtfully integrate AI to support efficiency, preserve clinical judgment, and enhance equity.

Population-health-oriented neuropsychology also requires confronting longstanding biases in assessment. Research by Manly (2020), Cacho-Tena et al. (2024) and others illustrates the limitations of race-corrected norms and static demographic adjustments. Newer approaches such as performance-based premorbid estimates and regression-based normative models offer more individualized and culturally valid methods for interpreting cognitive performance. Continuing to expand diversity considerations beyond language and race to include built-environment factors and broader social determinants of health (SDOH) is also essential. Neuropsychologists must also improve the ways SDOH are systematically measured and applied in both research and clinical practice, moving beyond proxy variables like reading level or demographic labels.

Finally, advancing population health will require neuropsychologists to shift further "upstream." Beyond identifying those who screen positive for cognitive impairment, the field must develop and help implement interventions for at-risk individuals who screen negative yet remain vulnerable due to modifiable risk factors. In dementia care, this means adopting frameworks that address prevention and risk reduction across communities rather than solely diagnosing impairment once present (Bransby et al., 2024). Achieving this vision demands cross-sector collaboration with public health systems, policymakers, advocacy groups, and epidemiologists. The Minnesota Guidelines reflect this expanded scope by emphasizing systems-level competence, cultural responsiveness, and the use of technology and IS—positioning future neuropsychologists to lead efforts that improve cognitive health outcomes at the population level.

Key Points in Review

1. Continuing to expand neuropsychological models to better account for intersectionality of diversity factors, including emphasis on built environment/social determinants of health, acculturation, and language will be essential.
2. Neuropsychologists will need to continue to think about how they continue to move their work "upstream." While early assessment through risk stratification and triaging is important, considering interventions for those at-risk populations who screen negative is essential.
3. Continual evaluation of triage models in their effectiveness to create equitable access is essential. Combining IS strategies with data from community health assessments and public health creates a path forward for meaningfully improving neuropsychological services.

References

American Psychological Association. (2025). *Ethical guidance for AI in the professional practice of health service psychology* (Updated July 2025). https://www.apa.org/topics/artificial-intelligence-machine-learning/ethical-guidance-professional-practice.pdf

Amofa-Ho, P. A., Fiala, J. A., Levy, S., Ross, K. M., Walker, A. F., & Smith, G. E. (2025). Interrelationships of social determinants with cognition, vascular health, and physical functioning. *Brain and Behavior, 1*(2), 1–12. https://doi.org/10.1002/bsa3.70013

Appelbaum, S. A. (1970). Psychological reports: Tools of persuasion. *Professional Psychology, 1*(3), 24–26. https://doi.org/10.1037/h0029301

Bransby, L., Rosenich, E., Maruff, P., & Lim, Y. Y. (2024). How modifiable are modifiable dementia risk factors? A framework for considering the modifiability of dementia risk factors. *The Journal of Prevention of Alzheimer's Disease, 11*(1), 22–37. https://doi.org/10.14283/jpad.2023.119

Christ, S. E., Kanne, S. M., & Reiersen, A. M. (2023). Regression-based normative approaches in neuropsychological assessment: Methodological considerations and clinical implications. *The Clinical Neuropsychologist, 37*(2), 245–270. https://doi.org/10.1080/13854046.2022.2051412

del Cacho-Tena, A., Christ, B. R., Arango-Lasprilla, J. C., Perrin, P. B., Rivera, D., & Olabarrieta-Landa, L. (2024). Normative data estimation in neuropsychological tests: A systematic review. *Archives of Clinical Neuropsychology, 39*, 383–398. https://doi.org/10.1093/arclin/acad084

Donders, J. (1999). Time pressure and the neuropsychological evaluation. *The Clinical Neuropsychologist, 13*(4), 483–493. https://doi.org/10.1076/clin.13.4.483.7248

Freilich, B. M., Scharaga, E., & Holtzer, R. (2025). Montefiore Einstein Robust Geriatric Normative Project: Robust Age- and regression-based demographic norms for the repeatable battery for neuropsychological status and select neuropsychological tests in older adults. *Archives of Clinical Neuropsychology, 40*(5), 1011–1029. https://doi.org/10.1093/arclin/acaf010

Gasquoine, P. G. (2022). Performance-based alternatives to race-norms in neuropsychological assessment. *Cortex, 148*, 231–238. https://doi.org/10.1016/j.cortex.2021.12.003

Grissom, N. M., & Reyes, T. M. (2019). Let's call the whole thing off: Evaluating sex differences in executive function. *Neuropsychopharmacology, 44*(1), 86–96. https://doi.org/10.1038/s41386-018-0179-5

Hannay, J. H., Bieliauskas, L. A., Crosson, B., Hammeke, T. A., Hamsher, K. de S., & Koffler, S. P. (1998). Proceedings of the Houston Conference on Specialty Education and Training in Clinical Neuropsychology. *Archives of Clinical Neuropsychology, 13*(Special Issue), 157–250.

Hardy, K. K., et al. (2017). Population-based neuropsychological models for medically vulnerable children. *The Clinical Neuropsychologist, 31*(7), 1326–1346.

Lanca, M. (2018). Integration of neuropsychology in primary care. *Archives of Clinical Neuropsychology, 33*(3), 269–279. https://doi.org/10.1093/arclin/acx135

Lanca, M., & Wilner, E. K. (2019). *Neuropsychology in the twenty-first century: The rise of multicultural assessments.* In K. M. Sanders (Ed.), *Physician's field guide to neuropsychology* (pp. 479–493). Springer. https://doi.org/10.1007/978-1-4939-8722-1_28

Manly, J. J. (2020). Racial and cultural bias in cognitive assessment. *Annual Review of Clinical Psychology, 16*, 24–52.

Mindt, M. R., Byrd, D., Saez, P., & Manly, J. J. (2010). Increasing culturally competent neuropsychological services for ethnic minority populations: A call to action. *The Clinical Neuropsychologist, 24*(3), 429–453. https://doi.org/10.1080/13854040903058960

Nielsen, T. R., Franzen, S., Watermeyer, T., Jiang, J., Calia, C., Kjærgaard, D., Bothe, S., & Mukadam, N., on behalf of the European Consortium on Cross-Cultural Neuropsychology (ECCroN). (2024). Interpreter-mediated neuropsychological assessment XE "Neuropsychological assessment" : Clinical considerations and recommendations from the European Consortium on Cross-Cultural Neuropsychology (ECCroN). *The Clinical Neuropsychologist*. https://doi.org/10.1080/13854046.2024.2335113

Nguyen-Martinez, A. L., Miao, I., Lesica, S., Patel, J., Tan, A., Samuel, A. R., Do, C., Hutaff-Lee, C., & Chen, J. (2025). Asian neuropsychologists: Current state, gaps, barriers, and future directions. *The Clinical Neuropsychologist, 39*(7), 1761–1789. https://doi.org/10.1080/13854046.2024.2438306

Oltra-Cucarella, J., Pérez-Elvira, R., Bonete López, B., de Andrade Moral, R., & García-Rubio, M. J. (2025). Regression-based normative data in neuropsychology: Using raw scores as observed response variables outperforms transforming for normality. *Psychological Assessment, 37*(9), 442–453. https://doi.org/10.1037/pas0001398

Postal, K., Chow, C., Jung, S., Erickson-Moreo, K., Geier, F., & Lanca, M. (2017). The stakeholders' project in neuropsychological report writing: A survey of neuropsychologists' and referral sources' views of neuropsychological reports. *The Clinical Neuropsychologist, 32*(3), 326–344. https://doi.org/10.1080/13854046.2017.1373859

Reyes, A., Fuchs, K., Penna, S., Waldron, E. J., Madore, M., Heffelfinger, A., Correia, S., Bristow, T., Whiteside, D. M., Stringer, A. Y., & Bordes Edgar, V. (2025). Proceedings of the Minnesota 2022 conference on clinical neuropsychology training guidelines. *The Clinical Neuropsychologist*, 1–28. Advance online publication. https://doi.org/10.1080/13854046.2025.2582538

Schretlen, D. J., Testa, M., & Pearlson, G. D. (2010). *Calibrated Neuropsychological Normative System: Professional Manual*. PAR.

Stricker, N. H., Holmes, C., & Iverson, G. L. (2025). Regression-based norms for remote cognitive assessments across platforms. *Journal of the International Neuropsychological Society, 31*(4), 414–426. https://doi.org/10.1017/S135561772500XXX

Stringer, A. Y., Fuchs, K., Bordes Edgar, V., Bristow, T., Correia, S., Penna, S., Reyes, A., Whiteside, D. M., Block, C., Bodin, D., Butt, S., Calamia, M., Didehbani, N., Dodzik, P., Dotson, V. M., Fernandes, M., Freece, K., Fuller, R., Getz, G., … Schmitter-Edgecombe, M. (2025). The Minnesota Conference proposed guidelines for education and training in clinical neuropsychology. *The Clinical Neuropsychologist,* 1–42. https://doi.org/10.1080/13854046.2025.2520957

Sue, D. W., & Sue, D. (2022). *Counseling the culturally diverse: Theory and practice* (9th ed.). Wiley.

Sweet, J. J., Klipfel, K. M., Nelson, N. W., & Moberg, P. J. (2021). Professional practices, beliefs, and incomes of U.S. neuropsychologists: The AACN, NAN, SCN 2020 practice and "salary survey." *The Clinical Neuropsychologist, 35(1),* 7–80. https://doi.org/10.1080/13854046.2020.1849803

Waggestad, T., Hestad, K., & Olsen, R. K. J. (2025). Regression-based normative data for the Trail Making Test across the adult lifespan. *Applied Neuropsychology: Adult, 32*(2), 123–132. https://doi.org/10.1080/23279095.2025.XXXXX

Xiao, Y., Behrman, J. R., & Liu, J. (2023). Social determinants of health and cognitive development in childhood: A population-based study. *The Lancet Child & Adolescent Health, 7*(6), 410–419. https://doi.org/10.1016/S2352-4642(23)00089-4

Yang, T. C., Chen, I. C., & Choi, S. W. (2025). Cumulative social disadvantage and cognitive decline among older adults. *Journal of Gerontology: Series B, Psychological Sciences and Social Sciences.* Advance online publication. https://doi.org/10.1093/geronb/gbadXXX

Index

M. Lanca and R. Fallows (eds.), *Advancing Neuropsychology Through Population Health*, https://doi.org/10.1007/978-3-032-22457-6

www.ingramcontent.com/pod-product-compliance
Ingram Content Group UK Ltd.
Pitfield, Milton Keynes, MK11 3LW, UK
UKHW020632260926
475829UK00003BA/46
* 9 7 8 3 0 3 2 2 2 4 5 6 9 *